The Cardiac Conduction System
in
Unexplained Sudden Death

by

Saroja Bharati, M.D. & Maurice Lev, M.D.

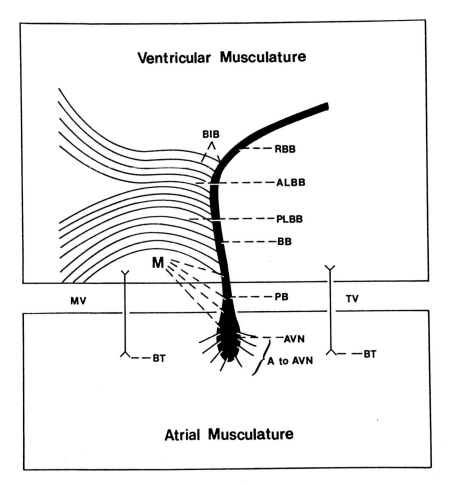

This schematic diagram may help the reader to understand the anatomic abnormalities or the pathological involvement of the peripheral conduction system which may be responsible for an arrhythmic event leading to sudden death. The diagram does not show all of the known anomalies and/or the pathology of the conduction system that may give rise to the arrhythmia. A to AVN = approaches to the atrioventricular node; AVN = atrioventricular node; BT = bypass tracts between the atria and ventricles; TV = tricuspid valve; MV = mitral valve; PB = penetrating part of the AV bundle; BB = branching part of the AV bundle; M = Mahaim fibers; PLBB = posterior radiation of the left bundle branch; ALBB = anterior radiation of the left bundle branch; BIB = bifurcating part of the AV bundle; RBB = right bundle branch.

The Cardiac Conduction System
In
Unexplained Sudden Death

by

Saroja Bharati, M.D.

Director
Congenital Heart and Conduction System Center
The Heart Institute for Children of the Christ Hospital
and Medical Center
Evangelical Health Systems
Oak Lawn, Illinois
and
Professor of Pathology
Rush Medical College, Rush University
Rush-Presbyterian-St. Lukes Medical Center
Chicago, Illinois

and

Maurice Lev, B.S., M.D., M.A.(Phil.)

Associate Director
Congenital Heart and Conduction System Center
The Heart Institute for Children of the Christ Hospital
and Medical Center
Evangelical Health Systems
Oak Lawn, Illinois
and
Distinguished Professor of Pathology, Medicine and Pediatrics
Rush Medical College, Rush University
Rush-Presbyterian-St. Lukes Medical Center
Chicago, Illinois

Futura Publishing
Company, Inc.
Mount Kisco, NY
1990

Library of Congress Cataloging-in-Publication Data

Bharati, Saroja.
    The cardiac conduction system in unexplained sudden death / by
Saroja Bharati and Maurice Lev.
        p.   cm.
    Supported by the National Heart, Lung, and Blood Institute of the
National Institutes of Health under projects HL-07605 and 30558.
    Includes bibliographical references.
    Includes index.
    ISBN 0-87993-362-3
    1. Cardiac arrest.   2. Heart conduction system.   I. Lev, Maurice,
1908–   .   II. National Heart, Lung, and Blood Institute.
III. Title.
    [DNLM: 1. Death, Sudden—etiology—case studies.   2. Heart
Conduction System—pathology.   WG 201 B575c]
RC685.C173B47   1990
616.1′23025—dc20
DNLM/DLC
    for Library of Congress   90-3881
                                            CIP

Published by
    Futura Publishing Company, Inc.
    2 Bedford Ridge Road
    Mount Kisco, New York 10549

LC #: 90-3881
ISBN #: 0-87993-362-3

Every effort has been made to ensure that the information in this book is as up to date and as accurate as possible at the time of publication. However, due to the constant developments in medicine, neither the author, nor the editor, nor the publisher can accept any legal or any other responsibility for any errors or omissions that may occur.

Printed in the United States of America.

Preface

Sudden unexplained death does occur in the young and healthy with or without prior history of arrhythmias. Although some might have had arrhythmias, the arrhythmias apparently did not disable them from the normal functions of everyday life and these young people were considered healthy. The cause of death, when not determined by the medical examiner and/or the pathologist, is assumed to be an arrhythmic event. The cardiac conduction system is then considered as a possibility for the arrhythmic event.

The cardiac conduction system is a specialized muscle and therefore requires a special kind of examination. A meaningful interpretation of the cardiac conduction system may be made only after serial section examination from the sinoatrial node and its approaches, the atrial preferential pathways, the atrioventricular node and its approaches, the atrioventricular bundle (penetrating, branching, and bifurcating parts), and the bundle branches, up to the level of the Purkinje network. This type of study takes a considerable amount of time.

In this book we have made an attempt to illustrate the findings of the conduction system in cases of unexplained sudden death. After having examined the conduction system in more than 100 hearts and finding some pathological and/or abnormal anatomical lesions in *all* the cases studied, we believe the findings may be responsible for an arrhythmic event. It is of interest that those who have previously studied the conduction system have also found lesions in most cases.

Thus it is clear that anatomical abnormalities or pathological lesions of the conduction system may remain quiet or elusive in nature for a considerable period of time, permitting a normal life pattern or even permitting extraordinary physical activities (as in cases of trained athletes). However, during a vulnerable period of time (altered physiological or metabolic states), these individuals may be prone to arrhythmias and sudden death.

We hope this book will enable the readers to understand or emphasize the pathology and/or the anatomical variations in various parts of the conduction system and will stimulate their interest in thinking in terms of developing new technologies to identify these lesions in the living. This in return may shed some light as to the mechanisms of sudden death in the young and healthy in the general population.

Saroja Bharati, M.D.
Maurice Lev, M.D.

Contents

Chapter 1

Introduction

We wish to thank each and every one who sent us hearts, the analysis of which constitutes the essence of this book. Such a listing, however, would be too long. Furthermore, we might inadvertently omit a few individuals, which for us would be a disaster. We also wish to thank some of the family members who insisted that we study the hearts of their loved ones who died suddenly.

Over the years, as pathologists, in our work on the conduction system in both congenital and acquired heart disease, we were incidentally confronted with the question of sudden unexpected cardiac death in some of these cases. More recently, various coroners and pathologists have sent us hearts from young people who had died suddenly and unexpectedly. These people had been living a normal life. Autopsies of these individuals disclosed no pathological change, grossly or histologically, that could be interpreted as a possible cause of death. Toxicologic examination done in all of the coroners' cases were neg-

ative. The hearts were sent to us for a study of the conduction system. In more than 100 cases, we found what we consider to be abnormalities in the conduction system and/or the surrounding myocardium. These changes were not found in similarly aged normal hearts.

The changes included either congenital or acquired abnormalities in and around the conduction system. We hypothesize that these changes and/or the anomalies of the myocardium and the conduction system may induce vulnerability of this system under certain conditions and may impair normal conduction and thereby permit reentry, abnormal automaticity, or fractionization of an impulse resulting in dysrhythmia. This may degenerate into ventricular fibrillation and sudden death. Furthermore, we speculate that these anomalies may remain innocuous in a normal healthy youngster for a long period of time. However, during an altered physiological or metabolic state, or in some genetically susceptible (weak) conduction system, these abnormalities may form a milieu for arrhythmogenicity and sudden death.

We wish to thank The National Heart, Lung and Blood Institute of The National Institutes of Health, Bethesda, Maryland, for the many years of support they have rendered for our project HL-07605 and 30558. Last but not least, we are greatly indebted to all of our technicians, photographers, artists, and secretaries in Chicago and New Jersey who worked with us and provided us with the histologic material, and the untiring secretarial help that made this book possible.

Especially we wish to remember the help of our technicians: Milorad, Mary, Mildred, Dena, Randi, Mark, Don, Mary Ellen, Debbi, Nancy, and many others.

Chapter 2

Definition of Sudden Death

In this book, sudden death implies that the individual died suddenly and unexpectedly, instantaneously or within 24 hours after the onset of symptoms without any evidence of trauma. Cardiac death implies that a complete autopsy was performed, including that of the brain and the spinal cord, and no findings could be found in any organ or in the epicardial coronary arteries to explain the cause of death. The assumption is further made that the cause of death lies in the heart, and the method of death was ventricular fibrillation or asystole. A further implication is that the death was electrical.

Thus, this book attempts to discuss the findings in the conduction system that might be related to such an electrical death. We studied more than 100 cases of sudden death, and we illustrate 75 cases in this book. The hearts of these patients were sent to us by medical examiners and other pathologists who could not ascertain the cause of death after complete autopsy and toxicologic examination. In each case, we examined the entire heart grossly and light microscopically, including the conduction system, all chambers, valves, myocardium of both the atria and the ventricles, the endocardium, and the epicardium and the atrioventricular (AV) rings. The method of examination will be described in detail later. However, we did not examine the spinal cord, stellate ganglion, and the nerve connections between them.

In the vast majority of cases, the heart was hypertrophied and enlarged in all chambers.

3

Chapter 3

Method of Examination of the Heart[1]

The heart and lungs are removed as a unit from the chest.

The Dissection of the Heart

External Examination

The unopened pericardium is examined first for defects, and then cut away. The direction of the base-apex axis of the heart is ascertained as to whether it points to the left or to the right or to the center of the body. This axis is a line drawn from the middle of the apex to the middle of the base. The shape of the heart is then noted, and its transverse diameter is compared in size to the inner transverse diameter of the chest.

The anterior descending coronary artery is then located. This roughly indicates the position and extent of the left and right ventricles. Of course, it is understood that we are not dealing with a transposition complex. The composition of the apex is now ascertained. The relative position and number of arterial trunks emanating from the heart are noted. The direction of the aortic arch, whether to the right or to the left of the trachea, is noted and the brachiocephalic arteries are traced from the aortic arch and their identity is established. The entry of the superior and inferior vena cava is seen.

The heart is now lifted anteriorly and to the right so that the entry of the pulmonary veins can be noted. The chest organs are now removed undissected in toto, with the abdominal aorta and part of the inferior vena cava and the superior vena cava attached to them. All the systemic and pulmonary veins are now traced into the right and left atrium.

5

Method of Opening the Heart

On opening the heart, the first cut (cut 1) is made from the left margin of the circumference of the opening of the inferior vena cava through the anterior wall of the right ventricle in an oblique manner, through the right atrial appendage up to its highest point. Care is taken not to approach in any way the linea terminalis of the right atrium. The second cut (cut 2) is made from the first cut through the right atrium and ventricle along the acute margin of the heart up to the apex. The third cut (cut 3) passes from the second cut through the anterior wall of the right ventricle along a line directly proximal to the anterolateral papillary muscle into the pulmonary trunk (Fig. 3–1) (cuts 1–3).

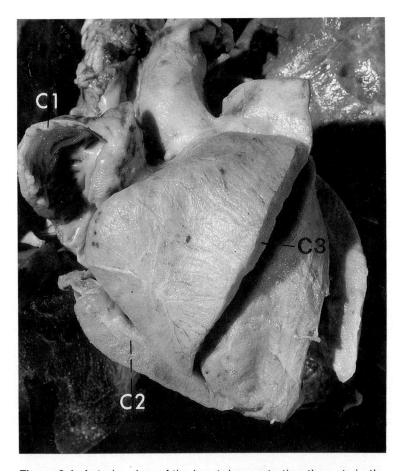

Figure 3-1: Anterior view of the heart demonstrating the cuts in the anterior wall, right side. C1 = cut from the inferior vena cava through the right atrial appendage; C2 = cut along the acute margin to the apex of the heart; C3 = cut through the anterior wall of the right ventricle, proximal to the anterolateral papillary muscle up to the pulmonary trunk (see text). (Reprinted with permission from Lev M, Bharati S: Lesions of the conduction system and their functional significance. *Pathol Annual* 1974; 9:169–171.)

The heart and lungs are now turned to the posterior surface, and a nick is made in the left atrial wall just distal to the entry of the pulmonary veins, close to the entry of the left pulmonary veins (Fig. 3–2) (cut 4). This cut is now extended into the entry of the four pulmonary veins. The next cut passes from the previous cut through the left atrium and ventricle along the obtuse margin of the heart to the apex, between the anterior and posterior groups of papillary muscles (Fig. 3–2) (cut 5). The next cut passes from the previous cut in the apex, paraseptally through the base (Fig. 3–3) (cut 6). As it passes through the aortic valve, the cut lies between the pulmonic valve and the left atrial appendage. It continues along the anterior (ventral) wall of the aorta in a curved manner between the exit of the brachiocephalic arteries and the attachment of the ligamentum arteriosum.

Internal Examination

The structures inspected in the right atrium are the linea terminalis, the junction of the superior vena cava with the right atrium, the limbus fossae ovalis, the mouth of the coronary sinus, the eustachian and thebesian valves, the endocardium, the thickness of the myocardium, the size of the chamber and the area between the coronary sinus and the septal leaflet of the tricuspid valve.

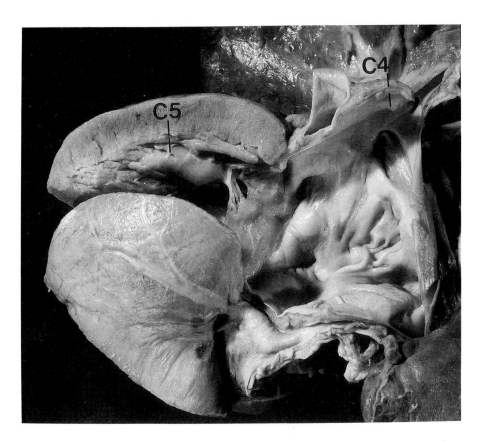

Figure 3-2: Posterior view of the heart demonstrating the left atrium and the obtuse margin. C4 = cut joining the left pulmonary veins to the right pulmonary veins; C5 = cut along the obtuse margin of the heart from the base to the apex (see text). (Reprinted with permission from Lev M, Bharati S: Lesions of the conduction system and their functional significance. *Pathol Annual* 1974; 9:169–171.)

The tricuspid orifice is now inspected. The size of the orifice is measured, its three leaflets inspected from the standpoint of size and thickness, the annular base, the leaflet structure, and the edge, with the corresponding chordae and papillary muscles.

The right ventricle is now studied. The demarcation between sinus and conus is noted. The trabeculated inlet and the configuration of the septal and parietal bands are studied. The size of the chamber, both conus and sinus, the muscle of Lancisi, and the thickness in these regions of the wall are noted. The efferent vessel of the right ventricle, its size, its valve, and its branches, are inspected up to the hili of the lungs, if we are dealing with the pulmonary tree. The size, length, and thickness of the ductus arteriosus are now observed.

The left side of the heart is now inspected for pathological change. The size of the left atrium, the thickness of the wall, the architecture of the endocardium, and the size of the left atrial appendage are noted. The mitral ori-

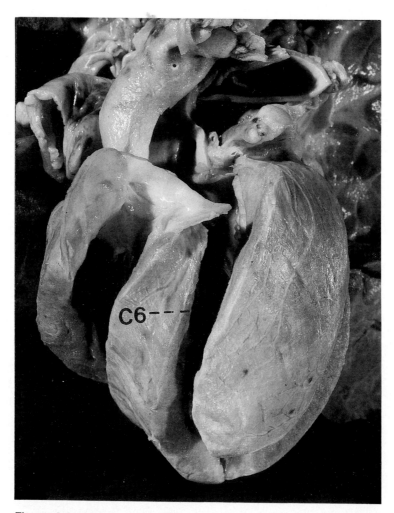

Figure 3-3: Anterior part of the ventricular septum demonstrating the paraseptal cut. C6 = cut along the anterior part of the septum, parallel to the anterior descending coronary artery from the apex to the base, up to the aortic valve (see text). (Reprinted with permission from Lev M, Bharati S: Lesions of the conduction system and their functional significance. *Pathol Annual* 1974; 9:169–171.)

fice is then measured, noting how much of the valve is occupied by the posterior leaflet and how much by the anterior leaflet. The size of these leaflets from the base to the periphery is ascertained. The thickness and configuration of the leaflets are noted. A careful study is made of the aortic-mitral annulus. Does it connect with the posterior aortic leaflet or with the left and right aortic leaflet?

The size and thickness of the left ventricle is now measured. The external configuration and trabeculation of the ventricular septum and the thickness and trabeculation of the endocardium, especially at the base of the septum, are noted. The membranous septum, including the ventricular and the right atrial component, is examined carefully, and its size, shape, and its relationship to the tricuspid, mitral, and aortic valves are noted. The size of the aortic orifice and the relative size of the three aortic cusps are ascertained. The location of the two coronary ostia, their size, and their position in the sinuses of Valsalva are noted. The thickness of the supravalvular ring and the size of the aortic ring at that level are noted. The coronary arteries are opened by dissection if a lumen is visible. Where a lumen is not visible, cross-sections are cut every one-fourth of an inch. The circumflexes, descending arteries, ramus anterior ventriculi sinistri, and ramus obtusi are routinely opened. The size of the right anterior ventriculi dextri is noted.

The various measurements of the heart are now taken; they are as follows:

RV-P = Thickness of the right ventricle at the pulmonic orifice.
RV-T = Thickness of the right ventricle at the tricuspid orifice.
RV-A = Thickness of the right ventricle at the apex.
LV-M = Maximum thickness of the left ventricle.
LV-A = Thickness of the left ventricle at the apex.
TV = Circumference of tricuspid valve.
PV = Circumference of pulmonic valve.
MV = Circumference of mitral valve.
AV = Cirumference of aortic valve.

TA = Measurement from the middle of the tricuspid valve to the apex of the right ventricle.
PA = Measurement from the base of the pulmonic valve to the apex of the right ventricle.
PRV$_1$ = Measurement from the midpoint of the posterior wall of the right ventricle to the lower septal band.
PRV$_0$ = Measurement of circumference at the junction of the medial and anterior leaflets of the tricuspid parallel to the pulmonic valve.
MA = Measurement from the middle of the posterior mitral valve to the apex.
AA = Measurement from the base of the aortic valve to the apex.
PLV = Perimeter of the left ventricle in a plane roughly parallel to the mitral and aortic orifice midway between the apex and these orifices.

Aging Changes of the Heart[2–4]

The above opened and measured heart is then compared with the normal aging changes in the heart which include, the epicardium, myocardium, endocardium, and valves at the gross level.

Method of Study of the Conduction System for Histologic Examination[1,5–11]

The heart, including a portion of the superior and inferior vena cava and the entire thoracic aorta, are now separated from the lungs.

The block containing the sinoatrial (SA) node is now fashioned (Fig. 3–4 A,B). A cut is made along the proximal margin of the right atrium through the right lateral wall of the superior vena cava. The next cut passes through the original cut, made in opening the heart, through the atrial appendage, over the hump of the appendage for a distance of about one-half inch into the superior wall. The final cut to form the block extends from the end of the

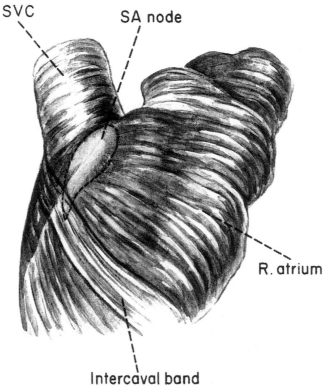

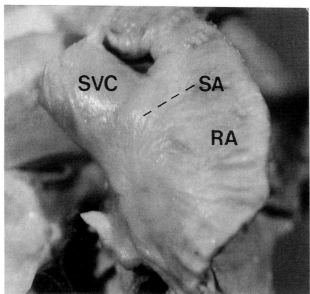

Figure 3-4: Block containing the SA node. Top: Diagrammatic sketch. Bottom: SA = sinoatrial node region in an infant; SVC = superior vena cava; RA = right atrium; SA = SA node; R = right atrium. (Reprinted with permission from Lev M: The conduction system. In: *Pathology of the Heart and Blood Vessels,* Gould SE (ed), 1968, Springfield, IL, Charles C. Thomas, and from Lev M, Watneal: Arch Pathol 1954; 57:168.

previous cut, along the superior wall of the right atrium along the apical aspect of the posterior crest. This cut then meets the first cut.

The next block contains the blood supply to the SA node—the ramus ostii cavae superioris. This consists of the distal portions of the anterior and lateral walls of the right atrium. The blood supply to the SA node is obtained with the superior and middle preferential pathways. Cuts are made paraseptally into the roofs of the right and left atrium to their terminals, care being taken not to cut the aorta. Cuts are then made into the opposite sides of the roofs of the atria to the atrioventricular (AV) grooves, and transverse cuts at the AV groove free both roofs of the atria. One of these blocks so fashioned contains the SA

nodal artery, dependent upon whether it arises from the main right or left circumflex. The atrial septum and its accompanying piece of atrial roof are now free to be cut into blocks to obtain the superior and middle preferential pathways.

The parietal walls of the right and left atria and ventricles are now separated from the atria and ventricles. To fashion the blocks containing the approaches to the AV node, the AV node bundle, and bundle branches, we proceed as follows (Figs. 3–5, 3–6, 3–7). A cut is made along a line just posterior to the moderator band and the right anterolateral papillary muscle at an angle of almost 45° to the septal band of the crista supraventricularis and passes below the crux. A second cut is

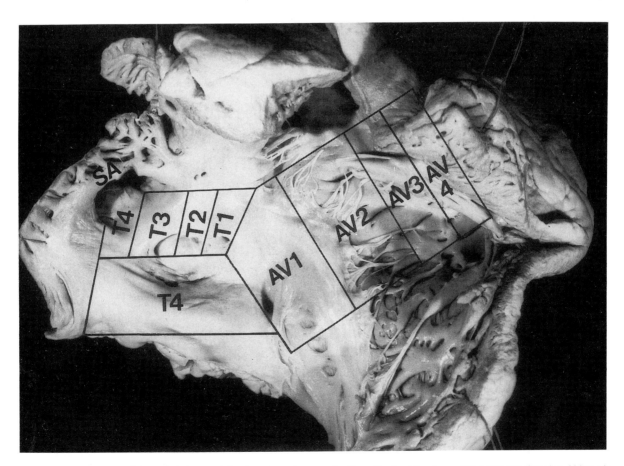

Figure 3-5: Right atrial and right ventricular view demonstrating the fashioning of the blocks for the AV node and its approaches (AV1), atrial preferential pathways (T1–T4), the AV bundle, and the bundle branches (AV2–AV4). (Reprinted with permission from Lev M, Bharati S: Lesions of the conduction system and their functional significance. *Pathol Annual* 1974; 9:169–171.)

made in the upper aspect of the atrial septum from the roof of the aorta to the center of the fossa ovalis. The third cut is made at right angles to the first cut along a line proximal to the insertion of the eustachian valve so that the coronary sinus region is in the block as well as the crux. A fourth cut is made through the lower part of the arch of the crista parallel to the baseline, making sure that the base of the aorta and most of the pars membranacea are in the block.

These blocks that contain the AV node, AV node bundle, and bundle branches are then subdivided into portions depending upon the pathology expected. Usually it is subdivided by cuts through the pars membranacea, prox-

imal to the insertion of the tricuspid valve, and through the muscle of Lancisi. Further cuts are made up to the moderator band (Figs. 3–5, 3–6).

The atrial septum is divided into blocks (Figs. 3–5, 3–7) housing the superior and middle preferential pathways, and the lower atrial septum (T4) if necessary.

These blocks containing the AV node, AV node bundle, and bundle branches are now sent through the Peterfi method which follows. This is a double-embedding method.

1. Wash in running water overnight.
2. Two changes in 80% ethyl alcohol in 24 hours.

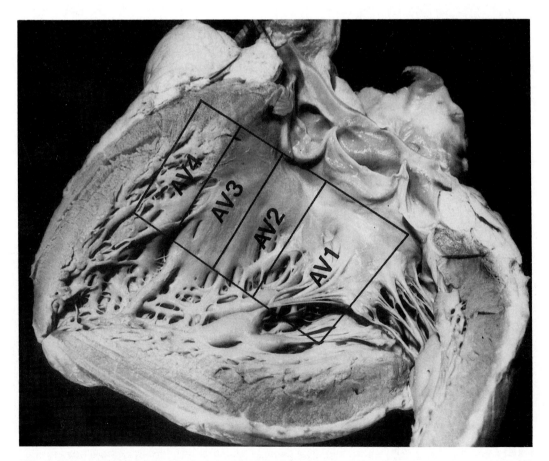

Figure 3-6: Left ventricular view of the blocks of the conduction system as depicted in Figure 3–5. (Reprinted with permission from Lev M, Bharati S: Lesions of the conduction system and their functional significance. *Pathol Annual* 1974; 9:169–171.)

3. Two changes in 95% ethyl alcohol, 6 to 8 hours.
4. Two changes in absolute ethyl alcohol, 16 to 20 hours.
5. Transfer to a 1% solution of celloidin in methyl benzoate until the tissue sinks. (Usually, it takes from 12 to 24 hours, depending upon the thickness and density of the tissue.)
6. A second change in a fresh solution of 1% celloidin in methyl benzoate. This is kept in from 3 to 30 hours, or 1 hour per millimeter of thickness. However, if the exigencies of time require a longer

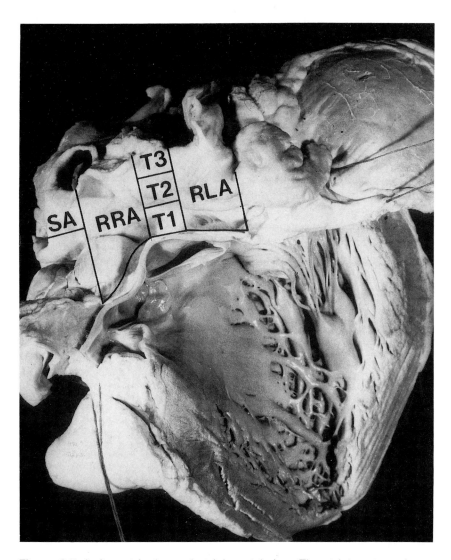

Figure 3-7: Left ventricular and atrial septal view. The atrial septum shows the blocks for the atrial preferential pathways as depicted in Figure 3–5. T_1-T_3 = atrial preferential pathways; RRA = roof of the right atrium; RLA = roof of the left atrium. Numbers indicate cuts and labels indicate blocks. SA = SA node; AV1 to AV4 blocks containing AV node and approaches, AV bundle, and bundle branches. (Reprinted with permission from Lev M, Bharati S: Lesions of the conduction system and their functional significance. *Pathol Annual* 1974; 9:169–171.)

period in the second celloidin, the tissue can be kept in this solution indefinitely.

7. Three changes of benzene for 2 hours each.

8. Three changes in melted tissue mat at 56° to 58° under vacuum. A vacuum-embedding oven may be utilized, and 1 hour for each millimeter is the time for embedding under vacuum in each change. In the first change, a vacuum of 10 to 15 inches of mercury (Hg) is used, which is built up in 20 to 30 seconds. In the second change, a vacuum of 20 inches of Hg is used, and is built up in 1 minute. In the third change, a vacuum of 25 inches of Hg is used, and is built up in about 1½ minutes. Care must be taken to release the vacuum slowly after each change.

9. Transfer the tissue from the last paraffin to a glass container, 3 by 4 inches, with a slightly narrower base than top, and lightly lined with glycerin and containing melted tissue wax (56° to 58°). Leave this in a vacuum of 15 inches of Hg for about 15 to 20 minutes. By this means, all air bubbles will be removed. The glass container with the tissue is then put in a pan of ice-cold water and the paraffin is allowed to solidify to form a thin film of about 3 mm. Then the tissue is correctly oriented for cutting and the paraffin is allowed to solidify completely. The block is placed in a refrigerator for about 15 to 20 minutes. Then the glass container is turned upside down and the block is ready for trimming and sectioning.

The block containing the SA node and its approaches may or may not be doubly embedded; it is sectioned as follows. The block is cut serially at 5- to 8-micron thickness, and every 80th section is retained for six sections, and every 20th section thereafter. The block containing the blood supply to the SA node is sectioned as follows. At this point, if the block is very large, it may be subdivided into two or three blocks by lines parallel to the acute mar-

ginal cut. Each of these blocks is sectioned with these latter cuts as base lines, at 7- to 8-micron thickness, and every 80th section is retained. The sections are alternately stained with hematoxylin-eosin and Weigert-van Gieson stains.

Blocks continuing the AV node, AV node bundle, and bundle branches are doubly embedded and serially sectioned at 6–8 microns and every 10th, 20th, or maximally 40th section is retained. All sections are stained alternately with hematoxylin-eosin and Weigert-van Gieson stains and sometimes Gomori trichrome.

Sections are then cut through the remainder of the walls of the heart. The blocks of these sections are not double-embedded. Two sections are taken from each block and stained with hemotoxylin-eosin and Weigert-van Gieson stains.

The total histologic study yields about 1,300 to 1,600 sections, and takes an average technician 6 weeks to 2 months to accomplish.

In sections that have gone through the Peterfi method of dehydration and embedding the celloidin must be removed. This is done as follows. After the paraffin has been removed with zylol, the sections are placed in 100% alcohol for 5 minutes. They are then placed in a mixture of equal parts of ether and absolute alcohol for 5 to 10 minutes. They then pass through 95% alchohol, 80% alcohol to running water, and are stained.

The above-described method of sectioning and sampling the entire heart yields qualitative data of changes in the atrial and ventricular endocardium, myocardium, and epicardium, the atrioventricular and semilunar valves, the entire conduction system, and the coronary arteries and veins. It yields semiquantitative data of everything but the valves, coronary arteries, and veins. It also localizes pathological changes in the ventricular myocardium according to wall and part of wall. It is self-evident that this method is not as good as some of the prevailing methods for the study of lateral wall infarcts. However, an attempt is made here to offer the most useful data for electrocardiographic correlation which are possible in a routine procedure. If this routine method seems too burdensome and lengthy, we feel it is still necessary to give a proper anatomical base for electrocardiographic interpretation.

Method of Study of the Heart and the Conduction System in Pre-Excitation

We make every attempt to retain the atrioventricular junction without opening the coronaries, and blocks are taken from the AV junction and completely serially sectioned. The approaches to the AV node, the AV node bundle, and bundle branches are taken into blocks and sectioned serially as above described.

Significance of Study of the Conduction System by Our Method[9–15]

The conduction system forms a curve or an arch and is not in a straight line. We, therefore, believe a semiquantitative analysis of the conduction system for correlative studies with electrocardiographic and electrophysiological studies can only be obtained if blocks were taken in such a manner that the entire conduction system can be followed from the beginning to the periphery. We believe in the

study of sudden death in pre-excitation; our task is to find the bypass pathways. Therefore, we study the AV rims completely and the conduction system as above described. Thus, we compromise to some extent in our study of the conduction system when we study hearts with pre-excitation.

Comparison of the Conduction System with Normal Control Hearts[16,17]

Having done the serial sections as discussed above, we now turn to compare the histologic findings of the conduction system with the normal control studies that we have done previously. These include the ages from birth to the ninth decade of life.

Limitation of Our Study

Although we are able to study the conduction system in an extensive manner, our studies are limited due to the fact that we do not use special histochemical staining or a special study of the nerves. Since blocks are taken and double-embedded, we are not sure, if special stains were indeed done in some of the sections, whether it would yield meaningful data.

Chapter 4

The Fibrous Skeleton of the Heart[18]

In order to understand the conduction system, the fibrous skeleton of the heart must be understood.

Anatomy (Fig. 4–1)

This consists of the central fibrous body (CFB), the pars membranacea, and the fibrous junctions of the right and left atria and ventricles. Since the tricuspid annulus lies somewhat more apical than the mitral annulus, there is a fibrous prong that proceeds from the CFB to the tricuspid annulus. Likewise, there is an aortic prong that proceeds from the base of the aorta to the CFB. In addition, the summit of the ventricular septum is considerably fibrous, which increases in thickness with advancing age.

Central Fibrous Body

The central fibrous body consists of a mass of connective tissue which joins the two AV annuli directly and the base of the aorta with the aid of the pars membranacea. It measures approximately 1 cm × 0.5 cm. However, the size varies considerably.

Membranous Septum

The membranous septum is more or less a rectangular form of connective tissue and is the distal extension of the CFB. There is a ventriculo-ventricular and left ventricular-right atrial component. The aortic-mitral annulus merges with the membranous septum, and the membranous septum proceeds to the base of

17

the noncoronary (posterior) aortic cusp. The membranous septum anteriorly extends to the junction of the noncoronary and right aortic cusp. Occasionally it may extend considerably anteriorly up to the base of the mid-part of the right aortic cusp. The aortic-mitral annulus, as it continues as the pars membranacea, joins the base of the noncoronary and left aortic cusp. Sometimes the membranous septum may be large and extend further posteriorly. Although the membranous septum measures approximately 0.8 to 1 cm × 0.6–0.8 cm, its size and shape varies considerably. The left ventriculo-right atrial component also varies considerably. It joins the right atrium at the

junction of the latter with the annuli of the septal and the anterior leaflets of the tricuspid valve.

Embryology

The CFB is formed by the fusion of the anterior and posterior endocardial cushions. This occurs at 10–11 mm of fetal length. With the absorption of the bulbus (14–17 mm of fetal length), the left side of the muscular bulbus comes into contact with the CFB. This bulbar portion atrophies to form the fibrous

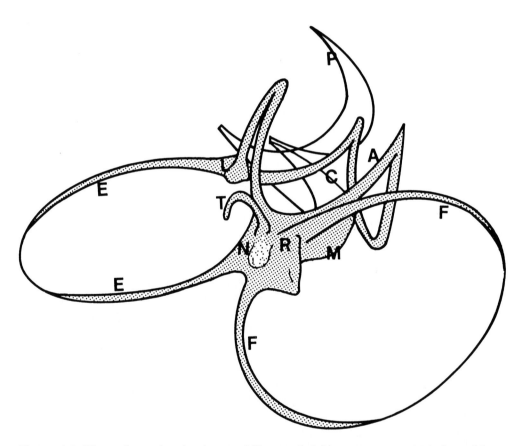

Figure 4-1: Three-dimensional schema of fibrous skeleton, as seen posteriorly and from the right (as conceived by Zimmerman and Bailey). L = left trigone; R = right trigone; A = scalloped line of root of aorta; C = conus tendon; P = scalloped line of root of pulmonary artery; T = tendon of Todaro; E-E = fila coronaria of mitral orifice; F-F = fila coronaria of tricuspid orifice; N = atrioventricular (AV) node; M = main AV bundle. (Reprinted with permission from Zimmerman J, Bailey CP: The surgical significance of the fibrous skeleton of the heart. *J Thorac Cardiovasc Surg* 1962; 44:701.)

prong connection of the aorta to the central fibrous body.

The pars membranacea is formed by the fused anterior and posterior endocardial cushions, aided by the bulbar cushions and the tissue from the summit of the posterior portion of the ventricular septum. This occurs at about 16–17 mm of fetal length. Up to about 20 mm of fetal length, the connections between the atria and ventricles are muscular. At about 30 mm, epicardial connective tissue in the coronary sulcus cuts into this muscle converting it into connective tissue with only remnants of muscle remaining. By 6 months after birth, these muscular remnants disappear.

Chapter 5

The Anatomy of the Conduction System[12,19]

Anatomy

The conduction system of the heart in man consists of the whole heart. However, in a limited sense, it may be said to consist of the sinoatrial (SA) node and its approaches, the atrial preferential pathways, the approaches to the atrioventricular (AV) node, the AV node, the penetrating portion of the bundle of His, the branching portion of the bundle of His, the right and left bundle branches, and the peripheral Purkinje nets (see color plates I and II).

SA Node

The SA node lies in the sulcus terminalis, extending from the hump of the atrial appendage to a varying distance downward, demarcated by the intercaval band. Grossly, in our hands, it is not dissectable. Histologically at the light level (Fig. 5–1 A,B), it consists of fusiform cells, with a diameter that is smaller than that of the atrial cells. The cytoplasm stains more lightly than that of the atrial cells, containing a smaller number of myofibrils, with scarce striations. No intercalated discs are visible at the light level. These cells lie in a sea of thick collagenous and thinner elastic fibers.

At the electron microscopic level, the cells show a smaller number of myofibrils, which are arranged in a disorderly manner, as compared to the atrial cells. The sarcoplasmic reticulum is scant and there is no transverse tubular system. The connections between the cells show desmosomes, with few fasciae adherentes and scant gap junctions. The center of the node is occupied by P or regular cells. Towards the periphery there are transitional cells that terminate in atrial cells.

Surrounding the SA node are ordinary atrial cells, but a few larger cells are present which bear some resemblance to Purkinje cells.

The blood supply to the SA node is by way of the ramus ostii cavae superioris, helped by other atrial branches and branches of the bronchial arteries. Nerve cells and fibers are present on the periphery, but only nerve fibers are found in the midst of the node.

Atrial Preferential Pathways

These pathways connect the SA node to the AV node (Fig. 5–2). They are part of the general musculature of the right side of the atrial septum. The upper pathway passes from the head of the SA node to the upper part of the atrial septum to the AV node. The middle pathway passes from the middle of the SA node through the proximal part of the right atrium along the limbus fossae ovalis to the AV node. The lower pathway journeys from the tail of the node along the linea terminalis,

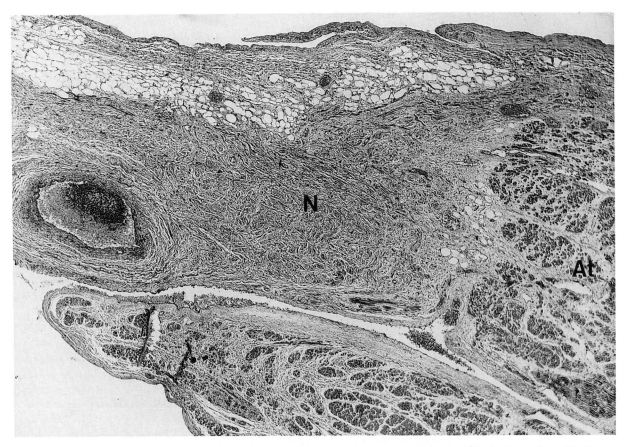

Figure 5-1A: Photomicrograph of the sinoatrial node with its approaches. Hematoxylin-eosin stain ×50. N = SA node; At = atrial muscle.

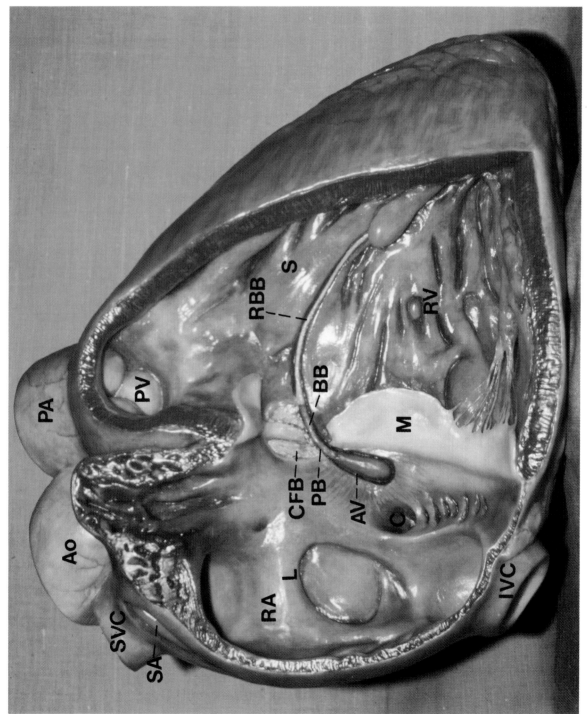

Color plate I: Diagrammatic sketch of the right side of the heart, showing the conduction system. RA = right atrium; RV = right ventricle; L = limbus fossae ovalis; C = coronary sinus; SVC = superior vena cava; IVC = inferior vena cava; M = medial leaflet of the tricuspid valve; AV = AV node; PB = bundle of His, penetration portion; BB = bundle of His, branching portion; RBB = right bundle branch; PA = pulmonary artery; Ao = aorta; SA = SA node; PV = pulmonary valve; S = septal band; CBF = central fibrous body.

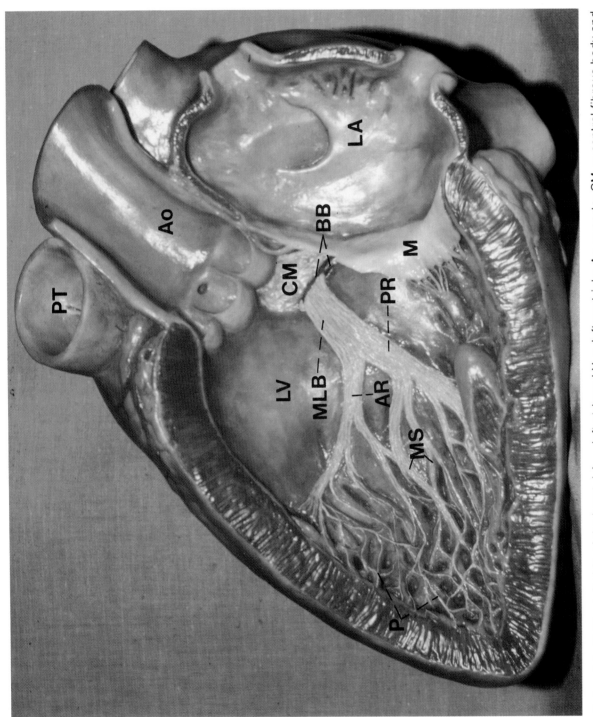

Color plate II: The left side of the heart. LA = left atrium; LV = left ventricle; Ao = aorta; CM = central fibrous body and pars membranacea; BB = bundle of His, branching portion; MLB = main left bundle branch; AR = anterior radiation of the left bundle branch; PR = posterior radiation of the left bundle branch; MS = midseptal fibers of the left bundle branch; P = peripheral Purkinje nets; M = mitral valve; PT = pulmonary trunk.

swings into the lower part of the atrial septum below the fossa ovalis to reach the coronary sinus area and then the AV node. These pathways consist of muscle of the same type as that found in the atrium. They are moderately sized typical working atrial cells among which are dispersed Purkinje-like cells.

AV Node

The AV node lies between the coronary sinus and the medial leaflet of the tricuspid valve (Fig. 5–3). Histologically at the light level, it consists of a meshwork of cells that are about the size of atrial cells and are distinctly smaller than ventricular cells (Fig. 5–4 A–C). The cytoplasm of the cells stains lightly, not as intensely as the atrial and ventricular cells. Striations and intercalated discs are seen at the light level. Mesothelial cells and spaces are seen between the nodal cells. The elastic and collagenous tissue is more copious than that of the atria and ventricles.

At the electron microscopic level, the AV node shows a smaller number of myofibrils and mitochondria, which are arranged in a helter-skelter manner. The sarcoplasmic reticulum is poorly developed and there is no transverse tubular system. Gap junctions are scarce but desmosomes are frequent. Fasciae adher-

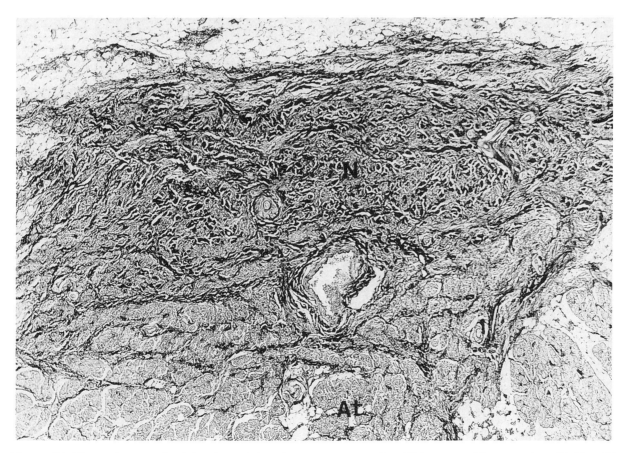

Figure 1B: Photomicrograph of the sinoatrial node, transverse section. Weigert-van Gieson stain ×57. N = SA node; At = atrial muscle. (Reprinted with permission from Lev M: The conduction system in the human heart. *Military Med* 1957; 120:262–268.)

entes are more frequent than in the SA node, but not as frequent as in the atrial and ventricular cells.

AV Bundle

The AV node now penetrates the central fibrous body to become the penetrating portion of the bundle of His (AV bundle) (Fig. 5–4C). The AV bundle and bundle branches are surrounded by a space (Fig. 5–5A) lined by mesothelial cells (Fig. 5–5B). The nature of

this space is today unknown. The cells of the bundle of His are arranged in longitudinal fascicles with some communication between the fascicles. The diameter of the cells of the AV bundle is greater than that of the AV node, but smaller than that of the ventricles. The cytoplasm stains lighter than that of cells of the ventricles, due to a smaller number of myofibrils. Striations and intercalated discs are seen at the light level.

At the electron microscopic level, the myofibrils and mitochondria are more plentiful than in the AV node, but are not as copious as in the ventricle. The arrangement of the

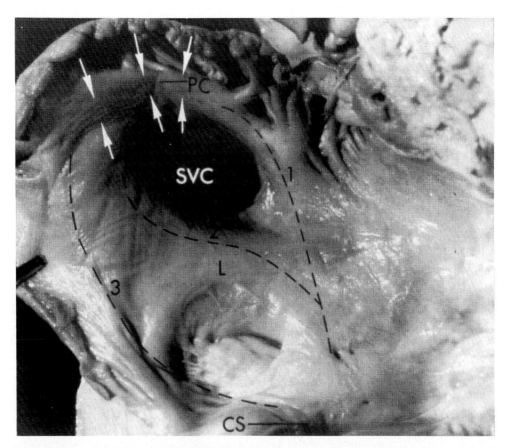

Figure 5–2: Atrial preferential pathways from the SA node to the AV node. Black lines point to the confluence of the anterior and middle preferential pathways. 1 = upper (anterior) preferential pathway; 2 = middle preferential pathway; 3 = lower preferential pathway (posterior); SVC = superior vena cava; PC = posterior crest; CS = coronary sinus. White arrows point to the position of the SA node. (Reprinted with permission from Bharati S, Lev M: Anatomy and histology of the conduction system. In: *Artificial Cardiac Pacing: Practical Approach,* 2nd Ed., Chung EK (ed), p 15, 1984.)

components is orderly. The connections between cells are by copious gap junctions, desmosomes, and fasciae adherentes.

The penetrating portion of the AV bundle now enters the lower confines of the pars membranacea and becomes the branching portion of the His bundle. Here it may proceed some distance before it becomes the latter when it gives off the fine fascicles of the posterior portion of the main left bundle branch (Fig. 5–6A). It then reaches the bifurcation or pseudobifurcation (Fig. 5–6B), which is the point where the right bundle branch and the remaining fibers of the left bundle are given off.

The right bundle branch (color plate I) is given off distal to the insertion of the medial leaflet of the tricuspid valve on the pars membranacea. It passes along the lower part of the septal band just below the muscle of Lancisi (Fig. 5–7) to reach the moderator band. In general, in the first portion, it is intramyocardial. In the second portion, it is usually intramyocardial (Fig. 5–8). In the third portion, it is subendocardial (Fig. 5–9). It ends at the an-

terolateral papillary muscle of the right ventricle where it divides into three portions. These supply this papillary muscle and the parietal and lower septal surface of the right ventricle. It is not certain how many fibers pass to the conus region.

The anterior radiation of the main left bundle branch is smaller than the posterior radiation (color plate II). The anterior radiation goes to the medial-basilar portion of the anterior papillary muscle. The posterior radiation goes to the medial-basilar portion of the posterior papillary muscle. Both radiations give off branches to the center of the septum (color plate II).

The term *Purkinje cell* in this chapter means only the large cells of the left bundle branch, and those of the third part of the right bundle branch. These cells are larger than those of the ventricular myocardium (Fig. 5–10). They are cross-striated with intercalated discs. At the electron microscopic level, these cells show an irregular arrangement of few mitochondria and myofibrils. Again there is no transverse tubular system. The connections

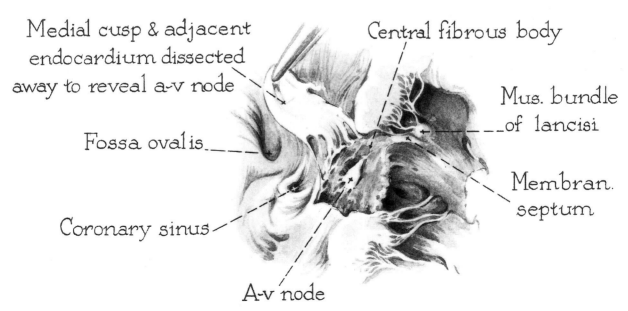

Figure 5-3: Diagrammatic sketch of the AV node with labels. AV = atrioventricular node; Mus. = muscle. (Reprinted with permission from Widran J, Lev M: The dissection of the human av node, bundle and branches. *Circulation* 1951; 4:863.)

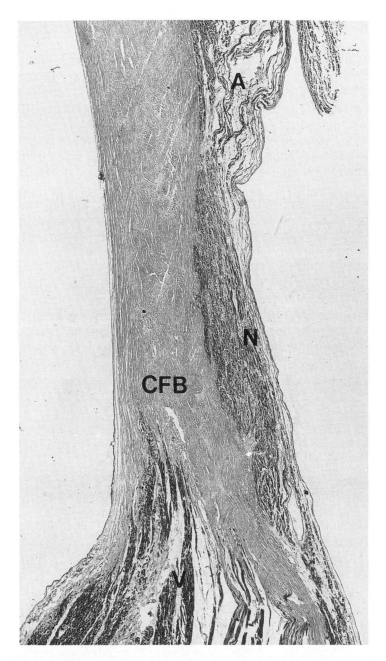

Figure 5-4A: Photomicrograph of the AV node. Hematoxylin-eosin stain ×15. N = AV node; V = ventricular myocardium; A = atrial musculature; CFB = central fibrous body.

between the cells, however, are well developed with many desmosomes, fasciae adherentes, and gap junctions.

The Purkinje cells that are subendocardial become transitional cells as they penetrate the myocardium and become regular working cells.

The blood supply to the AV node and bundle is by way of the ramus septi fibrosi reinforced by branches from the anterior descending coronary artery. The blood supply to the right bundle branch is by way of perforating branches from the anterior and posterior descending coronary arteries. A special large branch, the ramus limbi dextri, coming from the second anterior perforating artery, helps supply the midportion of the right bundle branch. The blood supply to the main left bundle is by way of branches from the anterior and posterior perforating arteries. The blood supply to the anterior radiation is by way of both anterior and posterior perforating arteries. That of the posterior radiation is in some cases by way of the posterior perforating artery and in others by way of both the anterior and posterior perforating arteries.

Copious nerve cells are found around the AV node. Nerve fibers are present in the AV node and bundle, and to a lesser extent in the bundle branches.

Histochemically, conductive cells have a well-developed anaerobic oxidative system, and a poorly developed aerobic one. This is the opposite for contracting cells. Certain cho-

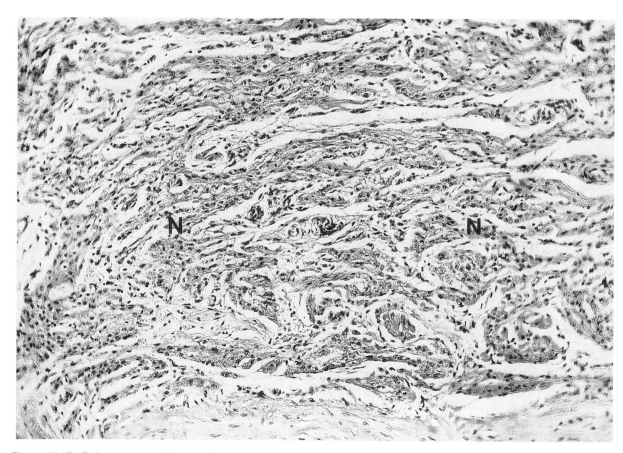

Figure 5-4B: Enlargement of Figure 5A. Hematoxylin-eosin stain ×90. N = AV node. (Reprinted with permission from Lev M: The conduction system. In: *Pathology of Heart and Blood Vessels,* 3rd Ed., Gould SE (ed), Springfield, IL, Charles C. Thomas, 1968.)

linesterases are found in the conduction system that are not found in the myocardium.

Paraspecific Fibers of Mahaim

These are fibers that pass from the AV node to the ventricle-nodoventricular, from the AV bundle to the ventricle-fasciculoventricular, and from the left bundle branch to the ventricular myocardium. No such cells are found between the right bundle branch and the ventricular myocardium in man.

Fibers of Kent

These fibers are normally present in some infants under the age of 6 months in the right and left AV rim communicating between atria and ventricles. On the atrial side they resemble atrial cells and on the ventricular side, they resemble ventricular cells.

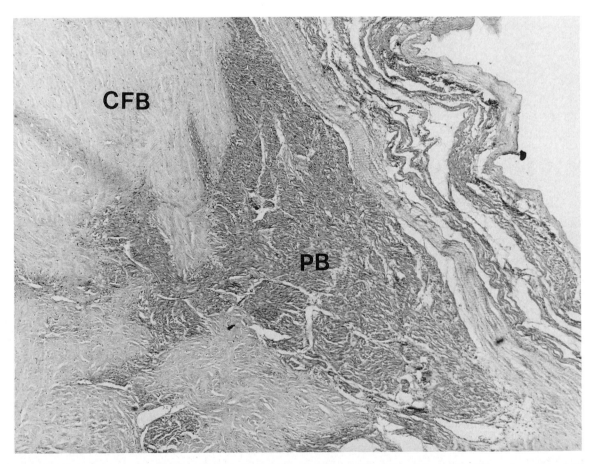

Figure 5-4C: AV node becoming the bundle of His. Hematoxylin-eosin stain ×45. PB = bundle of His, penetrating portion; CFB = central fibrous body.

Embryology of the Conduction System[20]

The SA node originates from the sinus venosus at about 7–10 mm of fetal length (crown-rump). The AV node originates at about 8–9 mm of fetal length from the posterior part of the musculature of the auricular canal. The AV bundle develops at about 10– 11 mm from the same source, either in situ or from the proliferation of the node. The left bundle branch is first seen at about 11 mm of fetal length. It originates in situ from the ventricular trabeculae, or from the proliferation of the bundle. It is completely developed by 16.5 mm. The right bundle branch originates at about 13 mm and can be traced to the moderator band at 22–25 mm.

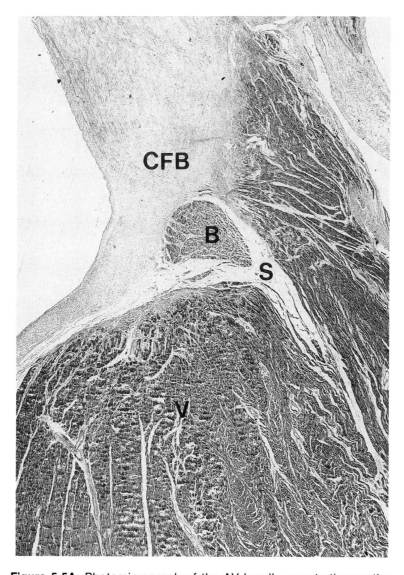

Figure 5-5A: Photomicrograph of the AV bundle, penetrating portion showing the space around it. Hematoxylin-eosin stain ×20. S = space; B = bundle, penetrating portion; V = ventricular septal musculature; CFB = central fibrous body. (Reprinted with permission from Lev M: The conduction system in the human heart. *Military Med* 1957; 120:266.)

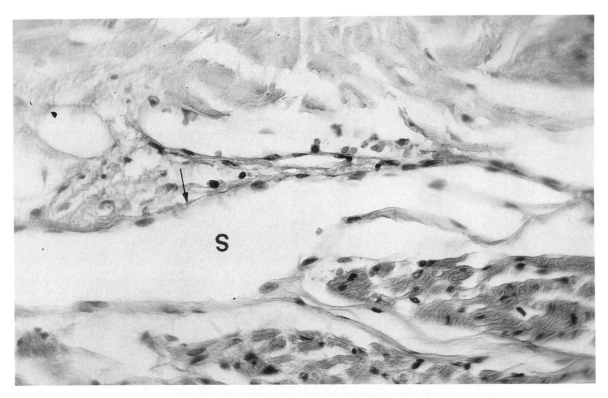

Figure 5-5B: Section of sheath and enclosed space that surrounds the bundle of His. Hematoxylin-eosin stain ×810. S = space. (Reprinted with permission from Lev M: The conduction system. In: *Pathology of Heart and Blood Vessels,* 3rd Ed., Gould SE (ed), Springfield, IL, Charles C. Thomas, 1968.)

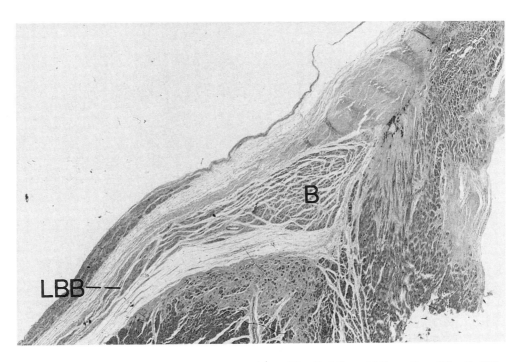

Figure 5-6: Photomicrograph of the branching (Fig. 5–6A) and bifurcating (Fig. 5–6B) portion of the bundle of His. Hematoxylin-eosin stain ×45 (A) and ×30 (B). B = branching portion of the bundle; LBB = posterior radiation of the left bundle branch; L = left side of bifurcation; R = right side of bifurcation; V = ventricular muscle. (Reprinted with permission from Lev M, Bharati S: Anatomic basis for impulse generation and atrioventricular transmission. In: *His Bundle Electrocardiography and Clinical Electrophysiology,* Narula OS (ed), Philadelphia, FA Davis, p 10, 1975.)

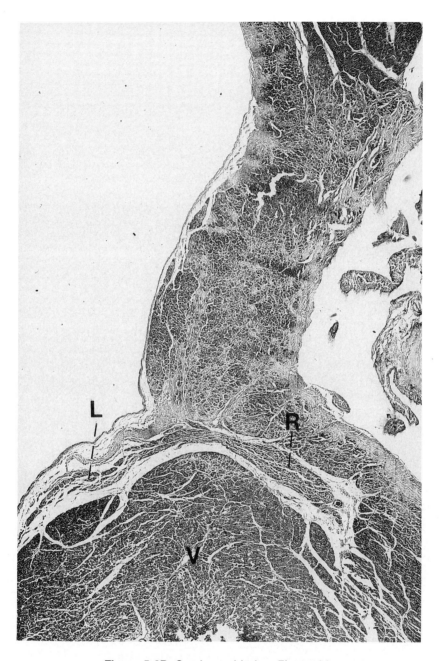

Figure 5-6B: See legend below Figure 6A.

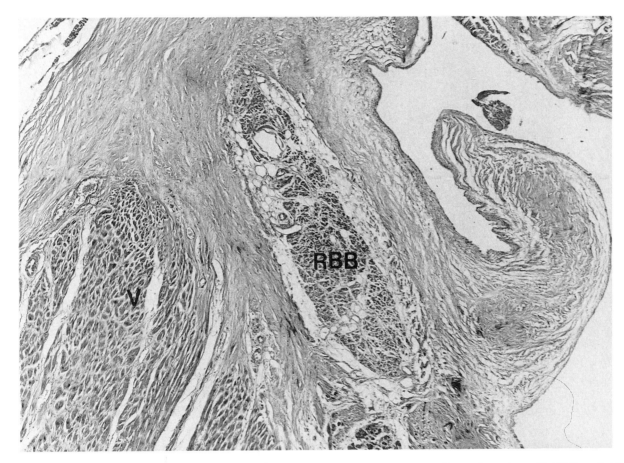

Figure 5-7: Photomicrograph of first part of the right bundle branch. Hematoxylin-eosin stain ×45. RBB = right bundle branch; V = ventricular myocardium. (Reprinted with permission from Lev M, Bharati S: Anatomic basis for impulse generation and atrioventricular transmission. In: *His Bundle Electrocardiography and Clinical Electrophysiology*, Narula OS (ed), Philadelphia, FA Davis, p 10, 1975.)

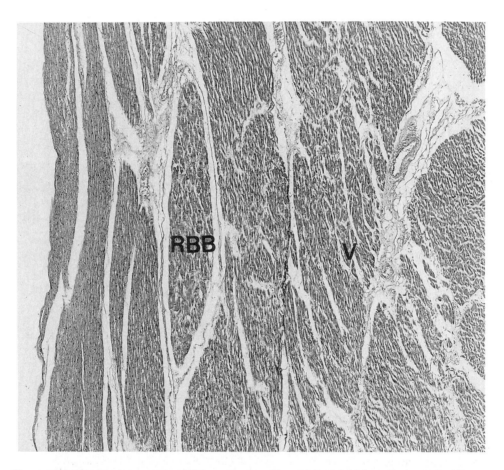

Figure 5-8: Photomicrograph of the second portion of the right bundle branch. Hematoxylin-eosin stain ×45. RBB = second part of the right bundle branch; V = ventricular myocardium.

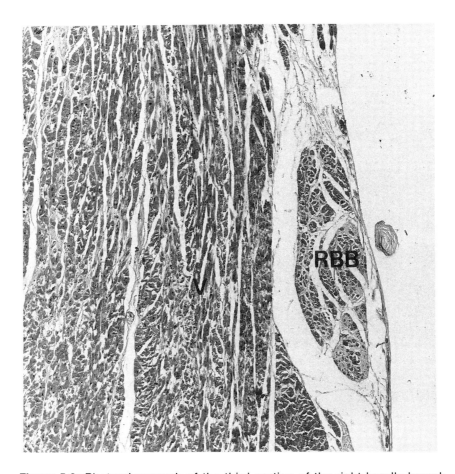

Figure 5-9: Photomicrograph of the third portion of the right bundle branch. Hematoxylin-eosin stain ×45. RBB = third portion of right bundle branch; V = ventricular myocardium.

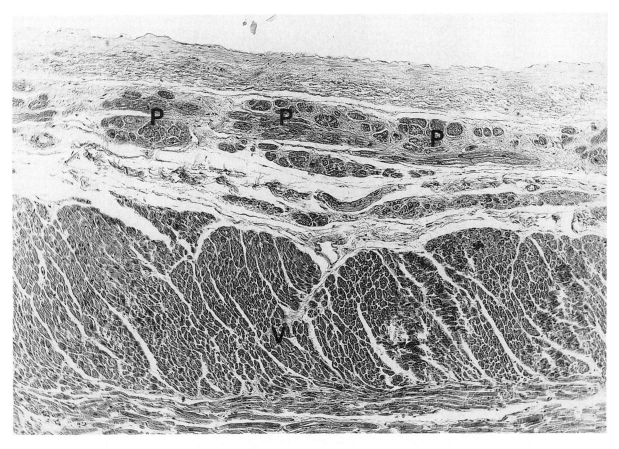

Figure 5-10: Peripheral portion of the left bundle branch. Hematoxylin-eosin stain ×100. P = Purkinje cells; V = ventricular myocardium.

Chapter 6

Historical Retrospect

Much work has been done in the past in recent times on sudden death. The following is a recording of such work, regardless as to whether conduction system studies were done. This, of course, does not cover all of the known literature in this field.

The authors who have contributed are: Bedford, 1933,[21] Koppisch, 1934,[22] Allen, 1944,[23] Helpern and Rabson, 1945,[24] Moritz and Zamcheck, 1946,[25] Richards, 1947,[26] Majoska, 1948,[27] Evans, 1949,[28] Sta Cruz, 1951,[29] Teare, 1958,[30] Sugai, 1959,[31] Aponte, 1960,[32] Burch and DePasquale, 1963,[33] Fraser, Froggatt, and James, 1964,[34] James, Rupe, and Monte, 1965,[35] Kuller, Lilienfeld, and Fisher, 1966,[36] James and Monto, 1966,[37] James and Birk, 1966,[38] Kuller, Lilienfeld, and Fisher, 1967,[39] James and Froggatt and Marshall, 1967,[40] Luke and Helpern, 1968,[41] James, 1968,[42] Green, Korovetz, Shanklin, DeVito, and Taylor, 1969,[43] James, 1969,[44] Anderson, Edland, and Schenk, 1970,[45] Goodwin, 1970,[46] James, 1970,[47] Schwartz and Walsh, 1971,[48] Haerem, 1972,[49] Ferris, 1973,[50] Valdes-Dapena, Greene, Basavarand, Catherman, and Truex, 1973,[51] Friedman, Manwaring, Rosenman, Donlon, Ortega, and Grube, 1973,[52] Anderson, Bouton, Burrow, and Smith, 1974,[53] Ferris and Kendeel, 1974,[54] James, Armstrong, Silverman, and Marshall, 1974,[55] Marshall and Shappell, 1974,[56] Ferris, 1974,[57] James, Marshall, and Craig, 1974,[58] Shah, Adelman, Wigle, Gobel, Burchell, Hardarson, Curiel, de la Calzada, Oakley, and Goodwin, 1974,[59] Pruitt, 1974,[60] Abildskov, 1975,[61] Lie, 1975,[62] Lie and Titus, 1975,[63] James and Marshall, 1975,[64] James, Marilley, and Marriott, 1975,[65] Gotoh, 1976,[66] Lie, Rosenberg, and Erickson, 1976,[67] James and Marshall, 1976,[68] Doyle, 1976,[69] James and Marshall, 1976,[70] Brechenmacher, Coumel, and James, 1976,[71] Voigt, 1976,[72] Gillette, Yeoman, Mullin, and McNamara, 1977,[73] James and Galakhov 1977,[74] James and Jackson, 1977,[75] James, 1977,[76] Lown, Verrier, and Rabinowitz, 1977,[77] Branch, Robertson, Beckett, Waldo, and

James, 1977,[78] James, Frogatt, Atkinson, Lurie, McNamara, Miller, Schloss, Carroll, and North, 1978,[79] James, 1978,[80] Thiene, Valente, and Rossi, 1978,[81] Fontaine, Guiraudon, Frank, Vedel, Grosgogeat, and Cabrol, 1978,[82] Meierhenry and Liu, 1978,[83] Haerem, 1978,[84] Davies and Popple, 1979,[85] Okada, 1979,[86] Lahiri, Balasubramanian, and Raftery, 1979,[87] Lown, 1979,[88] Southall, Arrowsmith, Oakley, McEnery, Anderson, and Shinebourne, 1979,[89] Kulbertus and Wellens, 1980,[90] Maron, Roberts, McAllister, Rosing, and Epstein, 1980,[91] Morales, Romanelli, and Boucek, 1980,[92] Waller and Roberts, 1980,[93] James, Pearce, and Givhan, 1980,[94] James and MacLean, 1980,[95] Krikler, Davies, Rowland, Goodwin, Evans, and Shaw, 1980,[96] Kuller, 1980,[97] Rossi, 1980,[98] Cheitlin, 1980,[99] Pedersen, 1980,[100] Davies, 1981,[101] Anderson, Bowie, Dempster, and Gwynne, 1981,[102] Fritchett, MacArthur, Oakley, Krikler, and Goodwin, 1981,[103] Smeeton, Anderson, Ho, Davies, and Anderson, 1981,[104] Rossi and Thiene, 1981,[105] Gallagher, Smith, Kasell, Benson, Sterba, and Grant, 1981,[106] Mirinato, Thiene, Menghetti, Buja, Nava, Cecchetto, and Rossi, 1981,[107] Virmani, Robinowitz, Clark, and McAllister, 1982,[108] Marcus, Fontaine, Guiraudon, Frank, Laurenceau, Malergue and Grosgogeat, 1982,[109] Hinkle, 1982,[110] Schroeder and Lyons, 1982,[111] Lown, 1982,[112] Schwartz, Montemerlo, Facchini, Salice, Rosti, Poggio, and Giorgetti, 1982,[113] Rossi, 1982,[114] Vesterby and Gregersen, 1982,[115] Wellens, Brugada, Fritz, and Bar, 1982,[116] Davies, Anderson, and Becker, 1983,[117] Rossi, 1983,[118] Sakurai and Kawai, 1983,[119] Baron, Thacker, Gorelkin, Vernon, Taylor, and Choi, 1983,[120] James, 1983,[121] Garson, Porter, Gillette, and McNamara, 1983,[122] Thiene, Pennelli, and Rossi, 1983,[123] Okada and Kawai, 1983,[124] Rossi and Thiene, 1984,[125] Furlanello, Bettini, Cozzi, Del Favero, Disertori, Vergara, Durante, Guarnerio, Inama, and Thiene, 1984,[126] Rossi, Piffer, Turolla, Frigerio, Coumel, and James, 1985,[127] Fuster, Steele, and Chesebro 1985,[128] James, 1985,[129] Driscoll and Edwards, 1985,[130] Joshi, 1985,[131] Meijler, Van Der Tweel, Herbschleb, Hauer, and Robles de Medina, 1985,[132] Surawicz, 1985,[133] Kir-

schner, Eckner, and Baron, 1986,[134] Galvaghan, Kelly, Kuchnar, Hickie, and Campbell, 1986,[135] Shah, Pahalajani, Gandhi, Pandey, and Punjabi, 1986,[136] Northcote, Flannigan, and Ballantyne, 1986,[137] Vikhert, Tsiplenkova, and Cherpachenko, 1986,[138] Shvalev, Vikhert, Stropus, Sosunov, Pavlovich, Kargina-Terentyeva, Zhuchkova, Anikin, and Maryan, 1986,[139] James, 1986,[140] James and Vikhert, 1986,[141] Coumel, Leclercq, and Leenhardt, 1987,[142] Dimsdale, Ruberman, Carleton, DeQuattro, Eaker, Eliot, Furberg, Irvin, Lown, Shapiro, and Shumaker, 1987,[143] Zipes, Levy, Cobb, Julius, Kaufman, Miller, and Verrier, 1987,[144] Corr, Pitt, Natelson, Reis, Shine, and Skinner, 1987,[145] Schwartz, Randall, Anderson, Engel, Friedman, Hartley, Pickering, and Thoresen, 1987,[146] Bigger, 1987,[147] Verrier, 1987,[148] Kligfield, Levy, Devereux, and Savage, 1987,[149] Wiedermann, Becker, Hopferwieser, Muhlberger, and Knapp, 1987,[150] Hattori, Murhohara, Yui, Takatsu, and Kawai, 1987,[151] Borhani, 1987,[152] Prystowsky, Fananapazir, Packer, Thompson, and German, 1987,[153] Furberg, 1987,[154] Amsterdam, 1987,[155] Andreoli, DiPasquale, Pinelli, Grazi, Tognetti, and Testa, 1987,[156] Nakamura, Takeshita, and Nose, 1987,[157] Kennedy and Fisher, 1987,[158] Surawicz, 1987,[159] Lehmann and Steinman, 1987,[160] Yee, Scheinman, Griffin, and Ebert, 1987,[161] Eldar, Sauve, and Scheinman, 1987,[162] Gillette and Hammill, 1988,[163] Okada and Gotoh, 1988,[164] Fontaine, Fontaliran, Limares-Cruz, Chomette, and Grosgogeat, 1988,[165] Inoue and Zipes, 1988,[166] Lemery, Brugada, Havenith, Barbour, Roberts, and Wellens, 1988,[167] Crozier, 1988,[168] Bhandari, Hong, Au, McKay, and Rahimtoola, 1988,[169] Skadberg, Braserud, Karwinski, and Ohm, 1988,[170] Baye's de Luna, Coumel, and Leclerq, 1989,[171] and Bharati and Lev.[172–210]

Concepts Developed

The concepts that these authors have developed concerning sudden cardiac death in which conduction system studies were not done are as follows:

1. The cause of death may not be disclosed by routine autopsy, gross and microscopic, and by toxicologic examination.
2. The most common cause of sudden cardiac death is coronary heart disease. This includes intramural coronary artery disease and origin of the left coronary artery from the right sinus of Valsalva.
3. Other diseases in which sudden cardiac death may occur are: (1) acute and subacute myocarditis, (2) syphilitic heart disease, (3) rheumatic heart disease, (4) rupture of the aorta, (5) diabetes mellitus, (6) hypertrophic cardiomyopathy, (7) polyarteritis nodosa, (8) congenital heart disease, (9) right ventricular dysplasia, (10) acquired aortic stenosis, (11) sarcoidosis, amyloidosis, hemochromatosis, (12) dilated or restricted cardiomyopathy, (13) mitral valve prolapse, (14) scleroderma, and (15) Whipple's disease.
4. In congenital heart disease (unoperated), sudden cardiac death may occur in: (1) congenital aortic stenosis, (2) ventricular septal defect with pulmonary vascular disease, (3) pulmonary stenosis and atresia, and (4) endocardial cushion defects.
5. Sudden cardiac death may occur in young athletes.
6. Sudden cardiac death may occur long after operations on tetralogy of Fallot and complete transposition of the arterial trunks and other malformations.
7. The basic cause of any sudden cardiac death may not lie in the heart but in the brain, spinal cord, or stellate ganglia.
8. The cause of sudden cardiac death may lie in the nerves of the heart.
9. Sudden cardiac death may be familial.
10. Sudden cardiac death may be due to abnormality in the platelets.
11. Sudden cardiac death may be due to Ebstein's disease.
12. Sudden cardiac death may be due to an enlarged pars membranacea.
13. Sudden cardiac death may be due to pre-excitation syndrome (Wolff-Parkinson-White [WPW] syndrome), actual or hidden.
14. Absence of a portion of the right ventricular myocardium may result in sudden death—Uhls' anomaly.

Mechanism of Sudden Cardiac Death

The mechanism of sudden cardiac death is the creation of ventricular fibrillation or asystole. In coronary heart disease, ventricular fibrillation may be instigated by frequent premature complexes which go into ventricular tachycardia and then degenerate into fibrillation. Factors influencing ventricular fibrillation are:

1. slow heart rate;
2. long QT interval;
3. electrocution;
4. hypokalemia;
5. acidosis;
6. sympathetic-parasympathetic imbalances with dominance of the sympathetic system—that is, there is adrenergic-cholinergic imbalance with exaggerated catecholamine action, increased oxygen consumption with increased chronotropic, and inotropic action. At the same time, there is a reduction of oxygen supply leading to muscle spasm and platelet aggregation. Cholinergic action exerted on specialized muscle severely inhibits automaticity leading to bradycardia and asystole; and
7. emotion.

In sudden cardiac death, there may be unequal and focal depletion of catecholamines. Stimulation of the left stellate ganglion may precipitate ventricular fibrillation. In ischemic myocardium, arrhythmias may arise from nonhomogeneous distribution of levels of hyperkalemia and acidosis. Where there is proximity between healthy and unhealthy myocardial tissue, ventricular fibrillation may be set up due to a re-entry phenomenon.

Conduction System Studies

In sudden cardiac death, conduction system studies have been performed by James and his associates,[34,35,37,38,40,42,44,47,55,58,64,65,68,70,71,74–76,78–80,94,95,121,127,129,141,142] Anderson and associates,[45] Ferris,[50,54,57] Lie,[62] Lie, and Titus,[63] Gotoh,[64] Lie, Rosenberg, and Erickson,[67] Rossi and associates,[81,98,105,114,118,123,125,127] Meierhery and Liu,[83] Davies and associates,[85,96,101,102] Okada and associates,[86,124] Anderson and associates,[102] Pedersen,[100] Smeeton and associates,[104] Vesterby and Gregerson,[115] Kirschner and associates,[134] Wiederman and associates,[150] and Bharati and Lev.[172–208].

James and his associates over the years studied the conduction system in a series of patients with sudden death. In 1964, with Fraser and Froggart,[34] he studied nine cases with congenital deafness, fainting spells, and sudden death. In two of these cases, the conduction system was examined. In case #1, he found local hemorrhage in the anterior internodal tract. The SA nodal artery was thickened. There was extensive hemorrhage at the junction of the SA node and right atrium. A few small arteries of the AV node were thickened and the bundle was congested. Ganglia in the atria showed hemorrhage. In case #7, both the SA and the AV nodal arteries arose from the right coronary artery. The SA nodal artery was thickened. At the junction of the SA node and the right atrium, there were large areas of replacement of nodal fibers by fat, hemorrhage, and granulation tissue.

In 1965, with Rupe and Monto, James[35] studied the conduction system in eight patients with systemic lupus erythematosus. In the heart, he found pericarditis. Adjacent to the SA node, he saw old, organizing, and re-

cent thrombi. The collagen was cystic. Scattered inflammatory cells were present between the AV node and the central fibrous body. This was especially evident in one case where there was complete AV block. In 1966, with Monto,[37] he studied the SA node, the AV node, and His bundle in three cases of thrombotic thrombocytopenic purpura. In the first case, the small arteries in all these regions showed changes with focal hemorrhage. In the second, multiple focal hemorrhages with occlusion of the arteries was seen. The third case, which had complete heart block, showed the bundle destroyed by edema and infarction. Occlusion of scattered arterioles was present in the SA and the AV nodes.

In 1966, James, with Birk,[38] studied the hearts of all six patients with polyarteritis nodosa. All cases showed a necrotizing angiitis of the SA node and, to a lesser extent, the AV node. This produced thrombosis and fibrotic occlusion with numerous small infarcts and hemorrhages. The endocardium beneath the sinus node showed old and recent mural thrombi.

In 1967, with Froggatt and Marshall,[40] in two athletes, 18 years old and 16 years old, with otherwise normal hearts, he found the following. In the first case, the sinus node artery was markedly narrowed. There were foci of scars, recent hemorrhage, and degeneration within the SA node and adjacent nerves and ganglia. The AV nodal artery was moderately narrowed with fibrosis of the AV node and His bundle. The weight of the heart was not given. The second case was that of a 15-year-old male. At the posterior margin of the AV node, there was recent necrosis with round cell infiltration. The sinus node artery was thickened and a major branch was occluded by medial hyperplasia and intimal proliferation.

In 1968, James[42] studied sudden infant death syndrome (SIDS) in babies. He found archipelagos of the AV node and bundle extending into the fibrous tissue of the central fibrous body, both in SIDS cases and in the normal babies. Occasional hemorrhages were present in the cardiac autonomic ganglia. In 1969, James[44] studied patients with arrhythmias in acute myocardial infarction. These patients had a moderate degree of coronary disease but no occlusion. They died suddenly and unexpectedly. The SA node was found to be involved due to advanced pericarditis. The maximum ischemic changes were found at the junction of the SA node and the right atrium.

In 1970, James[47] described the fetal and postnatal development of the conduction system. A process of postnatal molding goes on during the first 2 months of life. This includes cell death. In 1974, James with Armstrong, Silverman, and Marshall,[55] described sudden death in two young soldiers. In the first case, the heart was slightly hypertrophied and there was only one coronary ostium. Toxicologic examination was negative. Throughout both ventricles, there were extensive foci of round cell infiltration and focal necrosis. The SA node showed marked thickening and narrowing of the SA nodal artery with one small hemorrhage. The bundle of His revealed septated fibrosis and one small hemorrhage. In the second case, toxicologic examination was again negative. The weight of the heart was not given. The heart was negative pathologically aside from the conduction system. The AV nodal artery was markedly thickened. The midportion of the AV node showed several cystic spaces. The His bundle revealed edema, foci of hemorrhage and some fibrosis. The left bundle branch showed fibrosis at its origin. The central fibrous body was abnormally formed.

In 1974, James, with Marshall and Craig,[58] described a 19-year-old female patient, who died suddenly. She had a long history of paroxysmal atrial fibrillation. The heart showed nonbacterial endocarditis of the mitral and tricuspid valves. The SA nodal artery showed platelet and fibrin thrombi with virtual infarctions of the entire SA node. The AV node contained cells extending into the central fibrous body. The His bundle was fragmented with focal degeneration and edema extending into the bundle branches.

In 1975, James and Marshall[64] presented 22 cases with asymmetrical septal hypertrophy of the heart, which in each case was otherwise normal. Case #1 was a 22-year-old female. The heart weighed 390 grams. Many

small coronary arteries were narrowed. The central fibrous body contained cysts and an excess of nodal fragments adjacent to the node. Fibrosis of the ventricular septum was present. The sinus node was normal. Case #2 was that of a 59-year-old female. The heart weighed 434 grams. One-third of the SA node showed focal fibrosis and the posterior two-thirds was replaced by dense fibrosis. There were multiple narrow, small branches of the SA nodal artery. There were many narrowed, small coronary arteries in the heart. The septal myocardium contained several deep clefts. Case #3 was that of a 46-year-old male. The heart weighed 510 grams. There were many narrowed intramural coronary arteries. Many deep clefts were noted in the septal myocardium. The AV node was extensively fragmented in the central fibrous body. The sinus node showed moderate fibrosis. Case #4 was that of an 18-year-old male. The heart weighed 760 grams. The anterior two-thirds of the SA node was completely replaced by dense fibrosis. The AV node was extensively partitioned in the central fibrous body. The AV nodal artery was moderately narrowed. The right bundle branch showed extensive focal infiltration of fat.

Case #5 was that of a 23-year-old male. The heart weighed 580 grams. A single branch of the SA nodal artery was narrowed, as was one branch of the AV nodal artery. Numerous cysts were present in the central fibrous body. The anterior portion of the bundle of His showed fibrosis. Case #6 was that of a 71-year-old male. The heart weighed 690 grams. The SA node showed focal fibrosis. Moderate fibrosis was present in the AV node and the bundle of His. Fatty metamorphosis was also noted in the AV node. The AV nodal artery was markedly narrowed. Case #7 was that of a 39-year-old male. The patient had a family history of sudden death. The heart weighed 510 grams. The SA node showed fibrosis, as did the AV node focally. The bundle of His was extensively fragmented in the central fibrous body. It also showed fibrosis in its anterior portion. Case #8 was that of a 15-year-old male. The heart weighed 475 grams. The central fibrous body and the bundle of His presented numerous cysts. The AV nodal artery was narrowed by 50%.

Case #9 was that of a 72-year-old female. The heart weighed 440 grams. The small coronaries were narrowed throughout. The SA node showed focal areas of fatty metamorphosis and fibrosis in the anterior third which became marked in the middle third. The SA nodal artery was thickened. The bundle of His was the seat of focal fibrosis and marked fatty metamorphosis. Case #10 was that of an 11-year-old female. The heart weighed 250 grams. The SA node presented foci of fatty metamorphosis at its junction with the right atrium. The AV node and bundle were markedly fragmented throughout the central fibrous body. Case #11 was that of a 14-year-old male. The heart weighed 440 grams. The left half of the His bundle was undergoing absorption with replacement by fibroblasts. Elsewhere it showed fibrosis, which was also present in the beginning of the bundle branches. Case #12 was that of a 17-year-old male. The heart weighed 450 grams. The AV nodal artery was markedly narrowed, and the AV node showed fibrosis.

Case #13 was that of a 23-year-old female. There was a family history of sudden death. The heart weighed 425 grams. The small coronaries in the septum were narrowed. The AV nodal artery was narrowed by 50%. Case #14 was that of a 77-year-old male. The heart weighed 520 grams. There was patchy fibrosis of the ventricular septum. The SA node showed fibrosis and fatty metamorphosis virtually severing its connection to the atrium. The AV nodal artery was narrowed. There was fibrosis of the AV node and bundle of His. Both bundle branches showed fibrosis. Case #15 was that of a 4-year-old female. The heart weighed 175 grams. The SA nodal artery was narrowed by 50% and the AV nodal artery was slightly narrowed. There was marked fragmentation of the AV node and bundle of His in the central fibrous body. Case #16 was that of a 48-year-old female. The heart weighed 470 grams. Many small coronary arteries were narrowed in the septum, and the latter had numerous clefts. The SA node was virtually de-

stroyed by fibrosis, and the SA nodal artery was moderately narrowed.

Case #17 was that of a 30-year-old female. The heart weighed 500 grams. The SA node showed focal fibrosis in its anterior two-thirds. The AV nodal artery was markedly narrowed. The bundle of His was the seat of fibrosis and focal hemorrhage. Case #18 was that of a 14-year-old female. The heart weighed 530 grams. The SA nodal artery was slightly thickened. Large divisions of the AV node were present in the central fibrous body. The bundle of His showed slight fibrosis. Case #19 was that of a 26-year-old female. The heart weighed 250 grams. A number of clefts were present in the ventricular septum. The conduction system was normal with the exception of a small bundle of His.

Case #20 was that of a 47-year-old female. The heart weighed 500 grams. There was a large membranous septum. The small coronaries and the septum were thickened. Large foci of fatty metamorphosis were present at the junction of the SA node and the atrium. The AV node was fragmented in the central fibrous body. There were foci of fibrosis and fatty metamorphosis in the AV node and bundle of His. Case #21 was that of a 17-year-old male. The heart weighed 520 grams. There were many narrowed, small coronary arteries in the septum. The AV nodal artery likewise was markedly narrowed. The bundle of His showed mild fibrosis. Case #22 was that of a 13-year-old male. There was a family history of sudden death. The heart weighed 530 grams. Large clefts were found in the ventricular septum. The AV node was filled with cysts and was fragmented in the central fibrous body. Both bundle branches were honeycombed.

In 1975, with Marrilley and Marriott, James[65] studied the conduction system in a 17-year-old girl who died suddenly. She had a tall, thin habitus with long, thin extremities and a family history of seizures. Multiple premature beats were noted for many years. The heart weighed 270 grams. It was otherwise normal. The AV node exhibited numerous fronds and out-pouchings forming loop connections from one part of the node to another. Groups of AV nodal cells were attached to the crest of the ventricular septum. Fascicular ventricular fibers were also seen. The AV nodal artery was moderately narrowed.

In 1976, with Marshall, James[68] presented two cases of sudden death where toxicologic examination was negative. The first case was that of a 20-year-old boy. The heart was normal otherwise. Its weight was not given. The SA nodal artery was normal. The AV node was fragmented within the central fibrous body. Some of the fragments formed loops connecting one portion to another. Other fragments appeared isolated in the central fibrous body. The bundle of His had a long course with node-like cells in it. The second case was that of an 11-year-old boy who showed islands of cartilage in the central fibrous body. The AV node was again fragmented with numerous fronds and fragments in the central fibrous body. In some areas, there was resorptive degeneration of the AV node.

In the same year, James and Marshall[70] presented two cases of sudden death with grossly normal hearts. The first case was that of a 7-year-old male. The heart weighed 140 grams. The myocardium showed a few widely scattered foci of neutrophils and mononuclear cells. There was marked thickening of the sinus node artery by fibromuscular dysplasia. The bundle of His was to the right of the crest of the ventricular septum. The second case was that of a 64-year-old male. The weight of the heart was not given. Multifocal narrowing of the SA nodal artery and its branches was present, produced by fibromuscular dysplasia. The bundle of His showed focal scarring in its midportion.

In the same year (1976), Brechenmacker, Coumel, and James[71] presented another case of sudden death in a 1-year-old child. He had intractable tachycardia until his death. A cousin who is still living has the same problem. The boy in question had complete AV dissociation with a normal atrial rate but a ventricular rate of 20 beats per minute. Autopsy revealed an enlarged heart, grossly otherwise normal. The His bundle was split in its mid-

portion with several thin irregular longitudinal shreds with areas of focal degeneration. The AV node and bundle showed increased fibrosis.

In 1977, with Jackson, James[75] described a case of sudden death in a 20-year-old male 9 years after surgical repair of coarctation. Before and after surgery, he had paroxysmal atrial fibrillation, T-wave inversion, and persistent cardiac hypertrophy. The heart weighed 600 grams. Biventricular hypertrophy was present. The gallbladder was absent. The SA nodal artery showed focal fibromuscular dysplasia with narrowing. There was pericardial fibrosis over the heart including the SA node. The central fibrous body was thickened, especially on the left side, and the bundle of His was displaced towards the right. The AV node was split into upper and lower halves which were tenuously connected through the central fibrous body. The lower half was directly continuous with the myocardial cells of the interventricular septum. That same year, James, with Galakhov,[74] described two cases of benign tumor of the AV node with varying degrees of AV block who died suddenly. One was a 65-year-old woman and the other a 48-year-old woman. The weight of the heart was not given. The tumor (coelothelioma) replaced the AV node in both cases and was in the proximal part of the bundle in the second case.

In the same year, James[76] described a 30-year-old woman with sarcoid who died suddenly. She had recurrent ventricular arrhythmia and syncope. The SA and AV nodal arteries showed focal fibromuscular dysplasia with marked narrowing of the AV nodal artery. There was partial fat replacement of the bundle of His. Part of the small coronaries were narrowed in the myocardium.

In 1978, James, with Froggatt, Atkinson, Lurie, McNamara, Miller, Schloss, Carroll, and North[79] described eight patients with syncopal attacks and a long QT interval who died suddenly. Three were deaf and five had normal hearing. Case #1 was a boy who was diagnosed as having long QT interval at age 10 and who died at the age of 18. The His bundle was on the right side of the ventricular crest. There were small foci of inflammatory degeneration of the neural elements near the SA node, the internodal pathways, the AV node, His bundle, and the ventricular myocardium. Case #2 was a girl who was diagnosed at age 6 as having QT prolongation who died at age 9. Numerous foci of recent and old degeneration were found in the nerves and ganglia in the internodal pathways, the AV node, the His bundle, and ventricular myocardium. In addition, there was persistent fetal dispersion of the AV node and His bundle. The small arteries of the sinus node were thickened. Case #3 had blackout spells, and died at the age of 14. The nerves and ganglia showed focal degeneration around the SA and AV nodes as well as in the internodal pathways and the His bundle. Case #4 died at age 10, with a febrile convulsion. The nerves of the ventricular myocardium showed extensive focal degeneration and round cell infiltration. Case #5 was an 11-year-old with episodes of ventricular arrhythmia. He died in his sleep. There was focal degeneration within and near the SA node involving both nerves and ganglia. Both the SA and AV nodal arteries were moderately narrowed. Neuritis and neural degeneration was present in the myocardium. Case #6 was that of a 12-year-boy. Extensive neuropathological changes were present around the SA node, the AV node, and the His bundle. Case #7 was a 14-year-old female with syncopal attacks. There was no neuropathological abnormalities. Case #8 was a 3½-year-old with widespread neuropathological abnormalities.

In 1978, James[80] reviewed the pathological mechanisms responsible for sudden unexplained death including the neuropathological changes.

In 1980, James, with Pearce and Givhan,[94] described a 32-year-old man who died suddenly while driving. Atrial fibrillation had been present 3 months previously. The heart weighed 530 grams. A fibroma was present on the right side of the central fibrous body, and other fibromas were present on the mitral valve. The SA node showed perineural fibrosis. More extensive neural degeneration and ganglionitis were present adjacent to the SA node. Small foci of neuritis were present in the

ventricular myocardium and the AV node. In the same year, James and MacLean described a case of sudden death in a 17-year-old athlete.[95] He was known to have syncopal attacks, paroxysmal ventricular arrhythmias, and one attack of ventricular fibrillation. The weight of the heart was not given. It was normal on gross examination. Histologically, there was a focal infiltration and degeneration of the small nerves and ganglia throughout the heart including the AV node and around the SA node. There was fragmentation of the anterior portion of the AV node with loop formation within the central fibrous body. The bundle of His was on the right side. Edema and thickening of the epicardium were noted.

Thus, finishing the review of the work of James and his associates, we may now go back to others who have contributed during this period. In 1970, Anderson, with Edland and Schenk,[45] studied the conduction system in 18 cases of sudden infant death syndrome (SIDS) and used 12 cases of traumatic, infectious, and other types of disease as controls. He found focal intimal and medial hyperplasia of the AV nodal artery in 35% of the SIDS cases and in 10% of the controls. The incidence of any myocarditis and perinodal congestion and hemorrhage was the same in the SIDS cases as in the controls. In 1973, Ferris[50] studied 50 cases of SIDS. He found petechial hemorrhages in the region of the SA node and internodal conduction tissue. As far as we can tell, control tissue was not used in this work. In 1973, Valdes-Dapena, with Green, Basavarand, Catherman, and Truex[51] studied the conduction system in SIDS. They questioned whether the process of moulding took place in central fibrous body.

In 1974, Anderson, Bouton, Burrow, and Smith[53] studied 15 cot deaths along with 15 controls. Hemorrhages were present in the atrial myocardium and conduction system in both groups. He was unable to find the pathological changes described by James. He thus did not find the cause of cot death. In the same year, Ferris, with Kendeel,[54] found hemorrhages in 18 cases of SIDS versus two in controls.

In 1974, Ferris[57] cited four cases of sudden death. The first case was that of a 70-year-old male. The heart weighed 450 grams and was normal except for the conduction system. This showed recanalized occlusion of the AV nodal artery, with fibrosis and fatty degeneration of the nodal tissue. Case #2 was that of a 74-year-old female. She had repeated attacks of fainting spells and was diagnosed as having intermittent heart block. The heart weighed 420 grams. There was calcification of the mitral valve ring. Adjacent to the central fibrous body, there was a soft white necrotic nodule. Associated with this, there was extensive destruction of the AV node and bundle of His with an infiltration of lymphocytes, neutrophils, and giant cells. Case #3 was that of an 81-year-old woman with hypertension. The heart weighed 400 grams. Patchy ischemic fibrosis of the myocardium was noted with moderate narrowing of the coronary arteries. The central fibrous body was hard and somewhat nodular. The node and bundle of His showed extensive fibrosis. Case #4 was that of a 49-year-old woman who died suddenly. The weight of the heart was not stated. There was coronary narrowing in three vessels. The bundle of His showed hemorrhage.

Lie, in 1975,[62] and Lie and Titus,[63] in the same year, examined the conduction system in 49 cases of sudden death in coronary heart disease. Only two cases had acute lesions (infarction and hemorrhage) in the AV node and peripheral bundle branches. In both cases, the patient had a massive septal anterior myocardial infarct. The SA nodal artery was narrowed in 25%, and the AV nodal artery was narrowed in 50%.

In 1976, Lie, Rosenberg, and Erickson[67] examined the conduction system in 50 cases of SIDS, from birth to 2 years, and 24 controls. The histologic findings were almost identical in both groups, including hemorrhage in and around the conduction system. Moulding was identical in both groups, which began occurring the first year and completed in the second year. No cell death was apparent.

In 1976, Gotoh[66] studied the conduction system in seven cases of "Pokkuri" disease (sudden unexpected cardiac death of unknown origin in Japan). The hearts were normal in size or slightly enlarged with a dominant right coronary circulation. In six of these cases, there was fibrosis of the SA node and the junction of the node with the atrial musculature. The SA nodal artery had an abnormal course in six, and in three of these cases, the artery did not penetrate the node. In four cases, there were pathological lesions in the junctional system, two of which had fibrotic lesions in the distal part of the bundle of His and the proximal bundle branches, which were sandwiched in between the conal muscle and the summit of the ventricular septum, and two had lymphomatous partial interruption in the middle and distal parts of the His bundle. Simultaneous involvement of the SA node and the AV conduction system were present in four.

Voigt, in 1976,[72] did not know whether the changes we see in the conduction system in otherwise normal hearts are of importance and related to sudden death.

In 1978, Meierhenry and Liu[83] studied the conduction system in 12 dogs that died suddenly, or were vicious or had seizures. Seven of 12 dogs had narrowing of the lumen of small vessels in or near the AV bundle.

Rossi, Thiene, and their associates made multiple studies of the conduction system in various conditions. In 1978, Thiene, with Valenti and Rossi,[81] studied the conduction system in three cases of panarteritis nodosa. Case #1 was a 9-year-old female. The SA nodal artery was normal. The AV node showed severe fibrosis. In the central fibrous body, there were several gaps of fusion between the aortic and tricuspid rings. The pars membranacea was underdeveloped while the conal muscle was overdeveloped. The bundle of His took an intramyocardial course towards the left with the bifurcation on the left side. Case #2 was a 28-year-old male. The SA node showed a recanalized thrombus. There was coagulative necrosis of the approaches. The proximal part of the right bundle branch was intramyocardial. Case #3 was that of a 39-year-old male who had acute necrotizing angiitis with fibrinoid necrosis and leukocytic infiltration in the approaches to the SA node.

In 1980, Rossi[98] studied the occurrence

and significance of coagulative necrosis in the conduction system. In 5 of 18 hearts (15 from patients with early myocardial infarction), coagulative myocytolysis was found in the conduction system. This consisted of myofibrillar degeneration with contraction bands. In nine of these cases, the ordinary myocardium was also involved. He considered this as an exaggerated catecholamine action. In this process, there was disarray of myofilaments followed by conglutination of hypercontracted sarcomeres into coarse acidophilic bands across the cytoplasm and eventually cytolysis. This finding was present in pacemaker cells in the SA node, in some transitional cells, in the internodal tracts, and in a few cells in the AV node and the bundle branches. The His bundle was uninvolved.

In 1981, Rossi and Thiene[105] presented four cases of sudden cardiac death. The first case was that of a 25-year-old male. The heart weighed 360 grams. The right chambers were moderately enlarged. The main coronary arteries showed nonsclerosing atherosclerosis. An atrio-Hisian tract was demonstrated. Case #2 was that of a 29-year-old male. The heart weighed 375 grams. There was marked sclerosis of the major coronary arteries and of the main atrial branch of the right coronary artery. The SA nodal artery was stenosed by fibromuscular dysplasia. Some of the SA nodal fibers were vacuolated and atrophied. The atrial preferential pathways showed focal round cell infiltration. The third case was that of a 53-year-old male with Prinzemetal's angina. During cardiac catheterization, there was angina and spasm of the right coronary artery. The heart weighed 370 grams. The right coronary artery was 70% narrowed. Adjacent to the posterior septal perforating artery, a nerve showed intense lymphoid infiltration and segmental degeneration. The conduction system was normal. Case #4 was that of a 55-year-old man. The heart weighed 400 grams. The major coronary arteries were diffusely and severely stenosed. An early myocardial infarction was present in the ventricular septum and left ventricular free wall. The ganglia adjacent to the sinoatrial node showed severe degeneration, loss of neurons, accumulation of satellite cells, and obliterated empty neuronal spaces.

In 1982, Rossi[114] studied 13 cases of sudden coronary death. Anterior infarction was present in 38%, posterior infarction in 31%, septal involvement was present in 53%, obstruction of the left coronary artery in 31%, the right coronary artery in 23%, and both coronary arteries in 46%, obstruction to the SA nodal artery in 31%, and obstruction to AV nodal artery in 23%. Resultant changes in the SA node were present in 31%, and in the common bundle and bundle branches in 30%; the AV node generally escaped. Neural abnormalities were in the SA node in the ganglion plexus, in the ventricular neural network, and in the AV groove plexus in 92%. He also examined two surgically removed stellate ganglia, which showed focal inflammation and chronic neural changes. The changes in the nerves were vacuolar swelling of nerve sheaths, epiperineural edema, inflammation, hemorrhage, disruption of axons, neural degeneration, neural interstitial fibrosis, and proliferation of ganglion cells.

In 1983, Rossi[118] studied the pathological basis of cardiac arrhythmias. In SA node dysfunctions, he considered nerve degeneration as a basic cause. Nerves may be injured by pericarditis or epicardial tumor invasion. In sinus tachycardia, bradycardia, and arrhythmias, abnormalities in the nerve plexus had been seen. Dual SA nodes have been observed in single atrium, complex malformations, persistent left superior vena cava, and in asplenia. In atrial fibrillation, SA nodal fibrosis has been seen, and in others, pronounced sclerosis of the SA node has been shown. The sick sinus syndrome may be provoked by numerous diseases including arteriolar thickening or narrowing. Also, ventricular block may be congenital or acquired by various diseases. In ventricular tachycardia, re-entry occurs at the interphase between reversible myocellular damage and preserved muscle.

In 1983, Thiene, with Pennell and Rossi,[123] studied abnormalities in the conduction system in three young athletes who died suddenly. Case #1 was an 11-year-old female. The weight of the heart was not given. The heart was the seat of a micro-Ebstein, with a wide gap in the annulus of the medial leaflet; an atrial fascicle traveled laterally to AV junctional tissue on the right side and anastomosed with Mahaim fibers which reached the ventricular myocardium. Case #2 was that of a 24-year-old male. An atheromatous plaque obstructed the anterior descending coronary artery to the extent of 75%. The myocardium showed scattered myofibrillar degeneration with contraction bands and neutrophils. Nodoventricular fibers were present. The left bundle branch had Mahaim fibers to the septum. Case #3 was that of a 26-year-old man. The heart showed mild left ventricular myocardial hypertrophy and fatty infiltration. Scattered foci of myofibrillar degeneration with contraction bands were present in the myocardium. An atrio-Hisian tract was noted.

Rossi and Thiene, in 1984,[125] described three cases of downward displacement of the tricuspid valve and sudden cardiac death. Case #1 was an 11-year-old female. The weight of the heart was not given. A Kent bundle was found that bypassed the AV node and bundle of His, passed through the right annulus from atrium to the ventricular connection. Case #2 was that of a 69-year-old male, with diabetes, hypertension, and anteroseptal infarction and right bundle branch block pattern in the electrocardiogram. The weight of the heart was not given. There was severe coronary atherosclerosis. The AV node was displaced distally. A Kent bundle was present in the medial leaflet region. Case #3 was that of a 53-year-old male with a type B Wolff-Parkinson-White syndrome, and a left bronchus carcinoma who died suddenly. The weight of the heart was not given. A bundle of Kent was found bypassing the AV node. In all these cases, the central fibrous body and right annulus were abnormally formed.

In 1985, Rossi, in conjunction with Pipper, Turolla, Frigerio, and James,[127] described a case of sudden cardiac death in a 13-month-old male. The patient clinically had intermittent pre-excitation (Lown and Ganong-Levine), and paroxysmal junctional tachycardia. Multifocal Purkinje-like tumors were found in the conduction system. One was directly at the bifurcation. In addition, there was an accessory communication between the AV node and the bundle of His with a Purkinje tumor.

In 1969, Green, with Korovitz, Shanklin,

Devito, and Taylor,[43] studied a 15-year-old boy and his 14-year-old sister who died suddenly. There was a family history of sudden deaths. The boy showed a bundle with numerous spurious, blind-end branches as it passed through the pars membranacea. The atrioventricular node was indistinct, and the approaches seemed to give rise to the bundle of His. The nodal artery could not be identified. The heart of the sister was exceedingly small with a short bundle inserting into the right myocardium before it became separated from the bifurcation.

In 1983, Davies, Anderson, and Becker[117] devoted an entire chapter to studies of the conduction system in sudden death. They discuss sudden cardiac death in SIDS, in ischemic and nonischemic heart disease, heart disease in prolonged QT syndrome, in pre-excitation, and in cases without previous clinical data.

Davies studied 37 cases of sudden death and found major lesions in 11, including absence of the right branch and fibrosis of the bundle branches. Ten had Mahaim fibers. A totally normal conduction system was seen in 16 patients, and according to Davies, "Such detailed studies do not provide even a potential cause of death in many cases." He further states that in the United Kingdom, there is no recognized nomenclature or classification in adults analogous to sudden infant death or cot death, and therefore the pathologist feels obliged to classify unexplained sudden cardiac death as "ischemic" or "cardiomyopathy" in adults, precluding any accurate assessment of the frequency of the problem or its further study.[117]

Okada,[86] in 1979, reported on 20 cases of sudden death in the young, 5 months to 41 years of age. In case #1, who was 15 years of age, the coronary arteries were unbalanced. There was a large circumflex, and a normal anterior descending and a rudimentary right coronary artery. There was mild fibrosis of the AV node, moderate stenosis of the AV nodal artery due to marked hypertrophy, and fibrosis of the AV bundle. The AV node and bundle branches were normal. In case #2, who was 29 years of age, the conduction system showed nothing of note, as did the other cases of coronary ischemia. In a 27-year-old male, with the ECG showing right bundle branch block (RBBB) and left anterior descending (LAD), pathology was found in the sinus node. The sinus node artery did not penetrate the sinus node. The SA node showed marked fibrosis and fatty infiltration. The AV node was normal. The bundle of His was sandwiched between the top of the ventricular and conal muscle. The proximal part of the right branch and the anterior radiation of left bundle branch were interrupted by fibrosis. In six cases of Pokkuri disease, there was a varying degree of fibrosis in the SA node compatible with the sick sinus syndrome. Multiple premature branching was noted in four. In a 7-year-old boy who died suddenly, 6 years after a Mustard procedure, there was marked fibrosis of the SA node. In a case of WPW with a septal Kent bundle, the sinus node was markedly fibrosed. In a 7-year-old girl with Romano-Ward syndrome, there were hypertrophied and disarrayed Purkinje cells.

Okada, with Kawai, in 1983,[124] studied the pathology of the conduction system in sudden death. He compared 35 autopsied hearts where the patient died suddenly with 27 hearts matched for age and disease from patients who did not die suddenly. They were able to separate two types of sudden cardiac death: (1) a type related to the sinus node and (2) a type related to the AV conduction system. The former included Pokkuri disease and a part of hypertensive heart disease. The latter included myocardial disease and ischemic heart disease. Both types of sudden death showed varying severities of the conduction system lesions. The conduction system lesions were composed of both primary and secondary involvement, but in advanced cases they could not be divided so clearly. They concluded that an attempt should be made to suppress or interrupt a chain reaction in the conduction system in order to prevent sudden cardiac death.

Okada and Gotoh, in 1988,[164] studied the conduction system in nine cases of Pokkuri disease (sudden death of unknown etiology in young men). Case #1 was that of a 27-year-old male. The heart weighed 280 grams and was grossly normal. The SA node was severely fibrotic, with fatty metamorphosis around the SA node. The internodal tract showed hypertrophy of the myocytes. The branching bundle and proximal portion of anterior radiation of the left bundle branch and the right bundle branch were replaced by fibrosis. Case #2 was a 32-year-old male. The heart weighed 300 grams. Both ventricles were slightly dilated but not hypertrophied. The heart was otherwise normal. The SA node showed moderate fibrosis and adiposis and a 50% reduction of nodal cells. The approaches to the SA node were fibrosed and interrupted posteriorly. The branching bundle and proximal part of the right bundle branch were compressed by conal muscle. Case #3 was that of a 41-year-old male. The sinus node artery showed medial hypertrophy. The sinus node showed diffuse moderate fibrosis. The approaches to the sinus node showed marked fatty metamorphosis which was also present in the posterior internodal tract. The branching bundle and proximal part of the left bundle branch showed moderate fatty metamorphosis. There was mild disarray and fibrosis of the ventricular septum. Case #4 was a 22-year-old male. The free wall of the right ventricle showed marked fatty metamorphosis. The sinus node showed moderate fibrosis and fatty metamorphosis. The approaches to the SA node revealed marked fatty metamorphosis. The ventricular septum showed mild disarray and fibrosis.

Case #5 was a 21 year-old male with anxiety neurosis. The heart weighed 280 grams. There was marked fatty metamorphosis of the right ventricle. The SA node showed moderate diffuse fibrosis, and fatty metamorphosis. The ventricular septum showed disarray, fibrosis and fatty metamorphosis. Case #6 was a 33-year-old male. The heart weighed 320 grams. Both ventricles were dilated. The right ventricular wall was partly replaced by fatty metamorphosis in the outflow tract. The SA node showed moderate diffuse fibrosis. Case #7 was that of a 35-year-old male. The heart weighed 465 grams. The left ventricle was moderately dilated and hypertrophied. The penetrating bundle showed marked fatty metamorphosis. The right ventricular wall revealed marked fatty metamorphosis. Case #8 was that of a 24-year-old male. The heart weighed 340 grams. The SA node showed marked fibromuscular dysplasia. The AV nodal artery revealed moderate to marked hypertrophy. The right ventricle showed moderate fatty metamorphosis. Case #9 was that of a 28-year-old male. The heart weighed 330 grams. The right ventricle was focally replaced by fatty metamorphosis in the outflow tract. The AV bundle and proximal part of the bundle branches and the right ventricle showed marked fatty metamorphosis. The ventricular septum revealed a localized tumor-like growth of myocardium compressing surrounding tissue.

Pederson, in 1980,[100] studied the proximal part of the conduction system in seven cases of sudden death due to coronary disease with 31 controlled cases. No remarkable differences were found between the sudden death cases and the controls.

Anderson, in 1981, in association with Bowie, Dempster, and Gwynne,[102] studied the conduction system in two patients, a 40-year-old male and a 17-year-old female, who died suddenly. Their only significant finding was a nonatherosclerotic focal occlusion of the AV nodal artery. In the 40-year-old, the heart weighed 430 grams and was moderately hypertrophied. The patient was an alcoholic. The 17-year-old had schizo-affective psychosis. The heart weighed 230 grams. The heart was otherwise normal. The AV node and bundle showed fibrosis.

Smeeton, in 1981, in conjunction with Anderson, Ho, Davies, and Anderson,[104] described three cases of sudden death in patients with an enlarged pars membranacea. Case #1 was that of a 34-year-old female who was pregnant at the time of sudden death. The heart weighed 300 grams. The tricuspid valve was deficient, notably in the region of the commissure between the septal and anterior leaflets. The heart was otherwise normal. The penetrating and branching bundle were right-sided. The bundle was elongated. The left bundle branch showed complete interruption. Case #2 was that of a 38-year-old female. She had previously had an atrial septal defect re-

paired. This was followed by second-degree heart block. Then she had bradycardia and ventricular fibrillation, then a long QT interval. The heart weighed 380 grams. The membranous septum was fibrosed, suggesting that there may have been a small defect previously. The penetrating and branching bundles were converted into a long plate-like structure with a ring of incomplete constriction in the penetrating bundle. The structures were more to the right. The origin of the left bundle branch showed fiber loss. The branches of the nodal artery showed focal intimal thickening. There was a small perimembranous defect. Case #3 was that of a 50-year-old female who had palpitations since childhood and tachycardia in the last few years. The ECG showed sinus tachycardia alternating with atrial fibrillation and left bundle branch block pattern. The heart weighed 380 grams. The fossa ovalis was herniated. (The membranous septum was fibrosed, suggesting that there may have been a small defect previously.) The origin of the left bundle showed extensive loss of fibers throughout its course. The bundle in all three cases was elongated.

Vesterby and Gregersen, in 1982,[115] studied 21 cases of sudden death in coronary heart disease with matched controls for age and sex, including a study of the conduction system. They found three cases of infarction in the conduction system and one in the left bundle branch. Extensive fibrosis was present in the sinus node.

Kirschner and colleagues[134] investigated sudden cardiac death in 18 Southeast Asian refugees. The hearts were hypertrophied in all cases. Endocardial fibroelastosis was present in the septal portion of the left ventricular outflow tract in 12 hearts. Conduction system anomalies were present in all hearts but one. Persistent fetal dispersion or archipelago formation of the AV node in the central fibrous body were present in 14 hearts with similar dispersion of the AV bundle was present in 12. Eleven hearts with AV nodal dispersion also had one or more accessory conduction pathways. These included atrio-Hisian in three, nodal-ventricular in seven, fascicular ventricular in four, and it was within the node in three.

In hearts with no nodal dispersion, a fasciculoventricular pathway was present in one. One case had discontinuity between the AV node and bundle in association with nodal ventricular and fasciculoventricular pathways. In 14 of the 17 hearts with conduction anomalies, there were developmental anomalies at the conduction tissue. Six of these showed subaortic or subpulmonic components extending into and around the pars membranacea. In three, ventricular conal musculature was interspersed between aortic root and the bundle of His, shifting the root of the aorta to either the left or the right side of the crest of the septum. In five, variations in configuration of the pars membranacea and central fibrous body were present. Fibrosis of the summit of the ventricular septum was present in two and calcification at the aortic base was present in one.

Wiedermann, with Becker, Hopfeiwieser, Muhlbergier, and Knapp, in 1987,[150] studied the conduction system in a young, competitive athlete with Wolff-Parkinson-White syndrome. They found an accessory connection in the posterior septal region immediately posterior to the AV node.

Thus, abnormalities in some part of the conduction system were present in practically all cases, often producing sudden death.

Chapter 7

Our Findings in the Conduction System in Cases of Sudden Death

In our work, we first became cognizant of sudden, unexpected death in 1969.[172] A 46-year-old woman with smoldering, chronic idiopathic myocarditis also had complete AV block. She had a sudden syncopal attack and died. The heart weighed 270 grams. There were no remarkable changes in the heart grossly except that the left coronary ostium lay high above the sinus of Valsalva. The sinoatrial node showed a fine elastosis with a scattering of mononuclear cells in the periphery. Focal degeneration of muscle cells was present in the approaches to the AV node, with a fine infiltration of mononuclear cells. The AV node revealed a fine elastosis with a fine infiltration of mononuclear cells as did the AV bundle. The bifurcating bundle was the seat of fat tissue replacement on the right side and distinct degeneration of the muscle. The posterior portion of the main left bundle branch was severely destroyed at its origin and was partially replaced by linear formation of fibroelastic tissue. The right bundle was the seat of partial fat replacement. The end of the second and third portion of the right bundle showed frank necrosis.

In 1972, Gault, Cantwell, Lev, and Braunwald[173] studied a 16-year-old patient with alternating bidirectional tachycardia leading to death during attempted suppressive therapy. There was no prior clinical evidence of cardiac disease. At autopsy, there were fatty and mononuclear cell infiltrations in the AV node and the main left bundle branch. A similar arrhythmia had been documented in an 18-year-old sister who died suddenly 9 months after discovery of her arrhythmia. Autopsy revealed no gross cardiac abnormality, although her conduction system was not studied. A brother, 21 years old, and mother of the propositus, aged 45-years-old, also exhibited ventricular bigeminal rhythm, and a maternal uncle and grandmother had died suddenly, the latter with the knowledge of an irregular heartbeat.

In this present patient, there was distinct fatty infiltration of the approaches to the SA and AV nodes and the penetrating portion of the bundle of His. There was a fine infiltration of mononuclear cells in the SA and AV nodes and in their approaches and in the nerve trunks around the SA node and the penetrating branching portion of the AV bundle. The AV node was especially involved, showing, in addition, a proliferation of sheath cells. The main left bundle branch, the radiations, and the peripheral Purkinje cells showed distinct vacuolar degeneration with an infiltration of mononuclear cells.

In 1972, Bharati, with Chervony, Gruhn, Rosen, and Lev,[174] studied a young woman who had an obscure heart disease with mitral insufficiency and bradycardia. Subsequent to a traumatic incident, she developed multiple atrial arrhythmias with collapse, was resuscitated, but later died suddenly. The heart showed hypertrophy and enlargement of all chambers. At the junction of the left atrium with the inferior mitral leaflet, there was a white plaque-like formation. On section, this showed a tumor-like formation consisting of masses of calcified concretions surrounded by hyalinized connective tissue with arteriolosclerosis.

The SA node showed a large area of hemorrhage and necrosis, accompanied by macrophages, fibroblasts, and mononuclear cells. Fat tissue partially isolated the node from the adjacent myocardium. The epicardium showed chronic inflammation and hemorrhage. The approaches to the AV node revealed moderate thickening and narrowing. The remainder of the conduction system showed no change.

In 1973, Husson, Blackman, Rogers, Bharati, and Lev[175] examined the conduction system in one of three siblings with conduction disturbances who died suddenly. The patient was a 10-year-old with complete AV block and with a left bundle branch block pattern. The heart was immensely enlarged, with all chambers hypertrophied, especially the left ventricle. The endocardium of both atria and the left

ventricle was diffusely thickened and whitened and that of the right ventricle was focally thickened and whitened. The AV node was relatively short. The AV bundle, penetrating portion, showed slight fibrosis, loss of parenchyma, marked increase in spaces, and a slight infiltration of neutrophils. The branching portion was small with small cells lying adjacent to a space. The first part of the right bundle branch was absent. The left bundle branch was almost completely absent.

In 1976, Bharati, Bicoff, Friedman, Lev, and Rosen[176] studied a case of a 16-year-old girl who died suddenly. At autopsy, the sinoatrial node showed no change. In the approaches to the SA node, there was focal degeneration of atrial cells. In the approaches to the AV node, the atrial septum, at its distal portion, was occupied by a tumor mass which consisted of tumor cells arranged in masses, cysts, or lacunae. These cells differed very little in size and shape and exhibited no mitotic figures. The AV node was almost completely replaced by the tumor which was a mesothelioma.

In 1977, Bharati, with Ciraulo, Bilitch, Rosen, and Lev,[177] studied a 29-year-old female with Uhl's anomaly who developed complete AV block and died suddenly. The autopsy was limited to the heart and lungs. The lungs showed pulmonary edema, chronic basal hyperemia, and an infarct of the right lower lobe. The heart was enlarged, weighing 545 grams. The right atrium was hypertrophied and enlarged. The right ventricle was tremendously enlarged. The myocardium could not be recognized grossly in most areas. The septal and parietal bands were flat and atrophied. The endocardium of the distal, downstream, septal, apical, and anterior walls was covered with thrombic material. The amount of fat in the wall of the right ventricle was considerable, both in the conus area and in the apical region. The left atrium was hypertrophied and enlarged. The left ventricle was enlarged and its wall was thinner than normal. The ventricular septum was remarkable in depth for a distance of 3 cm from the posterior to the anterior wall. In this area, the anterior septum was paper-thin and translucent.

The sinoatrial node showed chronic epicarditis, moderate mononuclear cell infiltration in the node, and moderate hemorrhage. The approaches to the SA node revealed a considerable amount of mononuclear cell infiltration. The approaches to the AV node revealed a slight amount of mononuclear cell infiltration. The AV node showed an increase in the connective tissue, and the left bundle branch was replaced by connective tissue.

The right side of the ventricular septum was completely replaced by connective tissue and fat tissue with an infiltration of mononuclear cells. The summit was converted into a mass of granulation tissue. In most areas of the right ventricle, there was complete absence of muscle.

In 1979, Bharati, Molthan, Veasy, and Lev[178] studied the conduction system in two cases of sudden death, 2 years after the Mustard procedure. The first child manifested sinus rhythm alternating with junctional rhythm in the last year of life. The second child, 2 months before death, had first-degree AV block which progressed to second-degree, with 2:1 conduction alternating with the junctional rhythm with AV dissociation. The conduction system in both cases revealed the approaches to the SA node and AV nodes to be markedly fibrosed. In addition, in case #1, the SA node was interrupted by sutures, and in case #2, the SA node was considerably fibrosed.

In 1980, Bharati, with Lev, Denes, Modlinger, Whyndham, Bauernfeind, Greenblatt, and Rosen,[179] examined the conduction system of a patient with sarcoidosis who died suddenly. The heart weighed 359 grams. The left atrium and ventricle were slightly hypertrophied and the latter was slightly enlarged. In the posterobasal wall adjacent to the mitral valve, there was an aneurysm with a thickened endocardium. Granulomatous infiltration of the AV node, the His bundle, and bundle branches was present.

In 1980, Bharati, with Nordenberg, Bauernfeind, Varghese, Carvalho, Rosen, and Lev,[180] studied the conduction system in two boys 16 and 17 years of age, who had prolonged, unexplained sinus node dysfunction and who died suddenly. Study of the conduction system in the first case revealed degeneration and fibrosis of the approaches to the SA and AV nodes and the atrial preferential pathways. The second case revealed fatty infiltration of the approaches to the SA and AV nodes.

In 1980, Bharati, with McAnulty, Lev, and Rahimtoola,[181] studied a case of idiopathic hypertrophic subaortic stenosis who died suddenly. She was 25 years of age. Conduction system studies revealed that the common bundle was situated on the right side of the septum. This showed fibrotic changes distally. The beginning of the left bundle branch was markedly disrupted as it traveled over the septum. The right bundle branch was moderately fibrosed.

In 1983, Bharati, with Bauernfeind, Miller, Strasberg, and Lev,[182] studied three teenagers, 15, 17, and 19 years of age, who died suddenly. In case #1, (the 15-year-old), the heart weighed 300 grams. The SA node and the approaches showed fatty infiltration. The left bundle branch revealed moderate fibrosis, while the third part of the right bundle branch showed considerable fibrosis. The summit of the ventricular septum revealed considerable fibrosis on the right side.

In case #2, (the 17-year-old), the heart weighed 355 grams. The right ventricle showed hypertrophy and dilation. The whole region of the pars membranacea and the adjacent aortic leaflet of the mitral valve were thickened. The mitral orifice was enlarged. The posterior leaflet was enlarged and divided into three segments with redundancy of the entire leaflet. The approaches to the AV node showed distinct zones of mononuclear cell infiltration accompanied by fatty infiltration and fibrosis. Mononuclear cells were present in the penetrating portion of the AV bundle with an increase in collagen and elastic fibers. The branching portion of the bundle also showed an increase in collagen and elastic fibers. The right bundle branch showed fibrosis in the first and second parts. The summit of the ventricular septum revealed marked fibrosis more on the right side.

In case #3, (the 19-year-old), there was a history of early death in the family. Both sisters had mitral valve prolapse. The heart weighed 220 grams. There was slight hypertrophy and enlargement of the left and right ventricles. The mitral valve showed distinct prolapse of the posterior leaflet which was redundant and nodose. The SA node revealed a thrombus or embolus filling part of the SA nodal artery. The approaches to the SA node showed fatty infiltration. The AV node was somewhat compressed against the central fibrous body. The central fibrous body sent a thick prong of connective tissue to the tricuspid valve. The penetrating bundle was septated and the branching portion was short and showed fibrosis, as did the bifurcation on the right side. The summit of the ventricular septum revealed considerable fibrosis more on the right side, with thickening and narrowing of the large arterioles.

In 1983, Bharati, with Feld, Bauernfeind, Kattus, and Lev,[183] studied a 20-year-old woman who died suddenly. She had first become aware of recurrent, short episodes of palpitations at the age of 15. For the next 3 years, the patient had 17 further hospitalizations. The heart was dilated and weighed 290 grams. The right ventricle was tremendously enlarged and the musculature of the wall was extremely thin. Most of the wall was replaced by fat. The pulmonic valve was quadricuspid.

The sinoatrial node showed slight fatty infiltration with an infiltration of mononuclear cells in some nerve ganglia. The approaches to the AV node revealed moderate to severe fatty infiltration and vacuolization of muscle cells, and occasional arterioles were thickened. The penetrating bundle was markedly septated. In the branching bundle, moderate fibrosis was seen. The entire right bundle branch was intramyocardial. The summit of the ventricular septum showed distinct large and small areas of necrosis. The right side of the ventricular septum showed necrosis of muscle and considerable infiltration of mononuclear cells and severe fibrosis.

The anterior wall of the right ventricular sinus area was largely replaced by fat, as was the case elsewhere. The left ventricular myocardium showed focal areas of necrosis, fibrosis, and infiltration of mononuclear cells.

From 1983 to 1985, Bharati and Lev reviewed the changes in the conduction system

that may be found in sudden death in young people.[184–187] These are depicted in the following outline.

Classification of Lesions of the Conduction System in Sudden Death[185]

Lesions of the sinoatrial node
    Trauma
    Sick sinus syndrome
        Adolescence
        Old age

Lesions of the atrioventricular node and its approaches
    Tumor
    Fatty infiltration

Lesions of bundle of His
    Fragmentation
    Calcific impingement

Lesions of bundle branches
    Sclerosis of left side of cardiac skeleton in older age group
    Sclerosis of right side of caridac skeleton in the young
    Genetically abnormal bundle branches

Lesions of myocardium and/or conduction system
    Coronary disease
    Uhl's disease
    Idiopathic hypertrophic subaortic stenosis
    Myocarditis

Mitral valve prolapse

Accessory pathways

Sudden death in various postoperative congenital heart diseases
    Tetralogy of Fallot
    Mustard procedure for complete transposition

Lesions of nerves to conduction system

Abnormal formation of the central fibrous body with a right-sided or left-sided bundle of His

In 1985, Bharati, Krongrad, and Lev[188] studied the conduction system in 15 cases of SIDS with eight controls. No remarkable difference was found in the SA node and its approaches, in the atrial septum, in the central fibrous body, the AV node, and penetrating bundle. However, the branching bundle was more frequently on the left side in SIDS as compared to the controls. They advanced the theory that a bundle present on the left side and an intramyocardial right bundle branch might be more vulnerable to influences promoting arrhythmias in the transitional period of change from a newborn conduction system to an adult conduction system.

In 1985, Bharati, with Dreifus, Bucheleres, Molthan, Covitz, Issenberg, and Lev,[189] studied the conduction system in five cases of Romano-Ward syndrome and one case of Jervell and Lange-Nielson syndrome to determine the cause of the prolonged QT interval. The patients were 9 and 15 months and 2, 5, and 19 years of age. A sixth patient was a 16-year-old female who died suddenly. Several members of the family had a prolonged QT interval. All cases had fatty infiltration in the approaches to the AV node. In four cases, the AV bundle was lobulated with loop formation in one. In four, the AV bundle and bundle branches showed fibrosis. In two, the AV node was partially embedded in the central fibrous body. In all cases, the ventricular myocardium was inflamed. In three, the nerves in the atrial preferential pathways and the approaches to the SA node were infiltrated with mononuclear cells.

In 1986, Bharati and Lev[190] studied the conduction system in four cases of sudden death in young adults, 25, 24, 21, and 20 years of age. The heart was normal in size in two and slightly enlarged in two. No gross pathology was detected in any heart, and toxicological examination showed no cause of sudden death. In all hearts, the bundle showed loop formation. In two, the branching bundle was left-sided with the right bundle branch intramyocardial. In the other two, the bundle was markedly fragmented. Two had myocarditis and three had arteriolosclerosis at the summit of the ventricular septum. Three cases showed an infiltration of mononuclear cells in the nerves. Abnormal formation of the central fibrous body was present in all.

In 1986, Bharati and Lev[191] studied four cases of sudden death in congenital heart disease, many years after surgical correction. The first case was that of a 23-year-old who had a Hancock valve inserted from the right ventricle into the pulmonary trunk for tetralogy of Fallot with pulmonary atresia. He died suddenly 6 years after the operative procedure. The heart was enlarged, weighing 579 grams. All chambers were hypertrophied and enlarged. The tricuspid orifice was smaller than normal with a small accessory opening in the septal leaflet. The endocardium of the right atrium was diffusely thickened and whitened. The endocardium of the right ventricle was likewise distinctly thickened and whitened. The left ventricle was enlarged and hypertrophied. A ventricular septal defect had been closed by a prosthesis. The aorta emerged about 50% from the right ventricle before the closure of the defect. The aortic cusps were thickened, irregular, and nodose. The conduction system showed fibrosis and fatty infiltration of the approaches to the SA and AV nodes. There was marked edema of the atrial septum, the AV node, and left bundle branch, and marked fibrosis of the right bundle branch.

The second case was that of a 21-month-old child who had an atrial septostomy 2 days after birth for transposition of the great vessels, and a Senning procedure at 6 months of age. He died suddenly 15 months after the Senning procedure. The heart was enlarged and weighed 122 grams. The morphological right atrium received the pulmonary veins and the coronary sinus. The morphological left atrium received the superior and inferior vena cava. All chambers were hypertrophied and enlarged. Both atria showed fibroelastosis. The conduction system and the myocardium showed chronic myocarditis with maximal involvement of the right ventricle and the AV node. The atrial septum revealed marked fibroelastosis. There was edema and chronic inflammation of the approaches to the AV node. The sinoatrial node could not be identified.

The third case was that of a 30-year-old woman who had an ostium primum defect closed at the age of 13 and died suddenly 17 years later. The heart was enlarged. The region of the patch closure of the primum defect revealed an area of calcification. The mitral orifice was somewhat enlarged. Fibroelastosis was present in both atria and focally in the ventricles. The pulmonic orifice was enlarged and the valve showed thickening. The conduction system showed fatty infiltration of the head of the SA node. There was chronic inflammation and arteriolosclerosis of the approaches of the AV node. Partial fatty separation of the AV node from the approaches was seen. Fatty infiltration with fibrosis of the AV bundle was present. The summit of the ventricular septum showed marked fibrosis, arteriolosclerosis, and fatty infiltration.

The fourth case was that of a 9-year-old boy who died suddenly 4 years after patch closure of a ventricular septal defect and the introduction of a Hancock prosthesis to the pulmonary artery for double outlet left ventricle. The heart was enlarged, weighing 327 grams. All chambers were hypertrophied and enlarged. Originally, the ventricular septum presented a large defect in the anterior part. It entered the right ventricle in the region of the arch confluent with the aorta. Thus, the aorta emerged overriding from the left ventricle. The pulmonary trunk emerged also from the left ventricle confluent with the mitral valve. The defect was closed by a prosthesis which revealed calcification. The conduction system showed chronic inflammation in the approaches to the AV node. There was marked fibrosis and fibroelastosis in the atrial preferential pathways. The AV node showed fatty metamorphosis and partial separation of the node from the atrial musculature. There was marked fibrosis and lobulation of the penetrating bundle which was left-sided. The summit of the ventricular septum showed fibrosis. The central fibrous body and pars membranacea were deformed. Myocarditis was present in the right ventricle and ventricular septum. In all four cases, there was involvement of the nerves.

In 1986, Bharati and Lev[192] presented five more cases of sudden death, aged 14, 25, 28, 39, and 41 years. Here again, the heart was enlarged in all, but the hearts were otherwise normal, except in one case where vegetations were presented on the abnormally formed mitral valve. Toxicological examinations were negative in all five cases. The SA node showed fibrosis in three. The central fibrous body was abnormal in all five. The AV node was abnormally located in two and there was loop formation in the bundle in two. Node-like muscle fibers were present within the mitral valve annulus, which joined the AV node and the bundle in one case. An atrio-Hisian connection was seen in one. The sinoatrial node was divided into two components in one case. The branching bundle and the beginning of the bundle branches showed mild to moderate fibrosis in all five.

In 1988, Bharati, with Driefus, Chopskie, and Lev,[193] published the details of a 47-year-old trained jogger who died suddenly. He was known to have sinus bradycardia with first-degree AV block for 8 years and a type 1, second-degree AV block for 5 years. A pacemaker was inserted. The AV node was situated more to the left side of the atrial septum than usual, and made a tenuous connection with the atrium due to marked fatty infiltration. The AV node showed fatty metamorphosis, fibrosis, disarray of myocardial fibers, and mononuclear cell infiltration. The right bundle branch was fibrosed throughout. Increased aging changes of the left side of the summit of the ventricular septum were present.

In 1988, Bharati and Lev[194] studied the cause of sudden death in four cases of atrial septal defect of fossa ovalis type who died a few months to 9 years after the repair of the atrial septal defect. In two cases, there was a family history of sudden death. All four hearts were hypertrophied and enlarged. In case #1, there was a floppy mitral valve with diffuse fibroelastosis of the right atrium and ventricle. In case #2, there was a floppy mitral valve with focal fibrosis of the anterior wall of the right ventricle, which was devoid of muscle. In case #3, there was an aneurysm of the pars membranacea with subaortic stenosis, fenestration, and subluxation of the aortic valve. Case #4 did not show any abnormalities grossly.

In the conduction system, the following was found. The SA node in two showed sutures and chronic inflammation. The approaches to the AV node in all showed sutures with foreign body reaction. The atrial preferential pathways showed fatty metamorphosis in two with the foreign body reaction in one. The approaches to the AV node and the AV node revealed fatty metamorphosis in three. The AV bundle showed fragmentation and lobulation in one case and marked fatty metamorphosis in two. The left bundle branch revealed fatty metamorphosis in two with destruction in the other two. The summit of the ventricular septum showed fibrosis in all cases.

In addition to the above conduction system findings in cases of sudden death, we have studied the conduction system when death occurred suddenly and unexpectedly in known as well as in unknown diseases.

In 1974, Bharati, with Lev, Wu, Denes, and Rosen,[195] studied split His bundle potentials in two cases, one of whom died suddenly. The patient was a 67-year-old male with a history of congestive heart failure and a previous history of complete heart block. The electrophysiological studies revealed split His bundle potentials with intact AV conduction. The patient remained asymptomatic and was followed by the family physician. He died suddenly. An electrocardiogram showed complete heart block and an escape rhythm characterized by a right bundle branch block pattern, which later converted to normal sinus rhythm with first-degree AV block and right bundle branch block. At autopsy, severe congestion of the organs with severe generalized atherosclerosis was in evidence. The heart was enlarged, weighing 729 grams. There was marked calcification of the aortic and mitral valves. All the coronaries were calcified and narrowed. Calcific impingement on and degenerative changes within the bundle of His, with a healthy part of the bundle of His proximally and distal to the lesion, were noted. In addition, there was arteriolosclerosis.

Bharati, with Rosen, Miller, and Lev, in 1974,[196] studied the conduction system of a 2-year-old dog, who was well until 1 week prior to death. He was found to be in heart failure with a pulse of 30 to 40 per minute. The elec-

trocardiogram showed complete AV block, with an atrial rate of 88 per minute and a ventricular rate of 21 per minute, with a narrow QRS complex and left axis deviation. While an attempt was made to record the His bundle electrogram, atrial flutter was induced and AV block persisted. During the procedure, the dog went into ventricular fibrillation and died.

Only a remnant of the AV node was present, which had practically no connection with the surrounding atrial musculature. It made very little connection with the penetrating His bundle. The penetrating bundle was likewise markedly replaced by fatty tissue. The branching bundle was very abbreviated and showed fibrosis at the region of the junction with the left bundle branch posteriorly. The bifurcating bundle likewise revealed marked replacement by fat and vacuolization of the cells. The left bundle branch was replaced by fibroelastic tissue which extended throughout.

In 1975, Lev, with Bharati, Hoffman, and Leight,[197] studied the conduction system in a case of the peripheral type of rheumatoid arthritis with complete AV block. The patient was a 52-year-old male who had typical peripheral rheumatoid arthritis for 5 to 6 years before he developed complete heart block, with Stokes-Adams syndrome. The electrocardiogram showed complete AV block with widened QRS complexes. The heart was slightly enlarged, weighing 470 grams, with a thickened aorta. Both ventricles and the left atrium were somewhat hypertrophied and the left atrium was also somewhat enlarged. The tricuspid and mitral valves were diffusely thickened. The aortic valve was somewhat thickened at the base but the noncoronary aortic cusp especially was thickened throughout.

The SA node showed some thickening of the intima of the nodal artery. The approaches to the SA node revealed thickening of the small arteries and arterioles. The approaches to the AV node likewise showed intimal thickening and slight thickening of the ramus septi fibrosi. The AV bundle, penetrating portion, showed fibroelastosis with marked vacuolar degeneration. The AV bundle, branching part, revealed moderate to marked fibroelastosis on the right side. The junction of the left part of the bundle with the left bundle branch was almost completely replaced by fibroelastic tissue. At the bifurcation, there was a circular hyalinized mass of fibrous tissue which aided in the interruption. The first part of the right bundle branch showed marked fibroelastosis and arteriolar narrowing.

The patient received prednisone intermittently until a few months before the heart block developed, at which time the medication was discontinued. A pacemaker was implanted but later failed. A second pacemaker was implanted and this again failed. The patient died following an episode of irreversible pacemaker-induced ventricular tachycardia.

Bharati, with Towne, Patel, Lev, Rahimtoola, and Rosen,[198] in 1976, studied the conduction system of a 23-year-old previously healthy man who was stabbed in the anterior chest. This resulted in a ventricular septal defect and complete heart block. Despite a pacemaker insertion, the patient died suddenly 3½ years later. The patient was asymptomatic during this time period. The electrocardiogram revealed complete AV block with a QRS pattern of right bundle branch block. The His bundle recordings, 26 days after the stab wound, showed AV dissociation with split His potentials (P-H_1 interval of 100 ms and H_2-V interval of 40 ms). During the study, the escape QRS shifted from right to left bundle branch block with H_2 potentials still preceding each QRS interval and an H_2-V interval of 40 ms. Pathologically the heart was enlarged, weighing 680 grams. The tricuspid and mitral valves revealed sizable openings and a small ventricular septal defect involving the membranous portion and part of the muscular ventricular septum. The conduction system revealed the bifurcating bundle and the beginning of the right and left bundle branches to be replaced by fibrous tissue. In addition, the branching bundle was mostly replaced by fibrosis.

In 1979, Bharati, Bauernfiend, Scheinman, et al.[199] studied a 13-year-old asymptomatic boy who had a history of recurrent ventricular tachycardia and died suddenly. Clinically there was no organic heart disease and essentially the right and left heart catheterizations, including coronary arteriography, were normal. The electrocardiogram revealed the following: PR interval of 0.16, narrow QRS complexes with normal morphology except for Q- waves in lead 3, and left ventricular hypertrophy by voltage criteria. Ventricular tachycardia was characterized by rates of 150 to 220 beats per minute with left bundle branch block QRS morphology and AV dissociation with capture and fusion beats. Some rhythm strips demonstrated intermittent nonsustained bursts of ventricular tachycardia.

EPS studies showed normal PA and AH intervals but HV was prolonged (65 ms). AV nodal function was normal. Ventricular tachycardia could not be terminated with right ventricular incremental pacing and extrastimulus testing. The QRS pattern of the tachycardia was the left bundle branch type and most consistent with the tachycardia originating from the right ventricle, or via the right bundle branch. A left ventricular origin could not be ruled out since the tachycardia was self-limiting during sinus rhythm and could not be reproducible in the catheterization laboratory. The re-entry mechanism for the tachycardia could not be proven.

The conduction system findings showed that there was a right-sided His bundle that was markedly septated as it reached the bifurcation. What was on the right side became the right bundle branch. The atrioventricular node was partly engulfed within the central fibrous body and the node could not be well differentiated from the His bundle. The right bundle branch was divided into several segments. In addition, there was marked fatty infiltration of the atria and the right ventricle, with recent and old scars in the summit of the ventricular septum.

Bharati, with Granston, Liebson, Loeb, Rosen, and Lev,[200] in 1981, studied the conduction system in a 45-year-old physician who died suddenly. He had a long history of palpitations, and a 24-hour Holter monitor revealed frequent premature ventricular contractions and several episodes of tachycardia. He refused further medical care and died suddenly a year later. Pathologically the heart was enlarged. There was a floppy mitral valve that showed marked thickening redundancy, with calcification of the annulus. The conduction system showed marked fatty infiltration in the approaches to the SA node and the AV node. The atrioventricular node was compressed by the mitral valve under the calcification. The branching bundle was on the right side and what was on the right side became the right bundle branch. Some of the muscle fibers of the left bundle branch terminated just beneath the summit of the ventricular septum. In addition, there was marked premature aging phenomena on the summit of the right side of the ventricular septum with arteriolosclerosis.

In 1981, Bharati, with Strasberg, Bilitch, Salibi, Mandel, Rosen, and Lev,[201] studied the conduction system in two cases of idiopathic hypertrophy with fibroelastosis of the left ventricle with pre-excitation who died suddenly. One was a 13-year-old who had marked cardiomegaly. The heart weighed 480 grams. In addition, she had mitral annuloplasty at the age of 33 months. The mitral valve was markedly thickened with abbreviated chordae, as were the other valves. There were two small anomalous pathways in the right free wall. The other case, a 26-year-old male, also had a markedly enlarged heart, weighing 640 grams. In this case, there was no anomalous pathway in the right free wall. However, the right atrium was connected to the infundibular septum, anterior to the membranous septum, by way of an anterior AV node-like structure.

In 1984, Bharati, with Bump, Bauernfeind, and Lev,[202] studied a 36-year old female diagnosed to have myotonia dystrophica at the age of 30, and who died suddenly. Her father and brother also were found to have myotonia dystrophica. She had experienced progressive onset of muscular weakness during her childhood. Four years prior to death, she had brief episodes of paroxysmal palpitation and the electrocardiogram at that time revealed right bundle branch block, left anterior fascicular block, and first-degree AV block. Three years later, she had two more episodes of syncope and underwent further evaluation. A chest x-ray was found to be normal. A gated cardiac pool scan revealed reduced left ventricular ejection fraction of 36% with inferolateral akinesia and septal hypokinesia. An electrocardiographic monitoring revealed intermittent Mobitz type II, 2:1 and complete AV block, as well as nonsustained bursts of polymorphic ventricular tachycardia.

Electrophysiological studies showed 2:1 block distal to the bundle of His, normal PA and AH intervals with HV notably prolonged (135 ms). Spontaneous episodes of polymorphic ventricular tachycardia occurred during the electrophysiological study; however, they could not be induced. She was treated with a permanent ventricular demand pacer, which suppressed ventricular arrhythmias. She remained asymptomatic for 10 months and was admitted for left-sided pleurtic chest pain. Six hours after admission, she went into ventricular fibrillation and could not be resuscitated.

Postmortem examination showed bilateral pleural effusion, pulmonary venous thrombosis, and diffuse bronchiectasis. The heart was enlarged, weighing 414 grams. There was marked fatty infiltration of the approaches to the atrioventricular node, with fibrosis of the nerves. The AV node was situated adjacent to the aortic-mitral annulus. The penetrating bundle was fragmented and the branching bundle was fibrosed more anteriorly, with fatty infiltration on the right side of the bifurcation. The right bundle branch revealed fatty infiltration in the first part, with fibrosis in the second part, accompanied by fatty infiltration. The left bundle branch was destroyed almost completely in the beginning with fibrosis anteriorly.

In 1985, Bharati, Scheinman, Morady, Hess, and Lev[203] studied the conduction system in a 58-year-old woman who died suddenly, 6 weeks after an ablative procedure. She had recurrent atrial fibrillation refractory to all kinds of medications and therefore received two shocks of 500 joules (J), which produced complete AV block. This was accomplished by a percutaneous transvenous method. After 6 weeks, both 24-hour electrocardiogram recordings and exercise tolerance test showed infrequent premature ventricular Q complexes, third-degree atrioventricular block, and paced ventricular rhythm with 100% capture. She suddenly collapsed and was found to be in ventricular fibrillation and could not be resuscitated. Autopsy was limited to the heart, which weighed 434 grams.

There was marked fatty infiltration of the approaches to the AV node and almost complete separation of the AV node from the surrounding atrial musculature. A fibrosed atrio-Hisian connection was also found. Fibroelastosis with chronic inflammatory changes in the AV node, bundle of His, and the right and left bundle branches was present. In addition, marked inflammatory changes were present in the distal part of the atrial septum and the summit of the ventricular septum, with degenerative changes in the tricuspid and the aortic valves.

In 1987, Gallastegui, Hariman, Handler, Lev, and Bharati[204] studied a case of Kearns-Sayre syndrome who died suddenly. The patient was a 36-year-old male with electrocardiographic findings of bifascicular block (left anterior fascicular block and right bundle branch block). His cardiac catheterization revealed normal coronary arteries, decreased ejection fraction of 42%, and hypokinesia of inferior and anterior apical walls. The electrophysiological studies showed a prolonged HV interval of 80 ms. Despite a pacemaker insertion, he went into pulmonary edema and was hospitalized. During hospitalization, he suddenly went into ventricular tachycardia, which degenerated into ventricular fibrillation, and he died at the age of 37. The heart was greatly enlarged, weighing 625 grams. The approaches to the AV node showed hypertrophied myocardial cells with mononuclear cell infiltration and marked fatty infiltration with early necrosis of the myocardial cells. There was marked fatty infiltration of the AV node and the AV bundle. The branching portion of the AV bundle and the beginning of the posterior radiation of the left bundle branch were almost completely replaced by linear formations. The anterior radiation of the left bundle branch was markedly fibrosed with vacuolization and the right bundle branch revealed fibrosis and fatty infiltration.

In 1988, Brookfield, Bharati, Denes, Halsted, and Lev[205] studied the conduction system of a 15-year-old boy who died suddenly

while swimming. The family history revealed sudden death, involving three consecutive generations, including a brother. The patient had a history of exercise-related syncope for which he was treated with nadolol.

The heart was enlarged, weighing 333 grams. The pulmonary valve was quadricuspid. There was an accessory tricuspid valve and the mitral valve was thickened. The penetrating bundle was pushed to the left side of the summit of the ventricular septum by the right ventricular septal muscle which was hypertrophied. The bundle was lobulated and showed fatty and fibrous changes. These findings extended throughout the beginning of the bundle branches.

In 1989, Bharati, Scheinman, Estes, Moskowitz, and Lev[206] studied and presented the conduction system in three cases of intractable junctional tachycardia who died suddenly. Case #1 was a 6-month-old female, case #2 a 5-month-old male, and case #3 a 22-year-old female nurse. The latter had a pacemaker following surgical ablation of the AV node and died suddenly 7 months later while at work. All hearts were hypertrophied and enlarged. In case #1, the beginning of the AV node lay within the central fibrous body and there was a left-sided bundle of His. Acute necrosis was present in the summit of the ventricular septum adjacent to the AV node and bundle. In case #2, the coronary sinus was displaced cranially close to the central fibrous body, resulting in abnormality of the latter, and entrapment, distortion, and division of the AV node within the central fibrous body. In case #3, there was a left AV node connected to the atrial septum, and the right AV node formed the peripheral conduction system. The right AV node was completely interrupted by sutures and the penetrating and branching bundle was fibrosed.

In conclusion, (1) in all cases, abnormalities in the coronary sinus and/or the central fibrous body and/or the AV node are related to junctional tachycardia; and (2) before ablative procedures are undertaken, it might be useful to study clinically the anatomy of the atrial septum, and the coronary sinus.

In 1989, Bharati, Engle, Fatica, Bussell,

Sulayman, Lev, and Lynfield[207] studied and presented a case of sudden death in Kawasaki's disease in the early phase of the illness. Kawasaki's disease, or mucocutaneous lymph node syndrome of infants and young children, is characterized by acute febrile illness with mucocutaneous involvement and is associated with swelling of cervical lymph nodes. Sudden death occurs as a result of myocardial infarction or aneurysms in about 2% of cases during the 3rd and 4th week of the illness. However, sudden death in the early phase of the disease is rare. Despite this fact, the conduction system has rarely been studied histologically. We report a young child with this illness who died suddenly in the early phase of the disease. The conduction system was studied by serial section examination.

A 4½-year-old boy with mucocutaneous lymph node syndrome, Kawasaki's disease, had an unexpected cardiac arrest on the 13th day of his illness. He had no symptoms of heart failure and the electrocardiogram revealed no evidence of any arrhythmia but did show some nonspecific ST-T wave changes and rsr′ pattern in V_1. An echocardiogram 3 days prior to death revealed large right and left coronary arteries and some enlargement of the left ventricle with a moderately good ejection fraction of about 67%. Autopsy revealed an enlarged heart with aneurysms of the coronary arteries but no rupture. Serial sections of the conduction system showed diffuse periarteritis, neuritis, and myocarditis of the conduction system and the entire heart with diffuse chronic subendocardial inflammation.

In summary, sudden death in Kawasaki's disease may occur as a result of (1) myocarditis of the conduction system and the surrounding myocardium, (2) periarteritis, or (3) diffuse neuritis and, finally, (4) this case emphasizes that sudden death can occur in a relatively early phase of this disease unrelated to coronary aneurysm but as a lethal arrhythmia, secondary to myocarditis.

In 1989, Bharati and Lev[208] studied and presented the conduction system in 21 cases of sudden death (14 males stillborn to 40 years, and seven females 5 years to 40 years). All were clinically healthy except for three who

had arrhythmias, and two who had a history of familial sudden death. Autopsy and toxicological examination of the coronaries were normal in all cases. The heart was enlarged in 14, slightly enlarged in five, and was normal in two. Abnormalities of the tricuspid valve and mitral valve with prolapse were present in eight. The conduction system showed a narrowing of the SA or AV node arteries in five and sclerosis of the ventricular septum in five. The AV node was in tricuspid valve or mitral valve annulus in three. Marked fatty infiltration was present in and around the AV node in three, fibrosis of the node was present in two, and myocarditis of the node was present in two. The AV node lay within the central fibrous body in one. Acute myocarditis was present in a stillborn, lymphocytic myocarditis in one, granulomas with fibrosis of the conduction system in one, left-sided bundle in four, septated bundle in three, patchy fibrosis of the ventricular septum in 10, pressure of the conal muscle on the bundle in two, and fibrosis of the bundle and branches, with or without fat, in 10. The bundle was divided into a large right side, which became a right bundle branch and a discrete, small left bundle branch in one, and the bundle was in tricuspid valve annulus in one. Thus: (1) the conduction system and heart demonstrated varying pathological changes in all; (2) these changes are not present in normal controlled hearts; and (3) we conclude that these changes may form a milieu of arrhythmogenicity and sudden death in the young.

Summary

Thus, the review of the findings in our studies revealed the following: (1) There are cases with normal hearts grossly who die suddenly, (2) there are cases with incidental findings which appear to show no importance clinically who die suddenly; (3) there are cases with distinct disease entities who die unexpectedly; (4) there are cases who have congenital abnormalities of the conduction system who die suddenly; and (5) finally, there are other cases who have a combination of congenital abnormalities of the conduction system with associated acquired changes in the heart including the conduction system who die suddenly. Because of this array of findings, we felt we should study sudden unexpected death. The main theme would be what Lown has so aptly said:[112] "Sudden death does not necessarily imply an extension of a process, but it is within itself a disease entity which possibly may be avoided by proper therapy." In this chapter, we have not given all the details of the findings in the conduction system in each case. This would produce a book by itself. We urge the reader to read the original articles in the journals which would provide a better understanding of our findings.

Chapter 8

Illustrations of Our Work with Our Concept

In the following pages, we have given the brief clinical histories, morphologic heart findings, findings in the conduction system in 75 cases of sudden death, and our interpretation of the findings in each case. It must be understood that the findings in the conduction system may not be responsible for the sudden death of the individual. The cause of sudden death may lie in the brain, spinal cord, stellate ganglia, or in other unknown factors. Nevertheless, the conduction system findings cannot be overlooked in evaluating sudden death. This is especially true since some parts of the conduction system were involved in 100% of the cases in this series.

CASE #1[180]

A 16-year-old boy, asymptomatic, died suddenly. A murmur was heard at 11 months of age and he was diagnosed as having a small ventricular septal defect (VSD). At age 6, the murmur disappeared and at age 13, cardiac catheterization was normal. He was asymptomatic except for a single brief syncopal episode associated with convulsions at age 5 years.

ECG

At age 2, this showed sinus tachycardia, interrupted by sinus pauses of 1.3 to 1.4 seconds. At 7½ and 8½ years, this showed normal sinus rhythm. At age 13, the following were noted: brief runs of supraventricular tachycardia, followed by pauses of 1.5 to 1.7 seconds, terminated by junctional escape beats with rates of 40 to 50 beats/minute.

EPS

Sinus pauses up to 2.5 seconds in duration, absence of persistent bradycardia, and prolonged sinus nodal recovery time of 3,451 ms were present. He failed to keep up his medical appointment but was reported to have pulse rates of 70 to 90 beats/minute during a school examination.

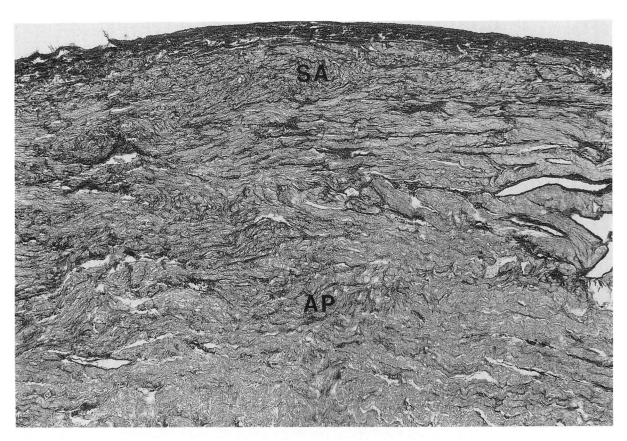

Figure 8-1: Sinoatrial node and approaches showing fibrosis of the approaches. Weigert-van Gieson stain ×45. SA = sinoatrial node; AP = approaches to the SA node.

Pathology: Gross

The heart was enlarged and weighed 325 grams. All chambers were hypertrophied and enlarged. The internal architecture of the right atrium was abnormal. There was no sharp line of demarcation between the sinus venarum and the right atrial appendage. The ventricular septum at its base presented a small defect measuring 1 mm in greatest dimension.

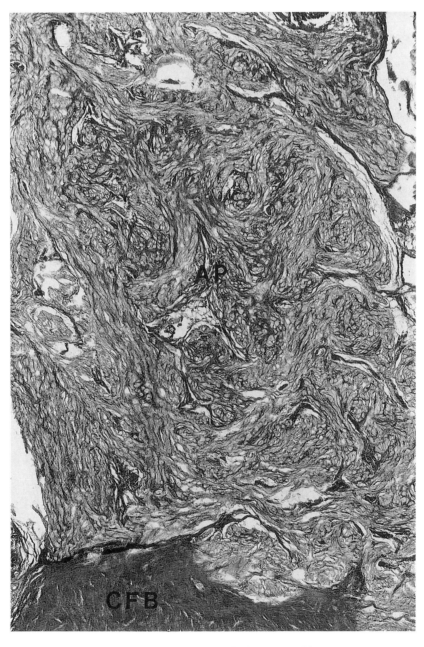

Figure 8-2: Approaches to the AV node. Weigert-van Gieson stain ×45. AP = approaches to the AV node; CFB = central fibrous body.

Microscopic Examination: Positive Findings

Approaches to the SA Node

The cells were enlarged. There was an increase in connective tissue (Fig. 8-1).

Atrial Preferential Pathways

There was diffuse fibrosis of the three pathways with marked swelling and vacuolization of the cells.

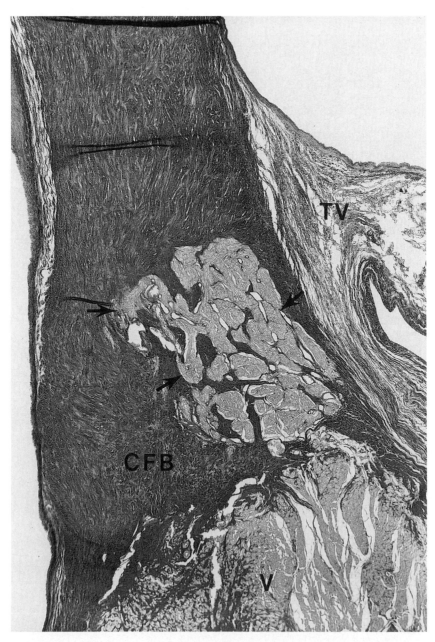

Figure 8-3: Bundle of His showing marked septation and fragmentation. Weigert-van Gieson stain ×30. CFB = central fibrous body; V = ventricular septum; TV = tricuspid valve. The arrows point to bundle.

Approaches to the AV Node

The cells were markedly swollen with diffuse fibrosis (Fig. 8-2).

AV Bundle, Penetrating and Branching

These were markedly septated (Fig. 8-3).

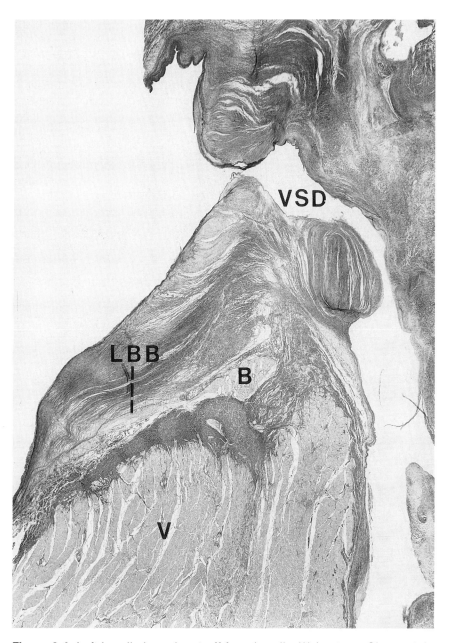

Figure 8-4: Left bundle branch cut off from bundle. Weigert-van Gieson stain ×17. V = ventricular septum; B = bundle; LBB = left bundle branch; VSD = Ventricular septal defect. (Reprinted with permission from Bharati S, Nordenberg A, Bauernfeind R, Varghese JP, Carvalho AG, Rosen K, Lev, M: The anatomic substrate for the sick sinus syndrome in adolescence. *Am J Cardiol* 1980;46:163–172.)

Left Bundle Branch

The left bundle branch was focally cut off from the bundle (Fig 8-4). Moderate fibrosis was present with disruption at the bifurcation.

Right Bundle Branch

Moderate fibrosis in the region of closing VSD was present.

Discussion

The patient was diagnosed as having sick sinus node dysfunction. The anatomic findings that might conceivably be related to this are fibrosis of the approaches to the sino-atrial (SA) node, of the atrial preferential pathways, and the approaches to the atrioventricular (AV) node. We do not know the cause of this fibrosis. It is possible that long-standing hypertrophy and enlargement of the atria secondary to hypertrophy and enlargement of the ventricles is due to a left-to-right shunt at the ventricular level, which may have produced the fibrosis.

What is the cause of sudden death? Speculation hinges on the septated and fragmented bundle of His.

CASE #2[192]

A 39-year-old female secretary woke up complaining of trouble breathing, and then collapsed.

Pathology: Gross

The heart was normal in size and showed no significant changes.

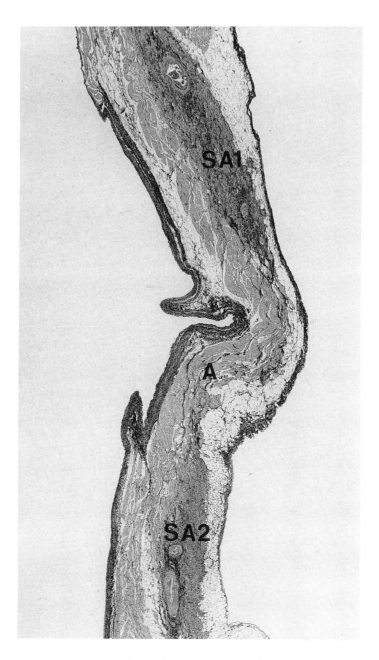

Figure 8-5: The SA node divided into two portions. Weigert-van Gieson stain ×15. SA1 = sinoatrial node 1; SA2 = sinoatrial node 2; A = atrial musculature.

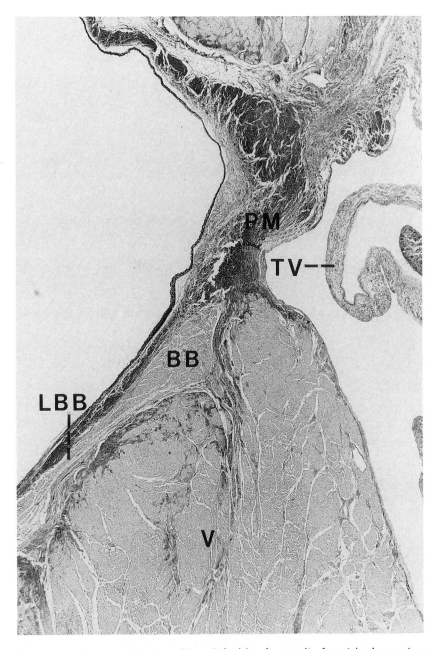

Figure 8-6: The branching bundle on left side of summit of ventricular septum with fibrosis of left bundle branch. Weigert-van Gieson stain ×30. PM = pars membranacea; BB = branching bundle; LBB = left bundle branch; V = ventricular septum; TV = tricuspid valve.

Microscopic Examination: Positive Findings

SA Node

The SA node was divided into two segments (Fig. 8-5).

AV Node

The AV node was embedded within the central fibrous body with arteriolosclerosis.

AV Bundle, Branching

The branching bundle was on the left side of the summit of the ventricular septum (Fig. 8-6).

Bundle Branches

The bundle branches showed moderate fibrosis.

Ventricular Septum

There was fibrosis of the right and left sides with arteriolosclerosis and myocardial disarray.

Discussion

The cause of sudden death in this healthy person may be related to the numerous abnormalities in the conduction system: (1) the division of the SA node into two components; (2) the embedding of the AV node in the central fibrous body; (3) the branching bundle lying on the left side of the summit of the ventricular septum; (4) the fibrosis of the bundle branches; and (5) the sclerosis of the summit of the ventricular septum.

CASE #3[174]

A 35-year-old female was in an automobile accident and was admitted to a hospital. She had lost consciousness for an unknown period of time. She had a fracture of the left clavicle, but not of the ribs, and multiple contusions.

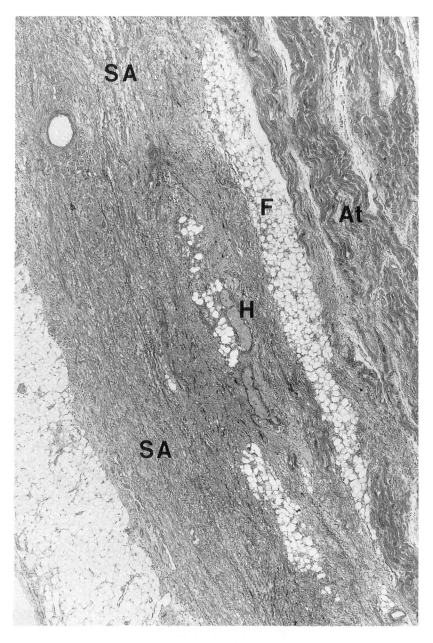

Figure 8-7A: The SA node, showing hemorrhage with partial isolation of the node by fat tissue. Hematoxylin-eosin stain ×39. SA = SA node; AT = atrial muscle; H = hemorrhage in SA node; F = fat.

ECG

Sinus bradycardia (50–60 beats/minute) with sinus arrhythmia and wandering of pacemaker from the sinus node to AV junction, biatrial enlargement, and nonspecific T-wave changes were present.

Course

Five days later she collapsed while walking and was found to be in ventricular tachycardia, AV dissociation, and she showed multiple cardiac arrhythmias including paroxysmal atrial tachycardia with varying block.

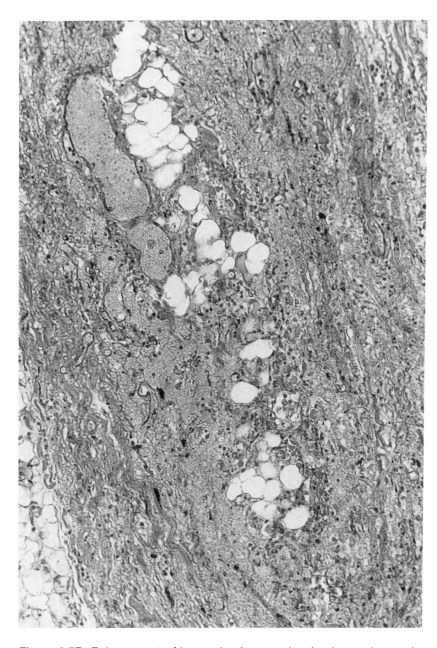

Figure 8-7B: Enlargement of hemorrhagic zone showing hemorrhage, pigment, and macrophages. Hematoxylin-eosin stain × 130.

She was treated medically and improved clinically and was ambulatory for a few days. Three weeks later she was found dead in bed. Four years before death, she was diagnosed as having cardiomyopathy but she was asymptomatic until the auto accident.

Pathology: Gross

The heart was enlarged and weighed 470 grams. There was hypertrophy and enlargement of both atria and ventricles, especially the left. The endocardium of the left atrium was thickened. At the junction of the left atrium with the inferior mitral leaflet close to the posterior commissure, there was a white plaque-like formation measuring 1.5 cm in greatest dimension. This plaque was firm, and on section showed a tumor-like formation measuring 0.3 to 0.4 cm in diameter. The mitral orifice was enlarged, but the valve showed no change.

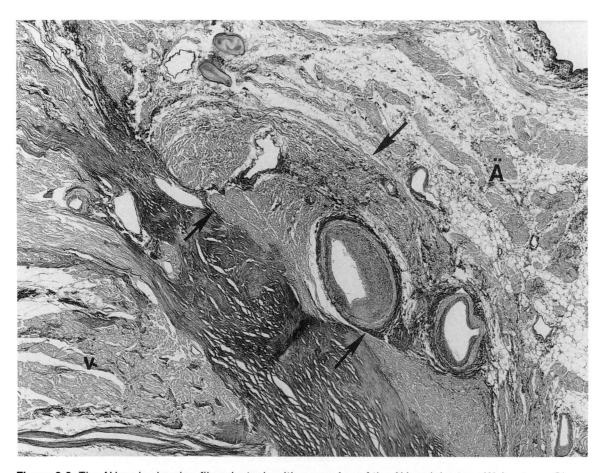

Figure 8-8: The AV node showing fibroelastosis with narrowing of the AV nodal artery. Weigert-van Gieson stain ×39. V = ventricular septum; A = atrial musculature. The arrows point to the node. (Reprinted with permission from Bharati S, Chervony A, Gruhn J, Rosen KM, Lev M: Atrial arrhythmias related to trauma to sinoatrial node. *Chest* 1972; 61:331–335.)

Microscopic Examination: Positive Findings

SA Node and Its Approaches

There was a large area of hemorrhage (Fig. 8-7 A,B) and necrosis in the SA node with macrophages, fibroblasts, and mononuclear cells. Fat almost isolated the SA node from the atrial musculature (Fig. 8-7A).

AV Node

The AV nodal artery showed moderate thickening and narrowing (Fig. 8-8). The AV node showed slight fibroelastosis (Fig. 8-8).

Ventricles

Focally there was marked proliferation of young fibrous connective tissue, especially in the left ventricle.

Mitral Rim

The tumor noted in the mitral rim consisted of osteoid tissue with areas of calcification. There was no evidence of malignancy.

Coronary Arteries

There was considerable atherosclerosis. The left circumflex was considerably narrowed.

Discussion

The cause of sudden death in this patient is related to: (1) the hemorrhage in the SA node; (2) the narrowing of the AV nodal artery; (3) proliferation of young connective tissue in the left ventricle; and (4) the osteoid tumor in the mitral valve.

CASE #4[194]

A 6½-year-old female child, asymptomatic, died suddenly at home, 3 months after surgical closure of an atrial septal defect of fossa ovalis type.

ECG

Before surgery, premature atrial contractions and nodal premature beats were present. After surgery, premature atrial contractions persisted. In addition, the ECG showed left ventricular hypertrophy, sinus arrhythmia, and occasional premature ventricular contractions.

Pathology: Gross

The heart was immensely enlarged. All four chambers were hypertrophied and enlarged. There was a floppy mitral valve with diffuse fibroelastosis of the right atrium and right ventricle.

Microscopic Examination: Positive Findings

SA Node and Its Approaches

The node presented sutures with marked chronic inflammatory changes, with foreign body granulomas (Fig. 8-9). The approaches showed foreign body granulomas, fibrosis, hemorrhage, and necrosis. The nerves were infiltrated with mononuclear cells.

Atrial Preferential Pathways

These showed chronic inflammation, foreign body reaction, and arteriolosclerosis.

AV Bundle, Penetrating

This was small with a large space around it and with moderate fibrosis.

Left Bundle Branch

Linear degeneration and fibrosis were present.

Right Bundle Branch

Moderate fibrosis was noted.

Summit of the Ventricular Septum

Moderate fibrosis was present.

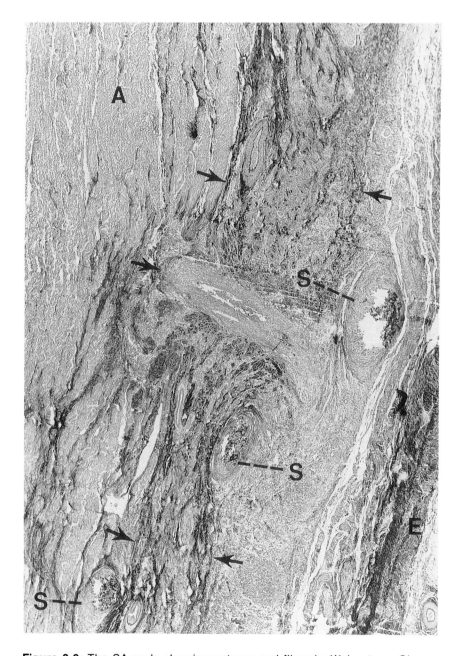

Figure 8-9: The SA node showing sutures and fibrosis. Weigert-van Gieson stain ×30. S = suture; A = right atrial musculature; E = thickened epicardium. The arrows point to the fibrosed sinoatrial node. (Reprinted with permission from Bharati S, Lev M: Conduction system in sudden unexpected death a considerable time after repair of atrial septal defect. *Chest* 1988; 94:142–148.)

Discussion

The sudden death of the child is most likely related to the sutures with marked chronic inflammation and foreign body granuloma in the SA node. However, the role of fibrosis in the bundle and bundle branches cannot be overlooked.

CASE #5[192]

A 41-year-old female nurse with a long history of arrhythmias passed out at the pool and could not be resuscitated. She had a history of mitral valve prolapse with regurgitation. Her identical twin sister, a nurse, has the same problem and is alive.

Pathology: Gross

The heart was enlarged and weighed 520 grams. All chambers were hypertrophied and enlarged. The region of the fossa ovalis in the right atrium showed several strands of tissue overlaying it. Hemorrhage was noted in the region where the AV node might be. The endocardium of the left atrium was thickened. The mitral valve had been removed by the prosector. According to him, it had been floppy with infective endocarditis superimposed. Several cuts were made in the left ventricle, revealing fibrotic patchy areas. In addition, there was a subendocardial hemorrhage in the region of the main left bundle branch and in the periphery. The membranous part of the ventricular septum was elongated and extended beneath the midportion of the right aortic cusp. The coronary arteries were patent throughout.

Microscopic Examination: Positive Findings

SA Node

This showed an increase in connective tissue.

Atrial Preferential Pathways

These showed marked fibrosis. In addition, node-like cells from the mitral valve annulus entered the central fibrous body and joined the AV node and the beginning of the AV bundle (Figs. 8-10, 8-11).

Approaches to the AV Node

Fatty infiltration was present. The AV nodal artery was normal.

AV Node

This was situated partly in the central fibrous body.

AV Bundle, Penetrating

There was moderate fatty metamorphosis.

Bifurcation

Linear degeneration of the left side and marked fatty metamorphosis of the right side with hemorrhage in between were noted (Fig. 8-12).

Left Bundle Branch

There was marked linear degeneration posteriorly with zones of hemorrhage. Purkinje cells were shrunken, and were smaller than myocardial cells.

Right Bundle Branch

Fibroelastosis was present further down.

Summit of the Ventricular Septum

There was marked fibrosis throughout (Fig. 8-13) with early necrosis of myocardium and a slight infiltration of mononuclear cells and arteriolosclerosis. A distinct myocarditis was present. Hemorrhage was present in many areas.

Left Ventricle

A florid myocarditis was present with myocardial necrosis.

Right Ventricle

This did not show myocarditis. Only fatty infiltration was present.

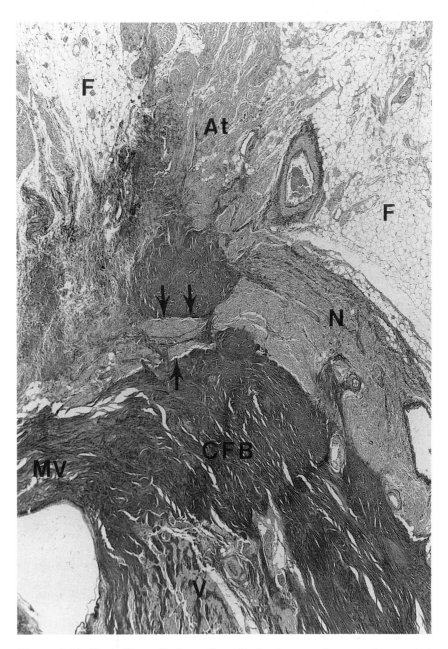

Figure 8-10: Node-like cells from the mitral valve annulus entering central fibrous body and joining the AV node and bundle. Weigert-van Gieson stain ×30. At = atrial musculature; N = AV node; CFB = central fibrous body; F = fat tissue; MV = mitral valve; V = ventricular septum. The arrows point to atrial musculature coming from region of mitral annulus and joining the AV node.

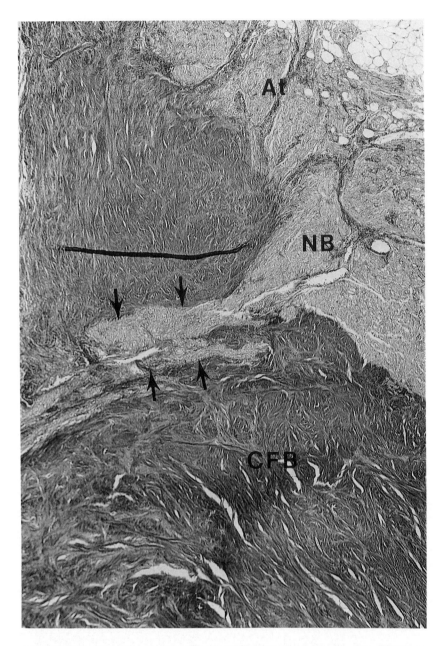

Figure 8-11: Atrial fibers reaching junction of AV node and bundle. Weigert-van Gieson stain ×45. At = atrial fibers; NB = junction of AV node and bundle; CFB = central fibrous body. The arrows point to fibers coming from mitral valve annulus.

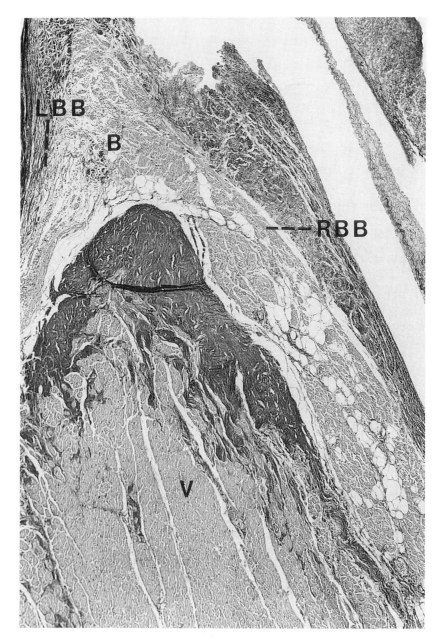

Figure 8-12: The bifurcating bundle showing fatty infiltration on the right side and linear degeneration on the left side. Weigert-van Gieson stain ×45. B = bifurcating bundle; RBB = right bundle branch; LBB = left bundle branch; V = ventricular septum.

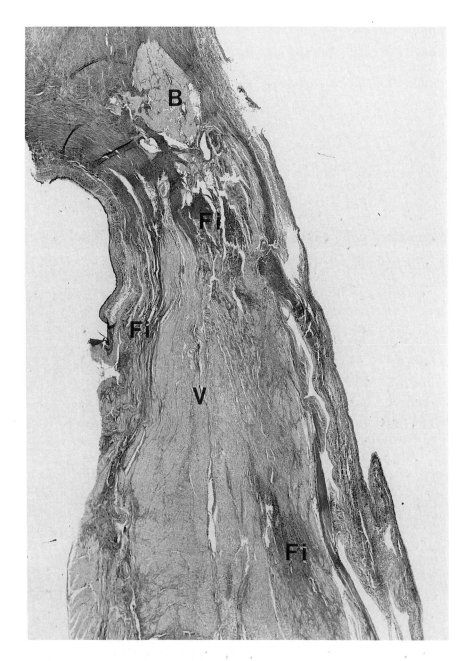

Figure 8-13: The ventricular septum showing marked fibrosis. Weigert-van Gieson stain ×14. B = bundle; Fi = areas of fibrosis; V = ventricular septum.

Discussion

This patient had a long history of arrhythmias and she was found to have mitral valve prolapse. Her sudden death may have been related to the mitral valve prolapse itself, or was related to the development of endocarditis on this mitral valve which was clinically silent. However, possible contributing factors to her sudden death were: (1) node-like cells from the mitral valve annulus joining the AV node; (2) the AV node was partly situated in the central fibrous body; (3) fatty infiltration was present in the AV node, the AV bundle, and the right side of the bifurcation; (4) degenerative changes were present in the bundle branches; (5) there was a distinct myocarditis in the summit of the ventricular septum, and there was florid myocarditis in the left ventricle.

CASE #6

A 25-year-old male collapsed while playing basketball and was found to be in ventricular fibrillation. Despite attempted defibrillation, he died.

Pathology: Gross

The heart was enlarged, weighing 725 grams. All chambers were hypertrophied and enlarged. The anterior leaflet of the tricuspid valve was divided into two parts, both parts being large, redundant, and thickened. Both leaflets of the mitral valve revealed distinct thickening and nodularity. Near the summit of the ventricular septum, there was an irregularly thickened fibroelastic ridge extending from the anterior part of the ventricular septum and extending into the posterior part of the mitral valve. The muscular ventricular septum was markedly thickened. Several scars were noted in the ventricular walls. The aortic valve showed distinct increased hemodynamic change. The coronary arteries emerged high, close to the junction of the noncoronary cusp. They were widely patent throughout.

Microscopic Examination: Positive Findings

Approaches to SA Node

The arterioles were thickened with small zones of hemorrhage. There was a generalized epicarditis and neuritis in the atrium.

Atrial Preferential Pathways and Approaches to the AV Node

There was marked fatty metamorphosis with fibrosis.

AV Node

The AV node was entrapped in the central fibrous body (Fig. 8-14). The central fibrous body showed arteriolar thickening.

AV Bundle, Penetrating and Branching

There was marked fibrosis with lobulation and loop formation (Fig. 8-15).

Left Bundle Branch

There was marked falling out of cells with atrophy of the remaining cells. (Fig. 8-16).

Bifurcation

Marked fibrosis was present on both sides with fatty degeneration of the right side and falling out of cells on the left side (Fig. 8-17).

Right Bundle Branch

Moderate fibrosis was present.

Left Ventricle

The muscle cells were hypertrophied with large areas of degeneration and fibrosis.

Right Ventricle

Occasional small subendocardial scars were noted.

Ventricular Septum

There were large areas of scar formation.

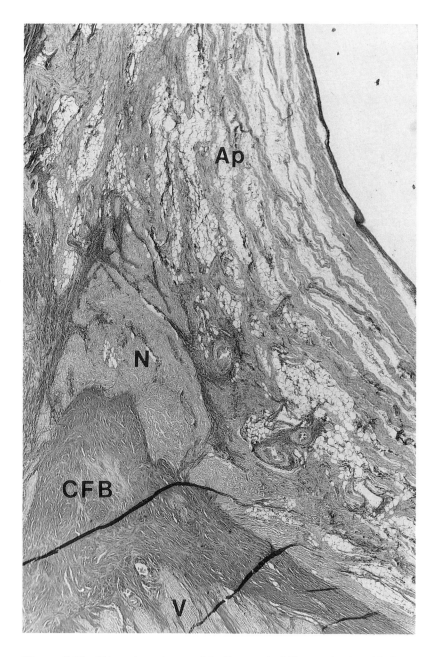

Figure 8-14: AV node entrapped in the central fibrous body with fatty metamorphosis and arteriolosclerosis of the approaches to the AV node. Weigert-van Gieson stain ×30. N = AV node; Ap = approaches to AV node; CFB = central fibrous body; V = ventricular septum.

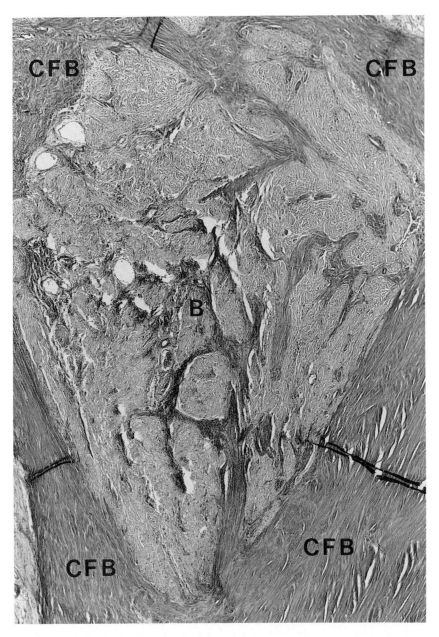

Figure 8-15: AV bundle, penetrating portion, showing marked fibrosis with lobulation and loop formation. Weigert-van Gieson stain ×45. B = bundle; CFB = central fibrous body.

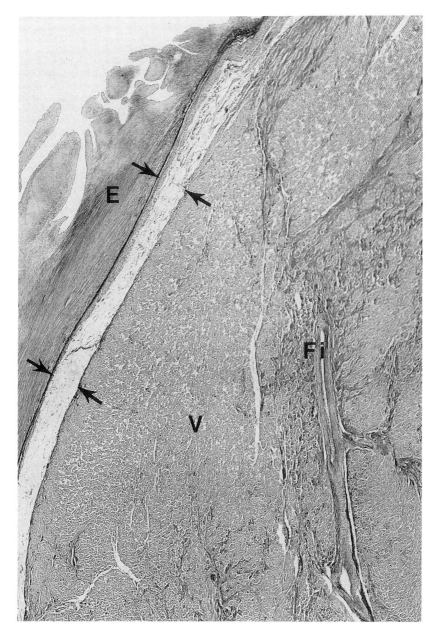

Figure 8-16: Left bundle branch, showing falling out of cells. Note the thickening of the endocardium and fibrosis of the septum. Weigert-van Gieson stain ×30. E = endocardium; V = ventricular septum; Fi = fibrosis. The arrows point to the left bundle branch.

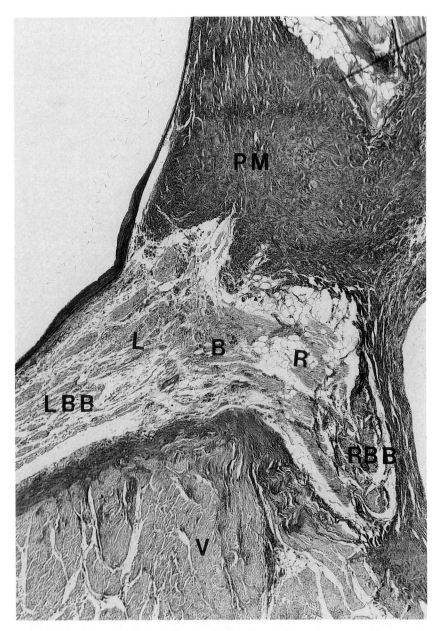

Figure 8-17: Bifurcating bundle, showing fibrosis in the center, falling out of cells on the left side, and fatty metamorphosis of the right side. Weigert-van Gieson stain × 45. V = ventricular septum; L = left side of bifurcating bundle; LBB = left bundle branch; R = right side of bifurcation; B = bundle; RBB = right bundle branch; PM = pars membranacea.

Discussion

The question is: Is this an atypical form of asymmetrical septal hypertrophy? The thickness of the septum was not appreciably greater than that of the parietal wall. The cause of sudden death may be related to: (1) fibrosis, lobulation, and loop formation of the AV bundle and the marked fibrosis on both sides of the bifurcation with fatty metamorphosis on the right; (2) the falling out of cells on the left side; or (3) the entrapment of the atrioventricular node in the central fibrous body could also conceivably lead to ventricular fibrillation and sudden death.

CASE #7

A 34-year-old trained bicyclist who since the age of 12 and throughout his adulthood actively participated in bicycling competition, collapsed suddenly while bicycling through town as part of a preliminary exhibition in preparation for races. Paramedics found him in coarse ventricular fibrillation. He went into fine ventricular fibrillation and died.

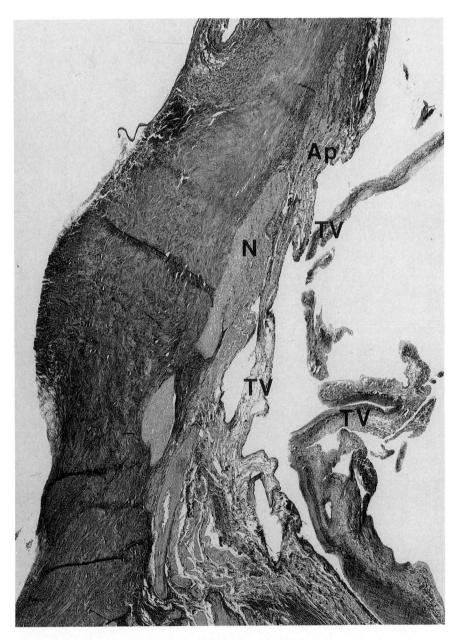

Figure 8-18: AV node within or directly adjacent to the tricuspid annulus. Weigert-van Gieson stain ×17. N = AV node; Ap = approaches to AV node; TV = tricuspid valve.

Pathology: Gross

The heart weighed 510 grams. There was a large area of thickening of the epicardium in the anterior wall of the right ventricle. The right atrium and both ventricles were hypertrophied and enlarged. The tricuspid orifice was enlarged and revealed increased hemodynamic change. There was fenestration in the aortic valve. There was some hemorrhage near the tail of the SA node.

Microscopic Examination: Positive Findings

AV Node and Its Approaches

The AV node lay within or directly adjacent to the tricuspid valve annulus (Fig. 8-18).

Bundle of His

This was at the left side and revealed hemorrhage.

Summit of the Ventricular Septum

Patchy fibrosis was noted on the left side.

Discussion

The AV node was separated from the tricuspid valve by atrial muscle which was part of the approaches to the AV node. Its situation directly adjacent to or in the tricuspid valve annulus constitutes an abnormality.

The sudden unexpected death in this trained bicyclist, who went into coarse ventricular fibrillation and then into fine ventricular fibrillation, may conceivably be related to irritation of the hemodynamically altered tricuspid valve on the AV node. Of course, the presence of the bundle on the left side in the hypertrophied heart may produce an irritation. The cause of the hypertrophy of the right atrium and both ventricles with scars in the myocardium is not explained by any findings in the heart. Is this related to exercise? How could exercise produce scars in the myocardium?

CASE #8[190]

A 20-year-old woman was found dead in bed. She had a history of transient arrhythmia during the year before she died.

Pathology: Gross

The heart weighed 380 grams. The eustachian valve was considerably enlarged. All chambers were slightly hypertrophied and enlarged. The coronary arteries were widely patent. There was a considerable amount of fatty infiltration in the epicardial surface on the anterior wall of the right ventricle.

Microscopic Examination: Positive Findings

Atrial Preferential Pathways and Approaches to the AV Node and AV Node

There was marked fatty infiltration (Fig. 8-19). There was arteriosclerosis and arteriolosclerosis of the ramus septi fibrosi (Fig. 8-19). The AV node in part was in the central fibrous body (Fig. 8-19).

Penetrating Bundle

This showed segmentation and loop formation.

Conduction System in General

Fibrosis was in evidence in the conduction system in general, which also showed a myocarditis.

Summit of the Ventricular Septum

There was a marked increase in fibrosis (Figs. 8-20, 8-21) with arteriolosclerosis.

Right Ventricle

Fatty infiltration was present.

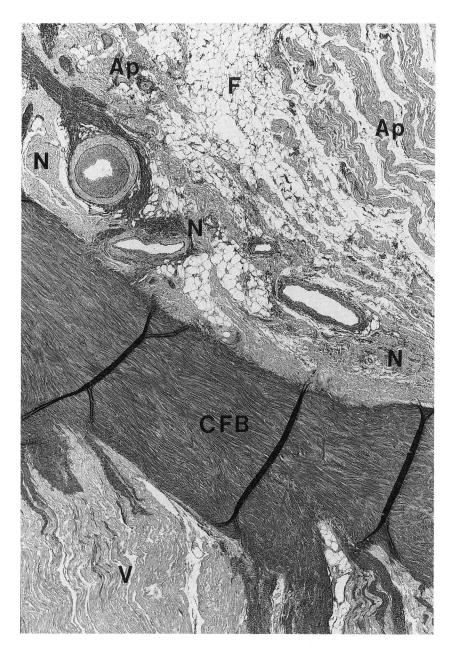

Figure 8-19: AV node, showing fatty infiltration of the approaches to the AV node and the AV node, with arteriolosclerosis of a branch of the ramus septi fibrosi. The AV node is partly within the central fibrous body. Weigert-van Gieson stain ×45. N = node; F = fat tissue; CFB = central fibrous body; Ap = approaches to the AV node; V = ventricular septum.

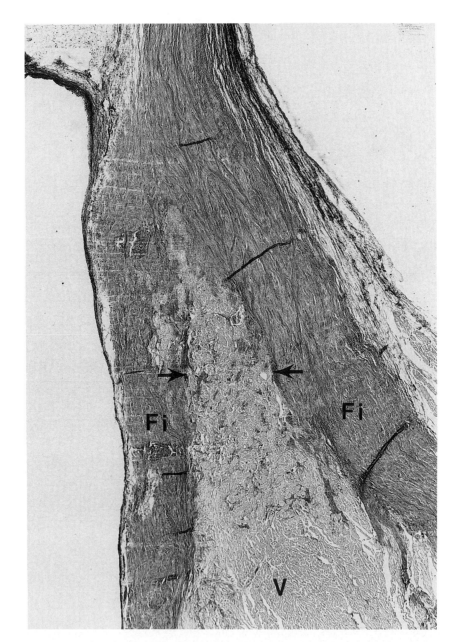

Figure 8-20: Summit of ventricular septum, showing marked fibrosis. Weigert-van Gieson stain ×45. V = ventricular septum; Fi = fibrosis. The arrows depict area enlarged in Figure 8-21.

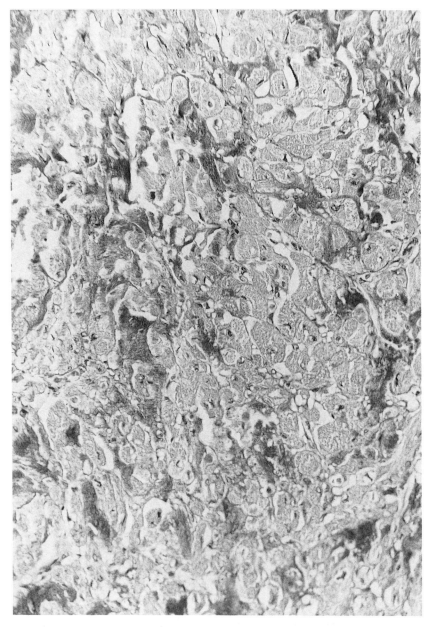

Figure 8-21: Enlarged area in ventricular septum depicted in Figure 8-20. Weigert-van Gieson stain ×300.

Discussion

The cause of death in this woman with transient arrhythmia may be related to (1) the fatty infiltration of the atrial preferential pathways, the approaches to the AV node and the AV node; (2) the marked sclerosis of the summit of the ventricular septum and the segmentation, loop formation, and fibrosis of the bundle of His. Another factor may be the atypical myocarditis of the conduction system.

CASE #9[190]

A 25-year-old male was found dead in his car on his driveway. He had no known history of drug or alcohol problems. A 2-year-old sibling had died of unknown cause previously and a 24-year-old brother had died suddenly of undetermined cause.

Pathology

The heart weighed 340 grams. The posterior leaflet of the mitral valve was somewhat enlarged and was divided into several segments. The coronary arteries were normal.

Microscopic Examination: Positive Findings

Sinoatrial Node

There was partial separation of the SA node from the right atrium by fat.

AV Node

The AV node was partly embedded in the central fibrous body.

AV Bundle

The AV bundle showed marked fragmentation (Fig. 8-22).

Left Bundle Branch

The beginning of the left bundle branch was partially destroyed (Fig. 8-23).

Summit of the Ventricular Septum

There was marked sclerosis and arteriolosclerosis (Fig. 8-22).

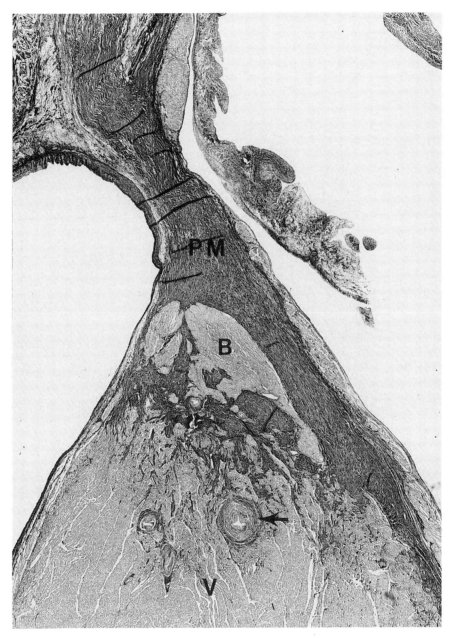

Figure 8-22: AV bundle, showing fragmentation. Note also the sclerosis of the summit of the ventricular septum with arteriolosclerosis. Weigert-van Gieson stain ×17. B = bundle; V = ventricular septum; PM = pars membranacea. The arrow points to thickened and narrowed arterioles.

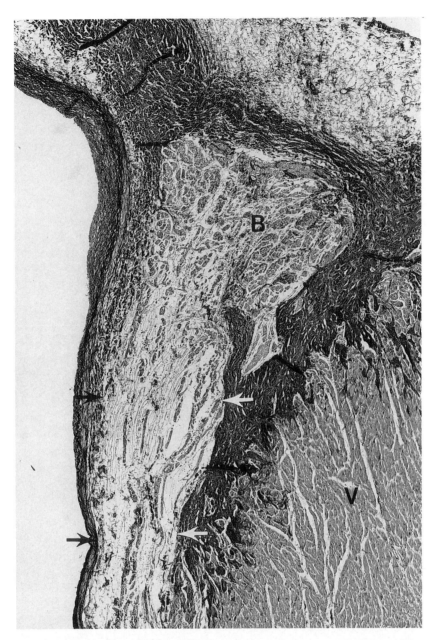

Figure 8-23: Partial destruction of the left bundle branch. Weigert-van Gieson stain ×45. B = AV bundle, branching; V = ventricular septum. The arrows point to the left bundle branch.

Discussion

This 25-year-old man who died suddenly had a family history of sudden death. The possible contributing factors to his demise are (1) fragmentation of the His bundle, and (2) partial destruction of the left bundle branch. Again we have marked sclerosis of the summit of the ventricular septum associated with arteriolosclerosis.

CASE #10[190]

A healthy 21-year-old male became involved in an argument in a bar and was later kicked against a cement wall and kicked in the head and neck. He collapsed and died. There were multiple abrasions and contusions which were not considered serious enough to have caused death.

Pathology: Gross

The heart was enlarged, weighing 397 grams. There was a small aneurysm of the fossa ovalis. The eustachian valve was prominent and showed marked fenestration. The right atrium and both ventricles were hypertrophied and enlarged. There was mild downward displacement of the medial leaflet of the tricuspid valve. The coronary arteries were normal.

Microscopic Examination: Positive Findings

Approaches to the AV Node

There was fibroelastosis in this area.

Atrioventricular Node

The AV node was in part within the central fibrous body.

AV Bundle, Penetrating

This was markedly lobulated with loop formation (Fig. 8-24).

AV Bundle, Branching

This lay distinctly on the left side of the septum (Fig. 8-25).

Ventricular Septum

There was marked fibrosis on the left side.

Bifurcating Bundle

The right bundle branch was intramuscular and fibrosed (Fig. 8-26).

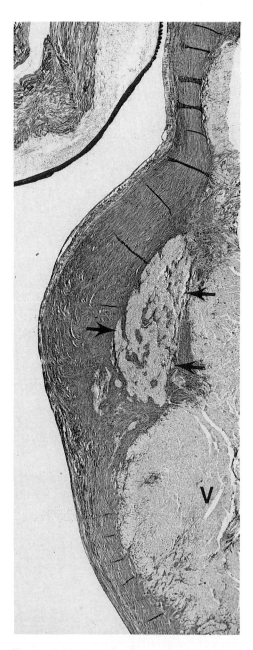

Figure 8-24: AV bundle, penetrating portion, showing lobulation with loop formation. Weigert-van Gieson stain ×17. V = ventricular septum. The arrows point to the bundle.

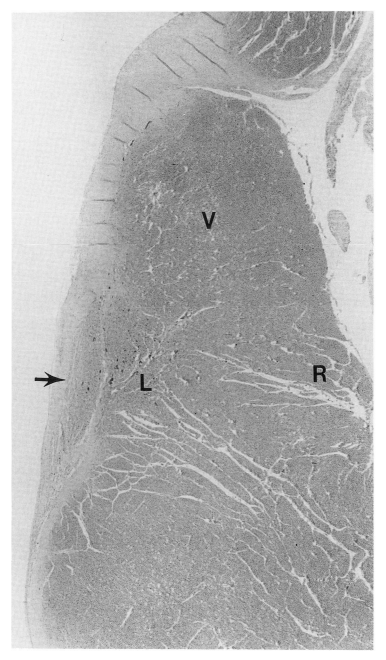

Figure 8-25: Branching bundle on the left side of the septum. Hematoxylin-eosin stain ×17.25. V = ventricular septum; L = left side of septum; R = right side of septum. The arrow points to the bundle.

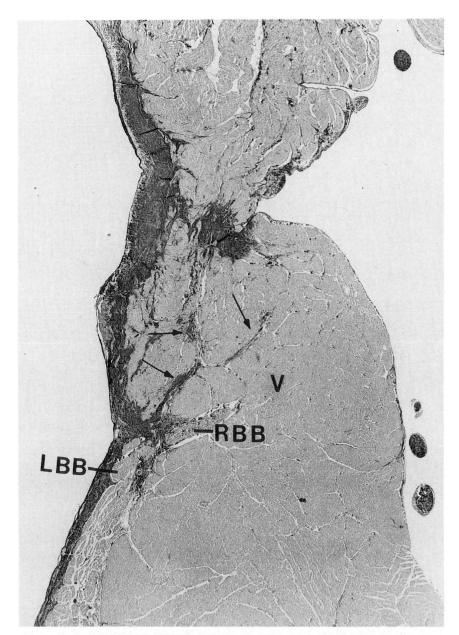

Figure 8-26: Bifurcating bundle on the left side showing fibrosis of the right bundle branch and focal fibrosis of the ventricular septum. Weigert-van Gieson stain ×22.5. V = ventricular septum; LBB = left bundle branch; RBB = right bundle branch. The arrows point to the focal fibrosis in the ventricular septum. (Reprinted with permission from Bharati S, Lev M: Congenital abnormalities of the conduction system in sudden death in young adults. *J Am Coll Cardiol* 1986; 8:1096–1104.)

Discussion

The outstanding finding in the conduction system in this case is the lobulation of the AV bundle with loop formation. However, the distinctly left-sided branching bundle may be a contributing factor in the cause of sudden death.

CASE #11²⁰⁰

A 45-year-old physician who had a long history of palpitations was found dead in bed.

ECG

Sinus rhythm, normal PR and QT intervals, inverted T-waves in lead III, and normal QRS morphology were present. A 24-hour Holter monitor revealed frequent premature ventricular contractions and several episodes of nonsustained (three to five beats) ventricular tachycardia.

Pathology: Gross

The heart weighed 483 grams. All chambers, especially the left atrium, were hypertrophied and enlarged. The posterior leaflet of the mitral valve was redundant, markedly thickened, nodose, and calcified at the annulus. The annulus of this leaflet was elongated and the valve was moored on the left atrial side (Figs. 8-27 and 8-28).

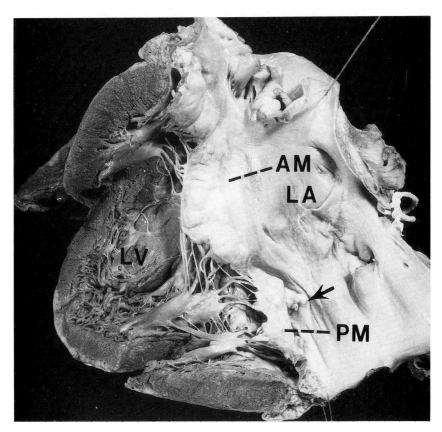

Figure 8-27: Gross view of the mitral valve showing billowing of the posterior and anterior leaflets, and elongation of the posterior leaflet with calcification of the annulus of the posterior leaflet. The calcification elevates the posterior leaflet and the calcification extends into the left atrium. LA = left atrium; AM = anterior leaflet; PM = posterior leaflet; LV = left ventricle. The arrow points to the calcification in the left atrium.

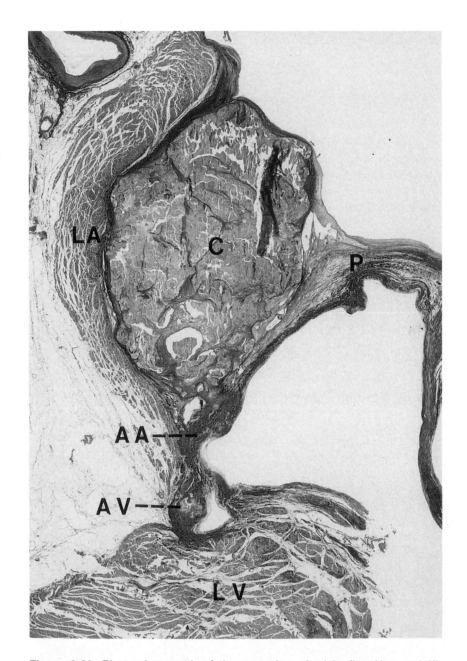

Figure 8-28: Photomicrograph of the posterior mitral leaflet. Note calcification of the annulus. The annulus is elongated and the calcific mass is embedded in the atrial side. Weigert-van Gieson stain ×9.75. AA = atrial side of annulus; AV = ventricular side of the annulus; C = calcific mass; LV = left ventricle; LA = left atrium; p = proximal portion of the mitral valve.

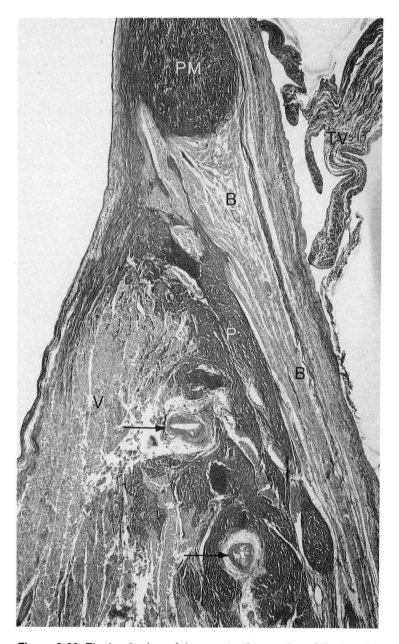

Figure 8-29: The beginning of the penetrating portion of the bundle of His extending downward on the right side of the summit of the ventricular septum. Note the marked fibrosis of the right side of the septum with marked arteriolosclerosis. Weigert-van Gieson stain ×30. PM = pars membranacea; P = prong of connective tissue to right side of summit of ventricular septum; B = bundle of His; V = summit of ventricular septum; TV = tricuspid valve. The arrows point to large arterioles.

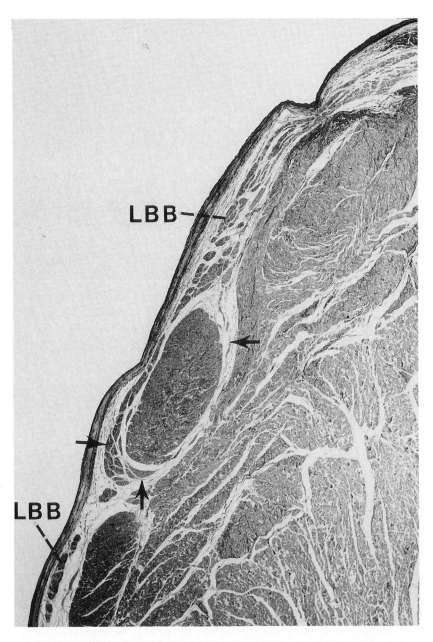

Figure 8-30: Left bundle branch encircling the myocardium. Weigert-van Gieson stain ×30. LBB = left bundle branch. The arrows point to fibers encircling the myocardium.

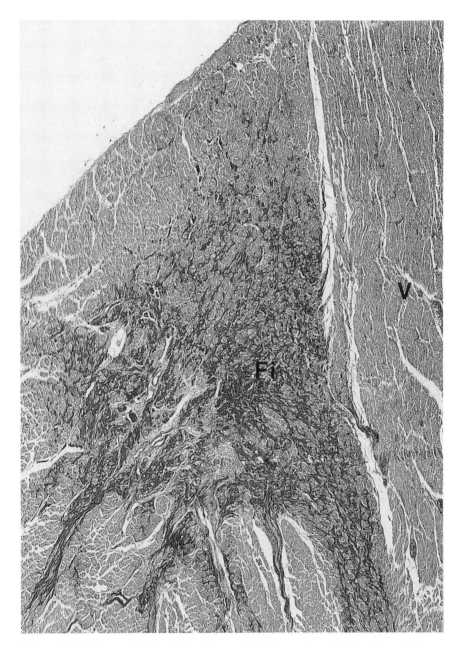

Figure 8-31: Zone of fibrosis in the ventricular septum. Weigert-van Gieson stain ×45. Fi = fibrosis; V = ventricular septum. (Reprinted with permission from Bharati S, Granston AS, Leibson PA, Loeb HS, Rosen KM, Lev M: The conduction system in mitral valve prolapse syndrome with sudden death. *Am Heart J* 1981; 101:667–670.)

Microscopic Examination: Positive Findings

Approaches to the SA and AV Nodes and Atrial Preferential Pathways

Marked fatty infiltration was present in these areas.

AV Node

The AV node was compressed either by the enlarged left atrium, the mitral orifice, or by the invasion of calcium in the abnormally formed central fibrous body.

Branching Bundle

The branching bundle was on the right side of the summit of the ventricular septum (Fig. 8-29).

Left Bundle Branch

Some of the fibers of the left bundle branch encircled the myocardium beneath the summit (Fig. 8-30).

Ventricular Septum

There was marked fibrosis and arteriolosclerosis of the right side of the summit. Scars were present throughout the anterior left ventricular wall (Fig. 8-31).

Discussion

In this case of a 45-year-old physician, we must assume that he had an arrhythmia. This arrhythmia may have been related to the prolapsed mitral valve. We do know that prolapsed valves may be related to arrhythmias and sudden death. It should be noted that the patient on Holter monitoring had demonstrated ventricular tachycardia some time ago.

Other factors in the conduction system in this case which may be related to arrhythmias and sudden death are: (1) compression of the atrioventricular node; (2) the marked fatty infiltration to the approaches to the SA and the AV nodes and the atrial preferential pathways; and (3) the marked sclerosis of the summit of the ventricular septum. We do not know whether the encircling of myocardial fibers by the left bundle branch, the position of the bundle on the right side, or the fibrosis of the left ventricular myocardium are related to the arrhythmia.

CASE #12[193]

A 47-year-old extremely active, entirely asymptomatic, trained jogger was found dead in bed. He was known to have sinus bradycardia with first-degree AV block for 8 years and a type I second-degree block 5 years prior to death. A permanent pacemaker was inserted and apparently he was then in good health and maintained his jogging program until he died suddenly.

Pathology: Gross

The pacemaker was tested and found to be functioning normally. The heart was enlarged, weighing 440 grams in a fixed state. All chambers were hypertrophied and enlarged. The eustachian valve formed a prominent membrane across the mouth of the inferior vena cava and the thebesian valve was considerably enlarged with several fenestrations. The space of His was aneurysmally dilated.

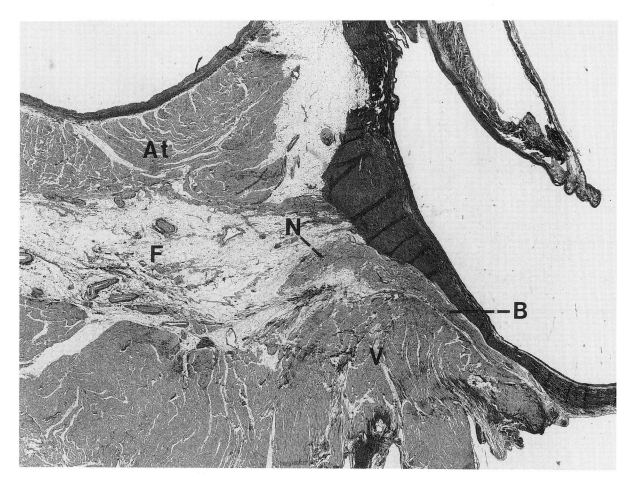

Figure 8-32: Obliquely horizontal section through the AV node and bundle of His. Weigert-van Gieson stain ×9.7. At = atrial septum; V = ventricular septum; N = AV node; B = bundle of His; F = fat tissue.

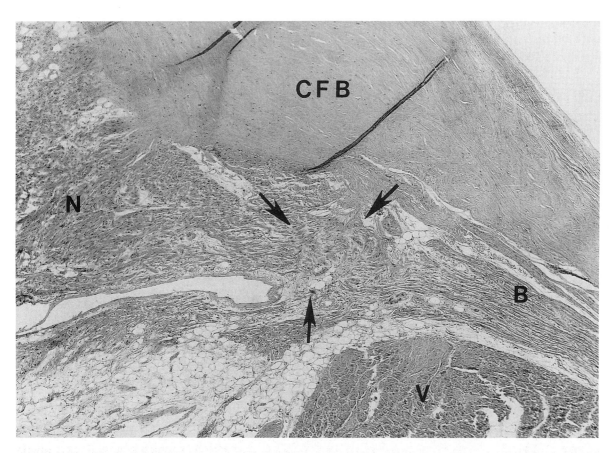

Figure 8-33: Enlarged magnification of part of Figure 8-32. Hematoxylin-eosin stain ×45. CFB = central fibrous body; N = AV node; V = ventricular septum; B = bundle of His. The arrows point to area of disarray. (Reprinted with permission from Bharati S, et al: Conduction system in a trained jogger with sudden death. *Chest* 1988; 93:348–351.)

The endocardium of the right atrium was thickened and whitened, especially in the region of the fossa ovalis. The tricuspid orifice was somewhat enlarged. The medial leaflet of the tricuspid valve was abnormally attached to the septal band and there were three muscles of Lancisi. The coronary arteries were wildly patent.

Microscopic Examination: Positive Findings

Approaches to the SA Node and AV Node and the Atrial Preferential Pathways

There was marked fatty infiltration and moderate fibrosis. The nerves showed distinct fibrosis.

AV Node

The node was situated more to the left of the atrial septum than usual. There was only a small, rare connection to the atrial musculature (Fig. 8-32).

AV Bundle

The node as it formed the bundle showed disarray (Fig. 8-33) of cells, with chronic inflammatory cells and fibrosis. In its midportion, the fibrosis increased and the bundle was shrunken.

Right Bundle Branch

This showed distinct fibrosis.

Summit of the Ventricular Septum

There was marked arteriolosclerosis.

Discussion

The first- and second-degree AV block in this active jogger is explained by the fatty infiltration of the approaches to the SA node, the atrial preferential pathways, and the approaches to the AV node and partial isolation of the AV node. His sudden death may be related to the disarray of the bundle of His, the fibrosis of the summit of the ventricular septum, and the fibrosis of the right bundle branch.

CASE #13

A 40-year-old female pediatric nursing co-ordinator was en route to California with a female friend to seek new employment. She collapsed and died suddenly in the passenger seat while her friend was driving.

Pathology: Gross

The heart was not weighed fixed, since the apical portion had been removed. According to the prosector, it weighed 380 grams fresh. The right atrium was enlarged with aneurysmal dilatation of the atrial appendage. The

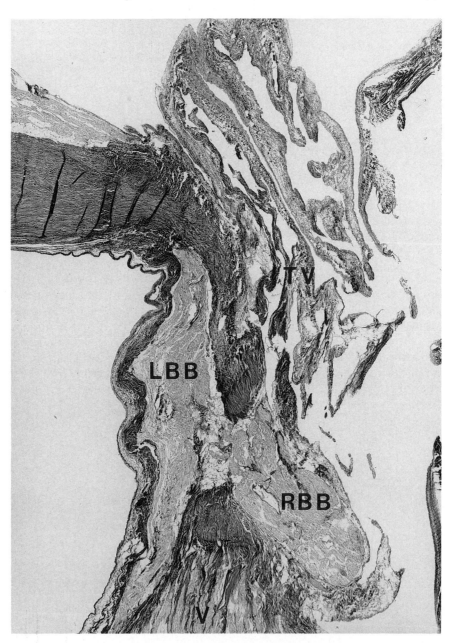

Figure 8-34: Bifurcating bundle showing right bundle branch within the tricuspid annulus. Weigert-van Gieson stain ×22. LBB = left bundle branch; RBB = right bundle branch; TV = tricuspid valve; V = ventricular septum.

pars membranacea was invaded by muscle. The aortic valve showed several fenestrations. There were focal areas of fibrosis in the wall of the left ventricle. The anterior descending coronary artery showed 60% narrowing according to the prosector.

Microscopic Examination: Positive Findings

Approaches to the AV Node

Fatty metamorphosis with almost isolation of the AV node by fat was present.

AV Bundle, Penetrating

This was very short and lay within the tricuspid annulus. It bifurcated into right and left bundle branches without forming a branching bundle.

Right Bundle Branch

This lay within the tricuspid annulus in its beginning (Fig. 8-34).

Ventricular Septum

Patchy fibrosis was present, mostly on the right.

Discussion

The narrowing of the anterior descending coronary artery may be a primary factor in the cause of death in this 40-year-old previously well female. Contributing factors were (1) fatty metamorphosis in the approaches to the AV node, and (2) the position of the penetrating bundle and right bundle branch in the tricuspid annulus.

CASE #14

An athletic 14-year-old boy, who practiced many sports, complained of chest pain while playing soccer, then collapsed and died suddenly.

Pathology: Gross

The heart was enlarged, weighing 475 grams. All chambers were hypertrophied and enlarged. There was a markedly hypertrophied combined eustachian and thebesian valve.

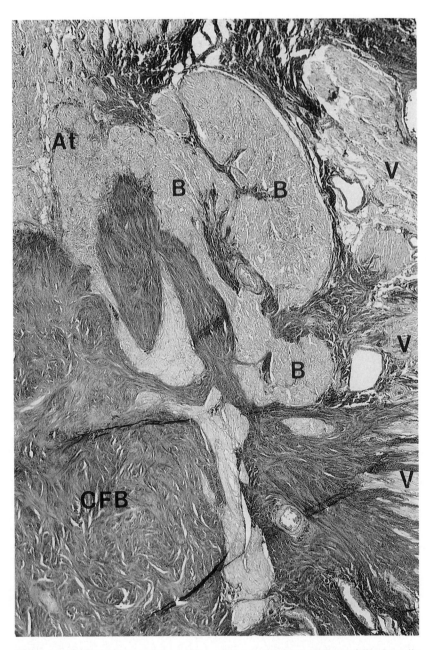

Figure 8-35: Atrio-Hisian connection, with marked lobulation of the bundle of His. Weigert-van Gieson stain ×45. At = atrial musculature; CFB = central fibrous body; V = ventricular musculature; B = bundle.

The architecture of the right ventricle was abnormal. Several anomalous muscle bundles of the right ventricle proceeded to the base of the anterior leaflet of the tricuspid valve. The endocardium of the left atrium was distinctly thickened, whitened, and geographic. The mitral orifice was enlarged. The posterior leaflet was distinctly enlarged from the annulus to the edge. It was divided into six segments which revealed increased hemodynamic change. The ventricular septum was distinctly thickened in the outflow tract. This thickening

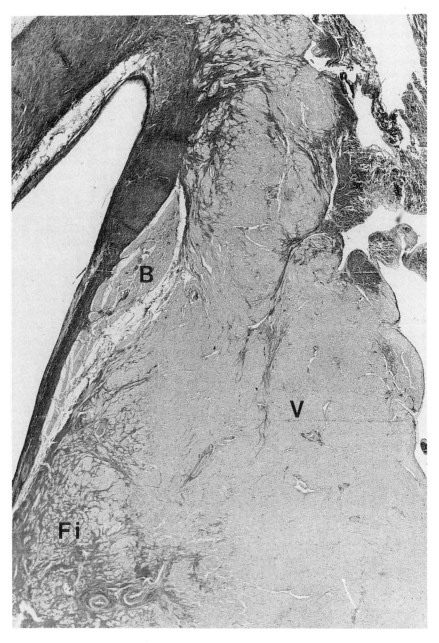

Figure 8-36: Left-sided branching bundle with slight fibrosis. Note the fibrosis in the left side of the septum. Weigert-van Gieson stain ×22.5. B = branching bundle; V = ventricular septum; Fi = fibrosis.

formed a bulge into the left ventricular cavity. A linear fibroelastic thickening was present about 1 cm beneath the aortic valve. The coronaries were patent throughout.

Microscopic Examination: Positive Findings

Approaches to the SA and AV Nodes

There was focal chronic epicarditis with fibrosis and arteriolosclerosis. Hemorrhages were also seen.

AV Node

This, in part, lay in the central fibrous body.

AV Bundle, Penetrating

A distinct atrio-Hisian connection (Fig. 8-35) was in evidence. The bundle was lobulated with loop formation (Fig. 8-35).

Branching Bundle

This was distinctly left-sided, showing slight fibrosis (Fig. 8-36).

Bundle Branches

They both showed fibrosis.

Summit of the Ventricular Septum

There was distinct fibrosis in the left side (Fig. 8-36).

Discussion

The sudden death of this 14-year-old boy during athletics may be related to the atrial-Hisian connection and/or the prolapsed mitral valve. However, we cannot overlook the lobulated penetrating bundle with loop formation and left-sided branching bundle and the fibrosis of the ventricular septum.

CASE #15[205]

An apparently healthy 15-year-old boy died suddenly while swimming. He had a strong family history of sudden death involving three consecutive generations, including a brother. The patient had a history of exercise-related syncope. A complete work-up 10 months prior to sudden death revealed a normal ECG, exercise-induced ectopy, normal intracardiac pressures and coronary arteries, mitral valve prolapse, pulmonary regurgitation by echocardiogram, and ventricular ectopy by electrophysiological studies. He was treated with nodalol 40 mg, which prevented the exercise-induced ventricular ectopy.

Pathology: Gross

The heart was enlarged, weighing 333 grams. All chambers were hypertrophied and enlarged. The atrial septum was abnormal. The limbus was situated more proximally than usual in the atrial septum. The septal leaflet of the tricuspid valve showed an accessory opening. All leaflets of the tricuspid valve were thickened. There were three muscles of Lancisi. A bulge was present on the right side of the ventricular septum at the upper part of the septal leaflet. The pulmonic valve was quadricuspid (Fig. 8-37), thickened, and nodular throughout. The mitral orifice was enlarged. The inferior leaflet of the mitral valve was mod-

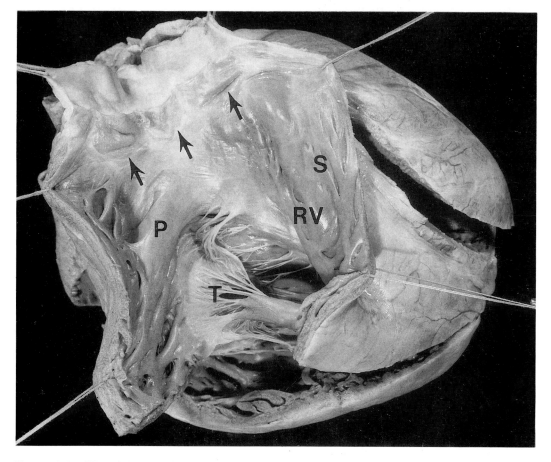

Figure 8-37: The right ventricle, showing quadricuspid pulmonic valve and three muscles of Lancisi. RV = right ventricle; P = parietal band; S = septal band; T = tricuspid valve. The arrows point to the quadricuspid pulmonic valve.

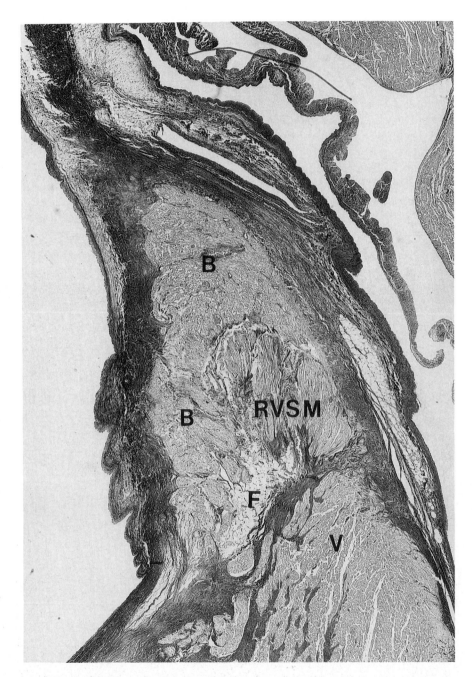

Figure 8-38: The right ventricular septal muscle invading and distorting the bundle of His. Weigert-van Gieson stain ×22.5. B = bundle of His; F = fibrous and linear change in the left bundle branch; RVSM = right ventricular portion of septal muscle; V = ventricular septum.

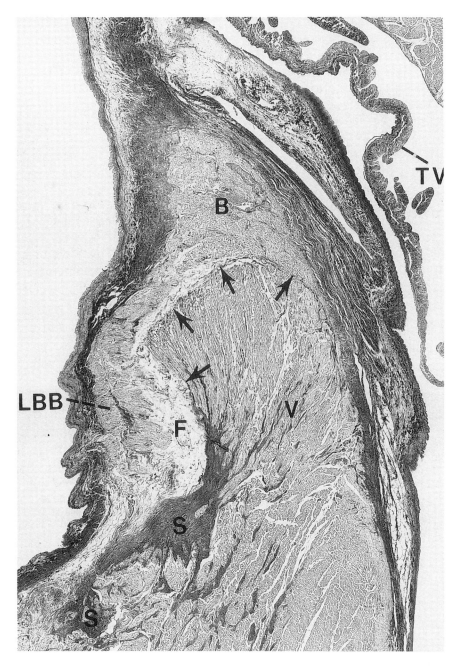

Figure 8-39: The right ventricular septal muscle pressing on and distorting the bundle and left bundle branch. Weigert-van Gieson stain ×22.5. B = branching bundle; LBB = posterior radiation of left bundle branch; F = fibrous and linear change in the left bundle branch; V = summit of the ventricular septum (right side); S = increased sclerosis of the midseptal area on left side; TV = tricuspid valve. The arrows point to pressure by the right ventricular septal musculature on the bundle at the level of the posterior radiation of the left bundle branch. (Reprinted with permission from Brookfield L, Bharati S, et al: Familial sudden death: Report of a case and review of the literature. *Chest* 1988; 94:989–993.)

erately elongated and divided into several segments which were thickened. The left ventricular apex was heavily trabeculated. Several chordae cris-crossed the base of the posterior papillary muscle. The membranous septum was enlarged both in its atrial portion and in its intercuspidal portion. The aortic valve showed generalized thickening and nodularity. The coronary arteries were normal.

Microscopic Examination: Positive Findings

Atrial Preferental Pathways and Approaches to the AV Node

There was moderate fatty metamorphosis and some areas of hemorrhage. The nerves showed distinct fibrosis. Arteriolosclerosis was also in evidence.

AV Bundle

As the bundle moved toward the left side of the central fibrous body, right ventricular septal musculature pressed on and deformed the structure (Fig. 8-38), producing dissolution of tissue, marked fibrosis, and fatty metamorphosis.

Left Bundle Branch

This again was pressed on and deformed by the right ventricular septal musculature (Fig. 8-39) with resultant dissolution of tissue, increase in spaces, fibrosis, and fatty infiltration. Further down, Purkinje cells were narrowed.

Summit of the Ventricular Septum

There was an increase in connective tissue. This began first on the right side, then became generalized to both sides (Fig. 8-39), which dipped deeper into the septum. Arteriolosclerosis was also noted.

Right Ventricle

There was moderate to marked fatty metamorphosis.

Discussion

The most likely abnormality having to do with the sudden death of this patient is the pressure of the right ventricular septal musculature on the bundle and the left bundle branch.

CASE #16

A 2-year-old male child developed an abnormal ECG pattern, 1 hour and 17 minutes after anesthesia was begun, during the course of surgery for an orchiopexy, and died sud-

denly. The child, during two pervious surgical procedures, at approximately 6 weeks of age and 3 months of age, developed tachycardia during the induction of anesthesia. The first time the heart rate was approximately 175 beats per minute, while the second time it

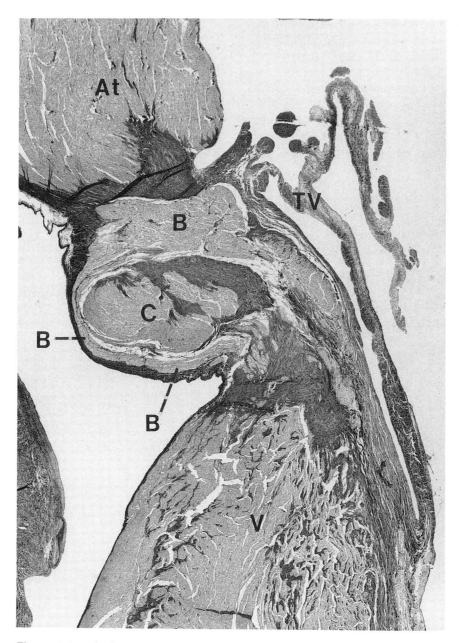

Figure 8-40 Penetrating bundle of His passing around conal muscle entrapped in the pars membranacea. Note the fibrosis of the summit of the ventricular septum. Weigert-van Gieson stain ×22. At = atrial muscle; B = bundle entrapping muscle (probably conal); C = conal muscle; V = ventricular septum.

went up to 212 beats per minute. However, on both occasions, he reverted to normal sinus rhythm after the full induction of anesthesia.

Pathology: Gross

The heart was enlarged, weighing 68 grams. There was hypertrophy and enlargement of the chambers. The eustachian valve was a prominent membrane that extended to the distal end of the linea terminalis. There was an aneurysm of the fossa ovalis and an atrial septal defect of the fossa ovalis type measuring 0.3–0.4 cm in greatest dimension. The endocardium of this chamber was distinctly thickened.

Microscopic Examination: Positive Findings

AV Node

This was segmented and lay within the tricuspid valve annulus.

Penetrating Bundle

This, with the left bundle branch, formed a loop around conal and ventricular muscle (Fig. 8-40).

Summit of the Ventricular Septum

There was a marked increase in connective tissue both on the right and on the left sides (Fig. 8-40).

Discussion

The sudden death of this child is probably related to the abnormality in the penetrating bundle. The role of the AV node lying in the tricuspid annulus and the fibrosis of the summit of the ventricular septum in a 2-year-old child are findings that cannot be overlooked.

CASE #17[182]

A 15-year-old boy had a history of premature right ventricular complexes for a number of years, but was apparently in good health. He suddenly collapsed while playing soccer.

Pathology: Gross

The heart weighed 300 grams. Diffuse fibrosis of the myocardium was seen by the coroner's physician at the gross level. All valves and the coronary arteries were normal. The heart was given to us in parts. Only the superior vena caval region, the sinoatrial nodal region, and atrioventricular node region, the bundle of His region, and the right and left bundle branches region were recognized.

Microscopic Examination: Positive Findings

Approaches to the SA and AV Nodes

Fatty infiltration was present.

Left and Right Bundle Branch

Moderate fibrosis was present.

Summit of the Ventricular Septum

Numerous areas of fibrosis were present especially in the right side (Fig. 8-41).

Left Ventricular Myocardium

Large areas of fibrosis were present beneath the epicardium (Fig. 8-42).

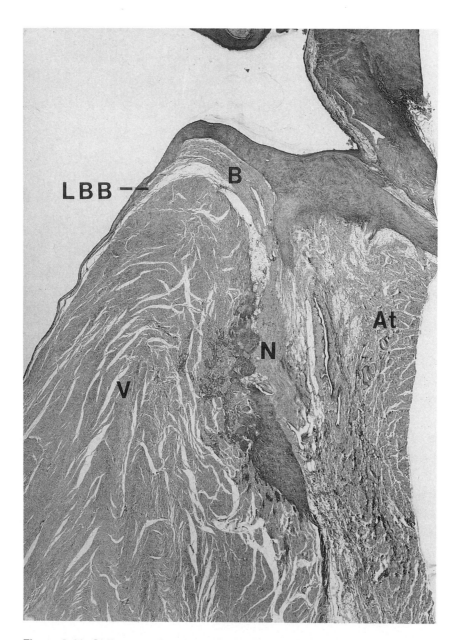

Figure 8-41: Oblique section through the AV node, bundle, and beginning of left bundle branch. Weigert-van Gieson stain ×10. At = atrial musculature; V = ventricular septum; B = bundle of His; LBB = left bundle branch; N = AV node. (Reprinted with permission from Bharati S, Bauernfeind R, Miller LB, Strasberg B, Lev M: Sudden death in three teenagers: Conduction system studies. *J Am Coll Cardiol* 1983; 1:879–888.)

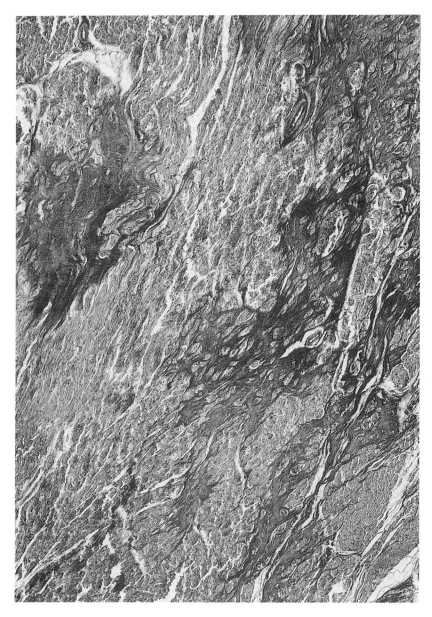

Figure 8-42: Enlargement of fibrosis on right side of septum. Weigert-van Gieson stain ×45.

Discussion

This is a case in which the fibrosis of the summit of the ventricular septum must be in- criminated in the production of arrhythmias. However, we cannot overlook the fatty infiltra- tion of the atria and the fibrosis of both bundle branches.

CASE #18[182]

A 19-year-old stable college student, while watching television, was startled when her mother entered the living room and she exclaimed that her mother had scared her because she thought she had gone to bed and didn't expect to see her come in the room. She then fell to the floor dead. She had recurrent dizzy spells a few days before death. Her father died suddenly at age 36 and his father died a few months later apparently of heart failure, with a history of repeated episodes of "passing out." Two of the father's sisters had heart problems. Her two younger sisters were diagnosed as having mitral valve prolapse, but are asymptomatic and are now on small doses of propranolol.

Pathology: Gross

The heart weighed 220 grams. There was slight hypertrophy and enlargement of the left

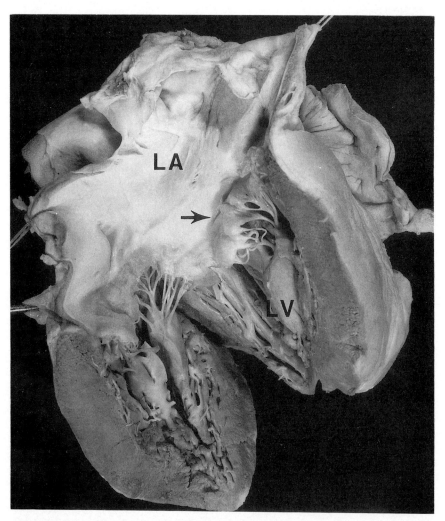

Figure 8-43: Left atrial and left ventricular view of the heart showing mitral valve prolapse. LA = left atrium; LV = left ventricle. The arrow points to the prolapsed mitral valve.

atrium and right ventricle. The mitral orifice was normal in size. The valve showed distinct prolapse of the posterior leaflet which was redundant and nodose (Fig. 8-43). This redundancy extended to the posterior part of the anterior leaflet. All other valves and the coronary arteries were normal.

Microscopic Examination: Positive Findings

SA Node

There was an organized thrombus or embolus (Fig. 8-44) filling part of the SA node artery. The arterioles were thickened.

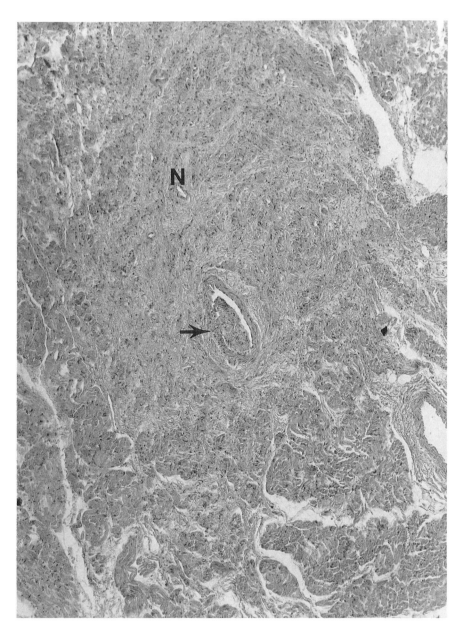

Figure 8-44: SA node, with organizing thrombus or embolus in artery. Weigert-van Gieson stain ×75. N = SA node. The arrow points to the artery.

Approaches to the SA and AV Node

Fatty metamorphosis was present.

AV Node

The AV node in part was in the central fibrous body.

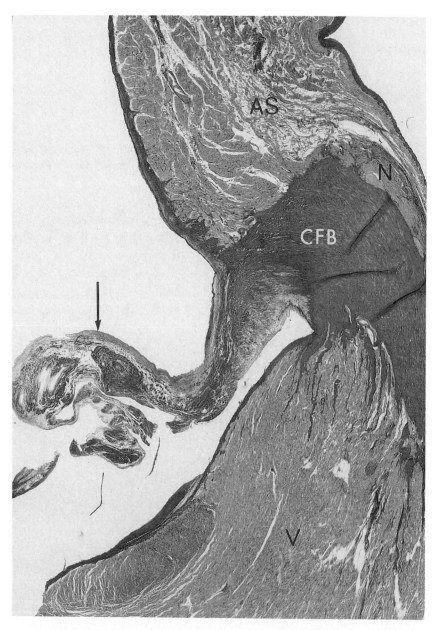

Figure 8-45: Prolapsed mitral valve, showing marked mixture of fibrosa and spongiosa. Weigert-van Gieson stain ×45. AS = atrial septum; N = AV node; CFB = central fibrous body; V = ventricular septum. The arrow points to the mitral valve.

Mitral Valve

There was a mixture of the fibrosa and spongiosa (Fig. 8-45).

AV Bundle, Penetrating

This was septated.

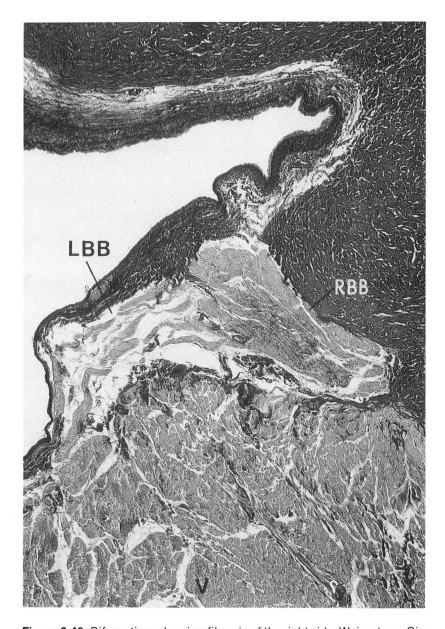

Figure 8-46: Bifurcation, showing fibrosis of the right side. Weigert-van Gieson stain ×45. LBB = beginning of left bundle branch; RBB = beginning of right bundle branch; V = ventricular septum. (Reprinted with permission from Bharati S, Bauernfi nd R, Miller LB, Strasberg B, Lev M: Sudden death in three teenagers: Conduction system studies. *J Am Coll Cardiol* 1983, 1:879–886.)

AV Bundle, Branching

Fibrosis was evident.

Bifurcation

Fibrosis was present on the right side (Fig. 8-46).

Central Fibrous Body

The central fibrous body sent a thick mass of connective tissue to the tricuspid valve.

Discussion

This 19-year-old female had dizzy spells a few days before her sudden death. There was a family history of sudden death.

The cause of sudden death may be related to the mitral valve prolapse. In addition, she had an organized thrombus or embolus in the SA nodal artery. Fatty metamorphosis was also present in the approaches to the SA and AV nodes, and the bundle was septated and fibrosed. Also, the right side of the bifurcation showed fibrosis. We would want to think that the mitral valve prolapse disrupts the fibrous skeleton of the heart to produce the changes in the conduction system, which in turn are related to arrhythmia and ventricular fibrillation, cardiac arrest, and sudden death.

CASE #19

Pathology: Gross

An 11-year-old female child, while attending class in school, collapsed and became unresponsive. The previous night, at a basketball game, she complained of being dizzy.

The heart was enlarged, weighing 230 grams. All chambers were enlarged with walls of average thickness. The posterior leaflet of the mitral valve was divided into two segments

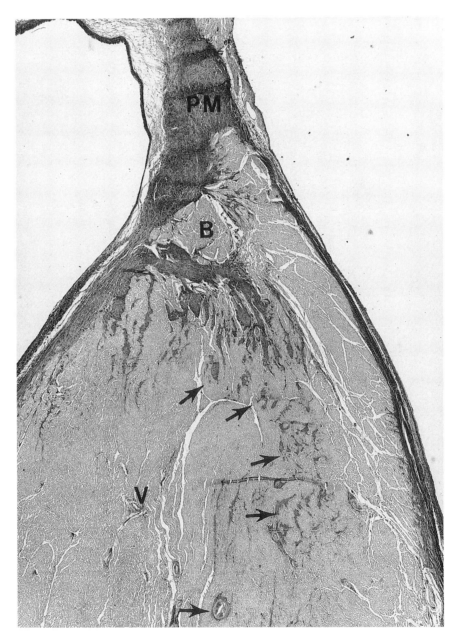

Figure 8-47: The summit of the ventricular septum, showing distinct fibrosis on the right side with arteriolosclerosis. Weigert-van Gieson stain ×22.5. B = bundle of His; PM = pars membranacea; V = ventricular septum. The arrows point to the arteriolosclerosis and fibrosis.

and was redundant. The membranous septum was enlarged with a small piece of conal muscle entrapped within the septum.

Microscopic Examination: Positive Findings

Penetrating Bundle

This was covered by conal muscle on the right side.

Summit of the Ventricular Septum

There was a distinct increase of connective tissue on the right side with arteriolosclerosis (Fig. 8-47).

Discussion

This is another case of prolapsed mitral valve and premature fibrosis and arteriolosclerosis of the summit of the ventricular septum. The thesis is evolving that any factor which disrupts the skeleton of the heart, such as prolapsed mitral valve, premature fibrosis of the summit of the ventricular septum, or invasion of conal or posterior ventricular septal muscle into the pars membranacea, may produce pressure upon or degenerative changes in the conduction system. We do not know whether these changes or the change in the summit of the ventricular septum are related to the assumed arrhythmia, ventricular fibrillation, and/or sudden death.

CASE #20[175]

This child was first referred at the age of 2 years for evaluation of a heart murmur. The electrocardiogram showed an axis +85°, complete AV block with an LBBB pattern, and a ventricular rate of 55/minute. The atrial rate was 110/minute. She remained asymptomatic for 8 years, with her ECG unchanged.

At age 10, while riding a bicycle, she had a Stokes-Adams attack and was taken to the hospital emergency room where she was noted to have ventricular fibrillation. Despite the successful cardioversion and insertion of

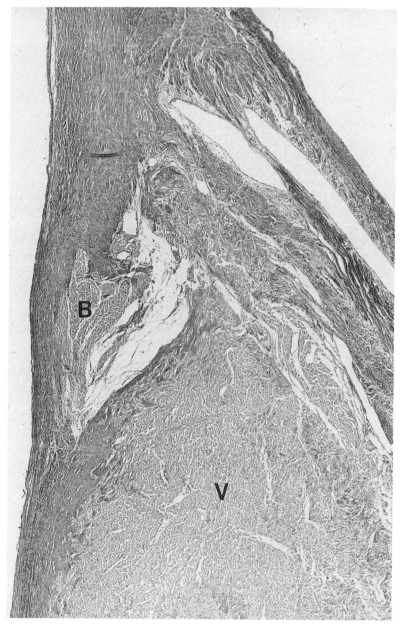

Figure 8-48: Atrophy of part of the branching bundle. Weigert-van Gieson stain ×39. B = bundle; V = ventricular septum.

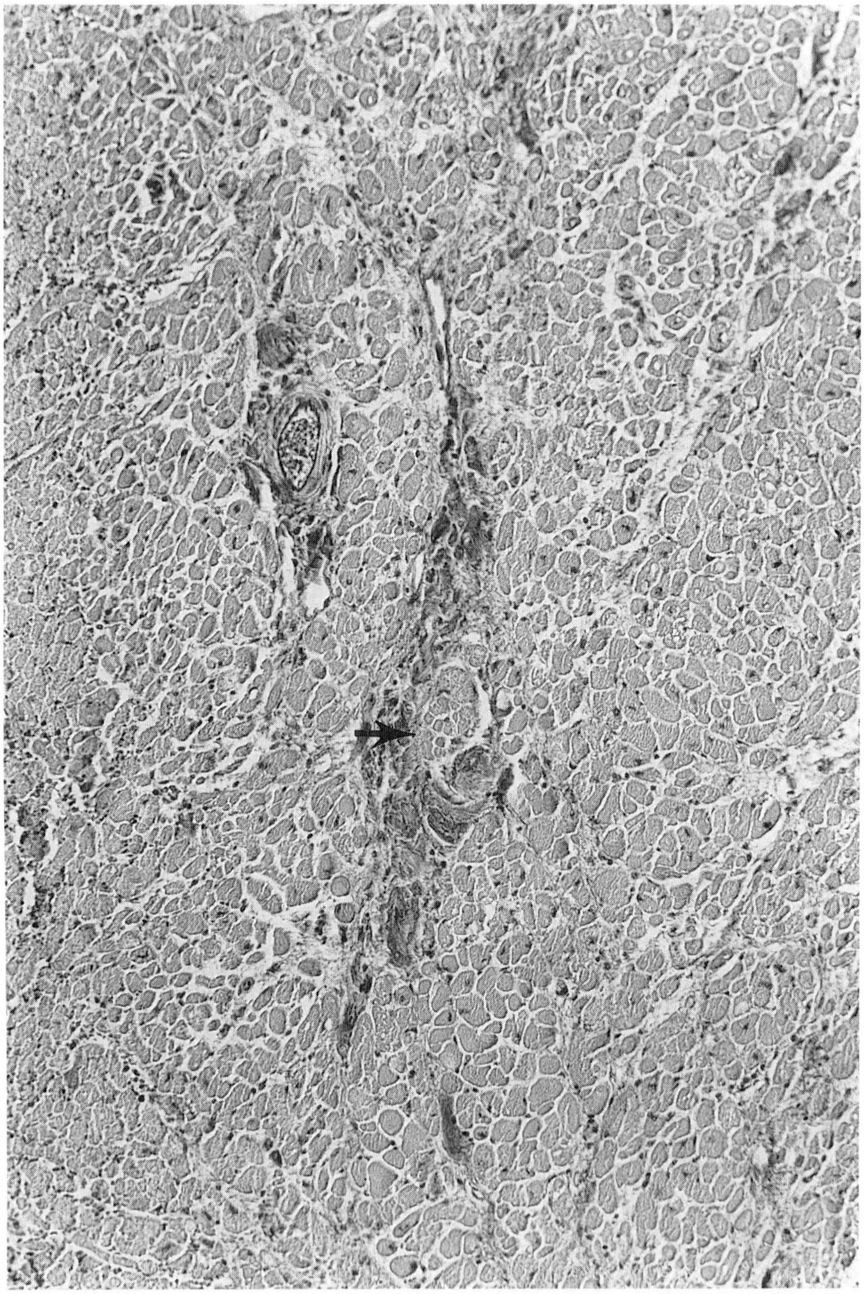

Figure 8-49: The beginning of the right bundle branch lying in scar. Weigert-van Gieson stain ×150. The arrow points to the right bundle branch. (Reprinted with permission from Husson GS, Blackman MS, Rogers MC, Bharati S, Lev M: *Am J Cardiol* 1973; 32:365–369.)

a temporary pacemaker, she died suddenly with ventricular fibrillation 48 hours later. A second sibling at age 15 years had a right bundle branch block with left axis and later developed complete heart block with a normal axis at age 17. Repeated Stokes-Adams attacks necessitated implantation of a permanent pacemaker and the patient is asymptomatic. Although both mother and father have normal ECGs, another sister, aged 17, asymptomatic, has normal sinus rhythm, normal AV conduction time, but prolonged intraventricular conduction time of 0.11 seconds with an incomplete right bundle branch block pattern.

Pathology: Gross

The heart was immensely enlarged and weighed 292 grams. All chambers, especially the left ventricle, were hypertrophied and enlarged. The endocardium of both atria and that of the left ventricle were diffusely thickened and that of the right ventricle was focally thickened and whitened. Additional endocardial plaques were found in the left ventricular endocardium.

Microscopic Examination: Positive Findings

Branching Bundle

This was partially atrophied and showed a large space (Fig. 8-48).

Left Bundle Branch

This consisted of only a few degenerated fibers peripherally; there were only a few Purkinje cells.

Right Bundle Branch

The first part was absent. The right bundle branch began at the end of the first part lying in a small scar (Fig. 8-49).

Myocardium

The left ventricular myocardium showed a distinct myocarditis.

Discussion

This 10-year-old child was a member of a family where she was one of three siblings with abnormal conduction systems leading to complete AV block with prolonged intraventricular conduction time. Sudden death in complete AV block may be anticipated. This patient developed ventricular fibrillation and died suddenly.

Conduction system studies revealed atrophy of the branching portion of AV bundle (Fig. 8-48), almost complete absence of the left bundle branch and complete absence of the first part of the right bundle branch (Fig. 8-49). In addition, there was a distinct myocarditis. The family history suggests that we are dealing with a genetically abnormally formed conduction system.

CASE #21[176]

An apparently healthy 16-year-old girl gave birth to a normal full-term infant. Immediately postpartum, her heart rate fell to 35 beats per minute and the ECG disclosed 2:1 AV block with intermittent complete heart block. She was discharged on a regimen of propranolol 10 mg three times a day. Six weeks later, an ECG disclosed complete heart

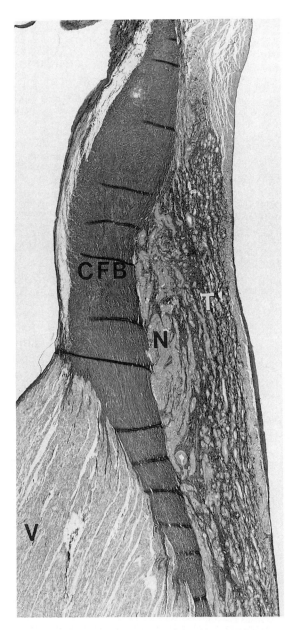

Figure 8-50: Mesothelioma of the AV node. Weigert-van Gieson stain ×14. CFB = central fibrous body; V = ventricular septum; T = tumor; N = AV node.

block with atrial rates between 70 and 100 beats per minute and a ventricular escape rate averaging 45 beats per minute with a narrow QRS morphology. A His bundle electrogram demonstrated complete block proximal to the His bundle recording site. Escape beats were all preceded by His bundle potentials with a normal H-V interval of 4 ms. Diagnostic cardiac catheterization disclosed normal pressures and output. The patient had asystolic cardiac arrest during diagnostic catheterization from which she could not be resuscitated.

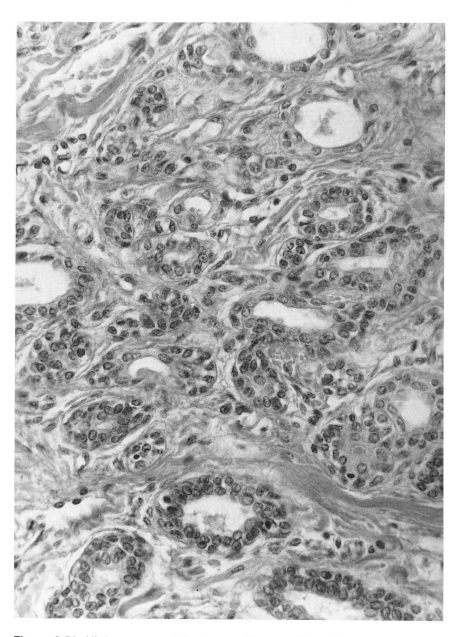

Figure 8-51: Higher power of the tumor. Hematoxylin-eosin stain ×375. (Reprinted with permission from Bharati S, Bicoff P, Fridman JL, Lev M, Rosen KM: Sudden death caused by benign tumor of the atrioventricular node. *Arch Intern Med* 1976; 136:223–228.)

Pathology: Gross

The heart weighed 270 grams. The right atrium and ventricle were hypertrophied. Part of the septal leaflet of the tricuspid valve was devoid of valvular tissue and adjacent to this there was a somewhat discolored area in the atrial septum that measured approximately 1.2 cm in greatest dimension. Otherwise the heart was grossly normal.

Microscopic Examination: Positive Findings

Approaches to the SA Node

There was focal degeneration of atrial cells.

Approaches to the AV Node

The atrial septum in its distal portion was occupied by a tumor mass. This consisted of tumor cells arranged in masses, cysts, and lacunae (Figs. 8-50, 8-51). These cells differed little in size and shape and exhibited no mitotic figures. The cells had oval nuclei, with a small amount of metachromatic staining cytoplasm lying in a sea of thick collagen fibers. The arterioles were noticeably thickened.

The AV node was almost completely replaced by the tumor. The penetrating portion of the AV bundle was partially replaced by tumor. The myocardium of the atria and ventricles showed focal acute degeneration of cells bordering on acute necrosis.

Discussion

This 16-year-old girl died suddenly during catheterization. She was known to have complete heart block and mesothelioma had almost completely replaced the AV node.

Here we have a perfect example of involvement of the conduction system in the cause of sudden death. However, the exact mechanism of the physiological events that was responsible for the sudden death is not known.

CASE #22[182]

A 17-year-old boy who was a trained athlete died suddenly during football scrimmage. Six months before his death, he was diagnosed as having a viral infection. Three days later, he went to football practice. Subsequently, he had no complaints and engaged in full athletics. A day or two before his death, he complained of muscle discomfort in his shoulder. He also had a head cold and was working out for more than an hour when he collapsed. Three weeks earlier, he had re-

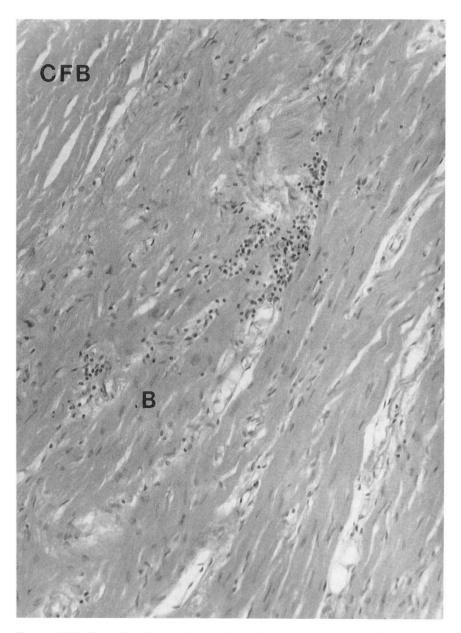

Figure 8-52: Chronic inflammatory cells in the penetrating part of the bundle of His. Hematoxylin-eosin stain ×150. B = bundle of His; CFB = central fibrous body.

ceived a thorough physical check-up and was reported to be in excellent condition.

Pathology: Gross

The heart weighed 355 grams. There was hypertrophy and dilatation of the right ventri-cle. The whole region of the pars membran-acea and the adjacent aortic leaflet of the mi-tral valve were thickened. For his age, the mi-tral orifice was somewhat enlarged. The posterior leaflet was enlarged and divided into three components. There was mild to mod-erate redundancy of the entire leaflet. The cor-onary arteries were normal.

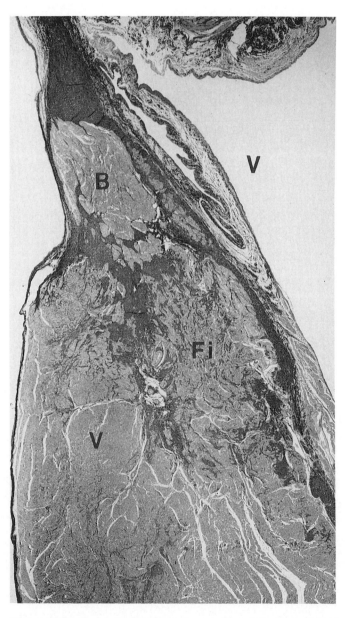

Figure 8-53: Summit of ventricular septum showing marked fibrosis, with more on right side. Weigert-van Gieson stain ×17. B = bundle; Fi = fibrosis; V = ventricular septum.

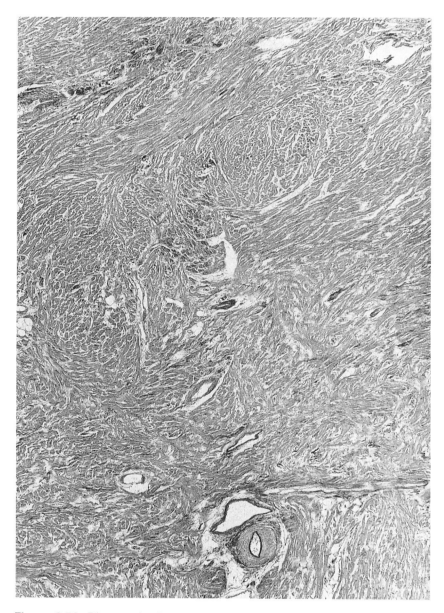

Figure 8-54: Disarray in the ventricular septum. Weigert-van Gieson stain ×45. (Reprinted with permission from Bharati S, Bauernfeind, Miller LB, Strasberg B, Lev M: Sudden death in three teenagers: Conduction system studies. *J Am Coll Cardiol* 1983; 1:879–886.)

Microscopic Examination: Positive Findings

AV Bundle, Penetrating Portion

Mononuclear cells were present, with an increase in collagen and elastic fibers. This was a distinct myocarditis (Fig. 8-52).

Right Bundle Branch

The first and second parts showed distinct fibrosis.

Summit of the Ventricular Septum

Marked fibrosis was present on both sides of the summit, especially on the right (Fig. 8-53). Focally, there was a pattern of disarray (Fig. 8-54).

Discussion

The sudden death of this 17-year-old boy may be related to (1) the prolapsed mitral valve, (2) myocarditis of the conduction system, (3) the marked fibrosis of the summit of the ventricular septum, (4) the focal disarray pattern, and (5) the fibrosis of the right bundle branch.

CASE #23[179]

A 34-year-old man of Italian ancestry collapsed and died suddenly while riding a bicycle. He was in good health until 3 years ago when he was diagnosed as having Mediterranean fever. A year later he was admitted for vertigo and syncopal episodes. Neurological evaluation was normal.

ECG

This showed RBBB with first-degree and intermittent third-degree AV block and recurrent paroxysmal unifocal ventricular tachycardia.

EPS

This showed normal sinus rhythm with prolonged AH (175 ms) and H-V (50 ms) intervals and extrastimulus induction of repetitive ventricular tachycardia. Left ventricular angiography revealed a well-delineated area of hypokinesia of posterior left ventricle with decreased left ventricular ejection fraction. Coronary angiogram showed normal coronaries.

Pathology: Gross

The heart weighed 359 grams. The left atrium and left ventricle were slightly hypertrophied. In the posterobasal part of the ventricular septum extending into the posterior basal wall adjacent to the mitral valve, there was an aneurysm (Fig. 8-55). The endocardium lining the aneurysm was thickened and included in the aneurysm. The myocardium of the basal part of the posterior wall was replaced by greyish-white tissue; the right aortic cusp was markedly fenestrated (Fig. 8-55). There was mild arteriosclerotic narrowing of the anterior and posterior descending coronary arteries. The endocardium of the sinus of the right ventricle close to the apex showed fibrous tubular formation indicating long-standing pacemaker presence.

Microscopic Examination: Positive Findings

Approaches to the SA Node

These were involved by sarcoidosis.

Approaches to the AV Node, AV Node, AV Bundle (Figs. 8-56, 8-57, 8-58) and Bundle Branches, and Ventricular Septum

These were involved by sarcoid.

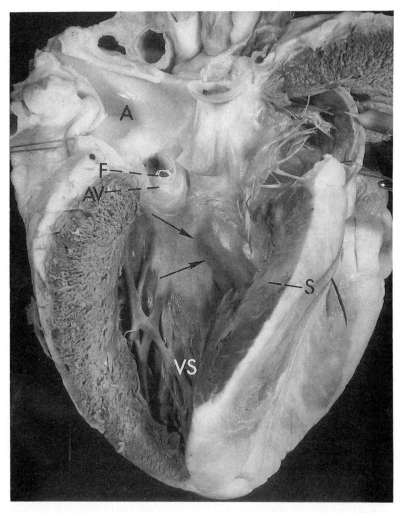

Figure 8-55: View of the outflow tract of the left ventricle and of the ascending aorta. Note the aneurysm in the basal part of the posterior ventricle septal wall and the posterior wall with sarcoidosis in the posterior wall. A = aorta; VS = ventricular septum; F = sarcoid in wall; S = sarcoid; AV = aortic valve. The arrows point to the aneurysm.

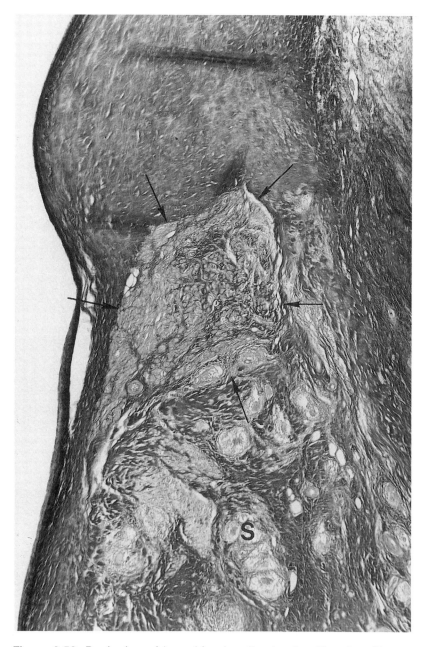

Figure 8-56: Beginning of branching bundle showing fibrosis, with sar-coidosis in the summit of the ventricular septum. Weigert-van Gieson stain ×45. S = sarcoid. The arrows point to the bundle.

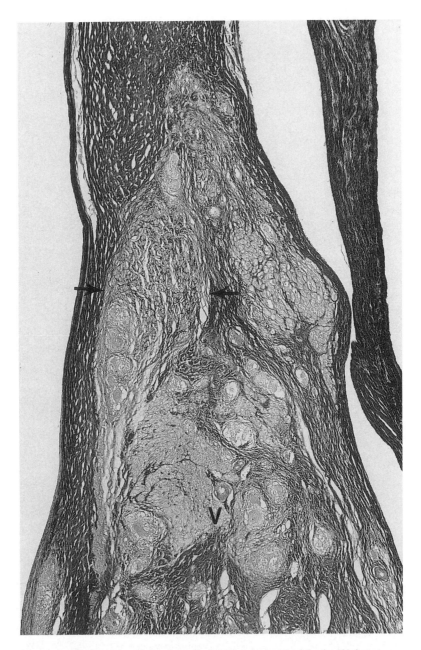

Figure 8-57: The branching bundle involved in sarcoidosis. Weigert-van Gieson stain ×45. V = summit of the ventricular septum. The arrows point to the branching bundle.

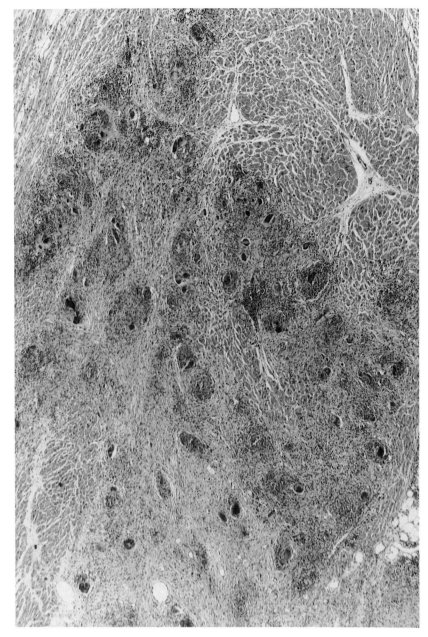

Figure 8-58: Posterior wall of the left ventricle involved in sarcoidosis. Hematoxylin-eosin stain ×45. (Reprinted with permission from Bharati S, Lev M, Denes P, Modlinger J, Wyndham C, Bauernfeind, Greenblatt M, Rosen KM: Infiltrative cardiomyopathy with conduction disease and ventricular arrhythmia: Electrophysiologic and pathologic correlations. *Am J Cardiol* 1980; 45:163–173.)

Discussion

This 34-year-old man had generalized sarcoidosis of the heart. His sudden death may be related to the generalized sarcoidosis of the conduction system, leading to ventricular fibrillation and sudden death.

CASE #24[201]

A 13-year-old girl had an unexpected cardiac arrest while in church and was found by paramedical personnel to have ventricular fibrillation and underwent defibrillation. She was hospitalized and remained in a coma for 18 hours. She then had another episode of ventricular fibrillation and died.

At age 1 year, she was noted to have cardiomegaly, mitral insufficiency, and pre-excitation. At age 33 months, she had mitral annuloplasty because of left ventricular failure. She did well subsequently until 6 months prior to death except for short brief episodes of palpitation (no documented arrhythmia).

Pathology: Gross

The heart was hypertrophied and enlarged in all chambers and weighed 580 grams. There was diffuse fibroelastosis of the left ventricle. All valve orifices were enlarged. The commissures of the tricuspid and pulmonic valves were widened and thickened. The mitral valve was irregularly thickened with shortened chordae. The aortic valve was markedly thickened with fenestration. The right coronary ostium was high. The coronary arteries were patent.

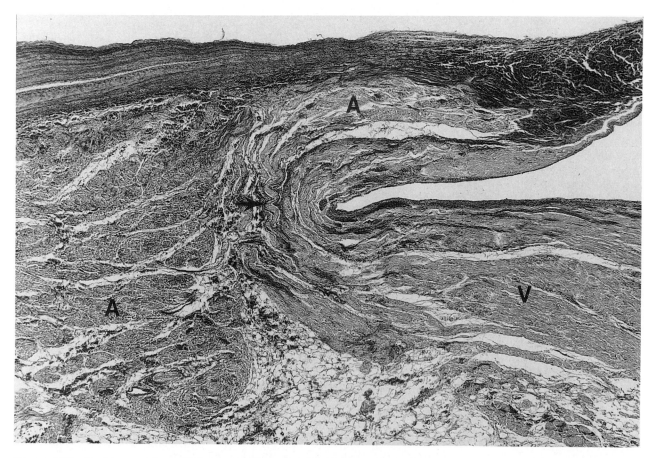

Figure 8-59: First bypass tract. Weigert-van Gieson stain × 40. A = atrial musculature; V = ventricular musculature. The arrow points to connection between atrial and ventricular musculature.

Microscopic Examination: Positive Findings

SA and AV Nodes and Their Approaches

Fatty infiltration was present.

Branching Bundle

Fibrosis at its junction with the left bundle branch was noted. The bundle was situated on the left side.

Left Bundle Branch and Right Bundle Branch

Fibrosis was present in both branches.

AV Rims

There were two small AV connections on the superior part of the free wall of the right atrium and ventricle (Fig. 8-59, 8-60). These connections consisted of "working" myocardial fibers with normal architecture with some increase in connective tissue.

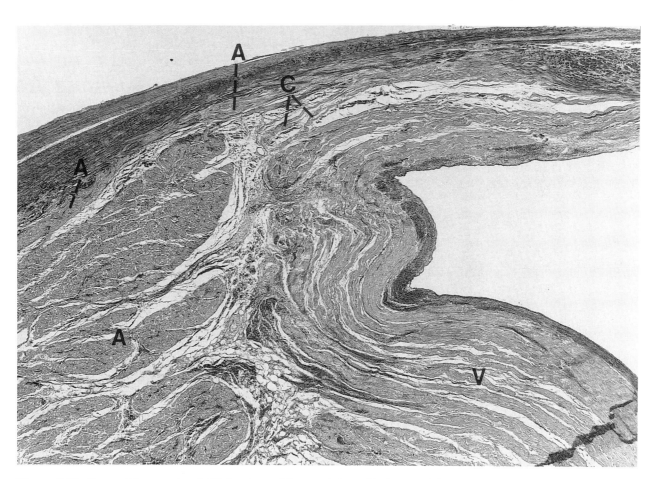

Figure 8-60: Second bypass tract. Weigert-van Gieson stain ×40. A = atrial musculature; V = ventricular musculature; C = connection between atrial and ventricular musculature. (Reprinted with permission from Bharati S, Strasberg B, Bilitch M, Salibi H, Mandel W, Rosen KM, Lev M: Anatomic substrate for preexcitation in idiopathic hypertrophy with fibroelastosis of the left ventricle. *Am J Cardiol* 1981; 48:47–58.

Discussion

Some people with Wolff-Parkinson-White syndrome are known to die suddenly. Presumably, the cause of death in these cases is the bypass tract. However, in other cases we have fatty infiltration in the SA and AV nodes and their approaches and fibrosis of the AV bundle and bundle branches. These may be added factors in the production of sudden death. We also cannot overlook the fibroelastosis of the left ventricle.

CASE #25[105]

A 67-year-old male was treated for congestive heart failure and became asymptomatic. Three months later, he developed se-

vere chest pain and died suddenly. The electrocardiogram revealed complete heart block with the escape rhythm characterized by right bundle branch block pattern. He later converted to sinus rhythm, first-degree AV block,

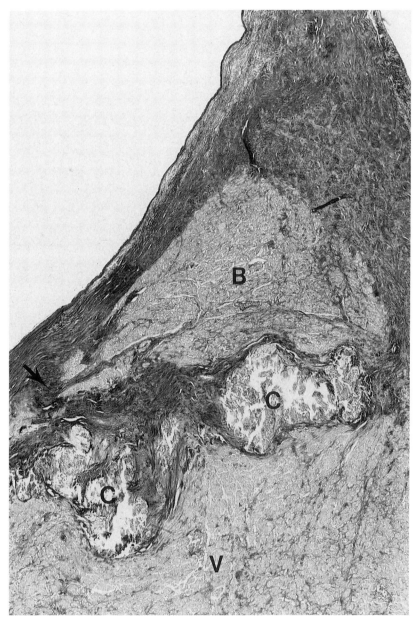

Figure 8-61: Bundle of His, branching portion, showing compression of the lower part by calcium. Weigert-van Gieson stain ×45. Note the left bundle branch interrupted by fibroelastic tissue. B = bundle of His; C = calcium; V = ventricular septum. The arrow points to interruption of the left bundle branch.

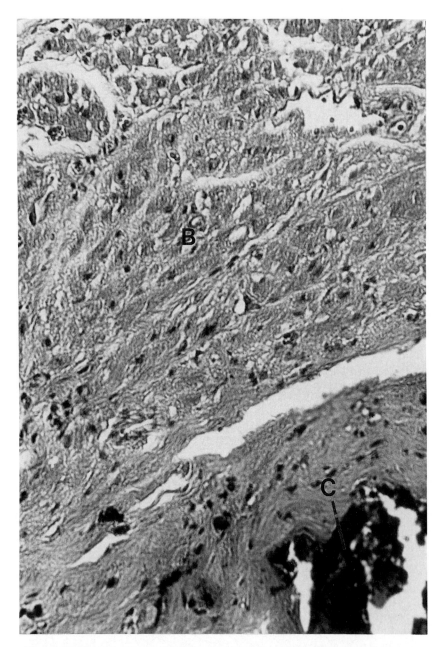

Figure 8-62: Lower part of the bundle of His, branching portion, lying adjacent to calcific mass. Note the degeneration of the adjacent His bundle. Hematoxylin-eosin stain ×300. B = bundle; C = calcium. (Reprinted with permission from Bharati S, Lev M, Wu D, Denes P, Dhingra R, Rosen KM: Pathophysiologic correlations in two cases of split His bundle potentials. *Circulation* 1974; 49:615–623.)

and right bundle branch block with QRS almost identical to the previous escape rhythm. EPS showed split His bundle potentials with intact conduction.

Pathology: Gross

The heart was hypertrophied and enlarged, weighing 729 grams. The right atrium and both ventricles were hypertrophied. The left atrium was hypertrophied and enlarged. The mitral valve was calcific at the base and line of closure and the chordae were thickened. The aortic orifice was narrowed by changes in the valve. These changes of the valve consisted of marked calcification in the body, the line of closure, the edge, the base, and upper margins of the sinuses of Valsalva. The pars membranacea was somewhat thickened. All the coronaries were calcified and narrowed.

Microscopic Examination: Positive Findings

Approaches to the SA Node and Atrial Preferential Pathways

These showed fatty infiltration.

Approaches to the AV Node

These showed moderate fibrosis. The ramus septi fibrosi was markedly thickened and narrowed. The central fibrous body and the base of the mitral valve were markedly thickened and showed arteriolosclerosis.

AV Bundles, Penetrating

Moderate fibrosis was present.

AV Bundle, Branching

Calcification of the summit of the ventricular septum produced pressure on the bundle with degenerative changes in the lower part (Figs. 8-61, 8-62).

Left Bundle Branch

This was severely separated from the bundle by fibroelastic tissue (Fig. 8-61). The more peripheral parts showed fibrosis and degenerative changes with fatty metamorphosis.

Right Bundle Branch

Marked fibrosis was present.

Myocardium

The posterior parts of both ventricles showed moderate fibrosis, small scars, and arteriolosclerosis.

Discussion

The sudden death of this 67-year-old man with coronary disease and an acute attack of precordial pain is common. This may be due directly to the coronary disease with fibrosis of the posterior walls of both ventricles. Yet it is of interest that we have calcific sclerosis of the summit of the ventricular septum with injury to the bundle and the left bundle branch. In addition, we have marked fibrosis of the right bundle branch, which may be due to the coronary disease. The fatty metamorphosis of the approaches to the SA and AV nodes may be implicated in arrhythmia and sudden death.

CASE #26[208]

A 72-year-old male had a history of syncopal attacks, bradycardia, and hypertension. He had a permanent pacemaker implanted. Four years later, he returned in congestive heart failure and bradycardia. He developed ventricular tachyarrhythmias and died suddenly.

ECG

Complete AV block with an atrial rate of 70 beats per minute and a ventricular rate of 50 beats per minute were present. There was also wandering of the supraventricular pacemaker with varying atrial cycles and P-wave contours. The QRS duration was greater than 0.12 seconds and usually of a right bundle branch block pattern. There was some variation in QRS configuration with occasional ventricular premature beats.

EPS Studies

Complete heart block, distal to the His bundle recording site with wide QRS pattern, was present.

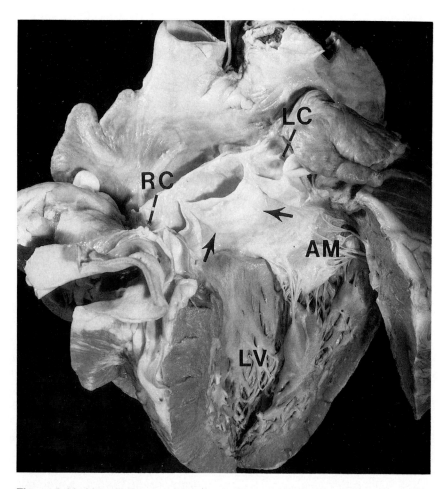

Figure 8-63: Monckeberg's sclerosis of the aortic valve (posterior noncoronary cusp). LV = left ventricle; AM = anterior leaflet of mitral valve; RC = right coronary ostium; LC = left coronary ostium. The arrows point to the noncoronary cusp of the aortic valve.

Pathology: Gross

The heart weighed 550 grams. All chambers, especially the left ventricle, were hypertrophied and enlarged. The coronary arteries were widely patent. Monckeberg's sclerosis of the noncoronary aortic cusp was in evidence (Fig. 8-63).

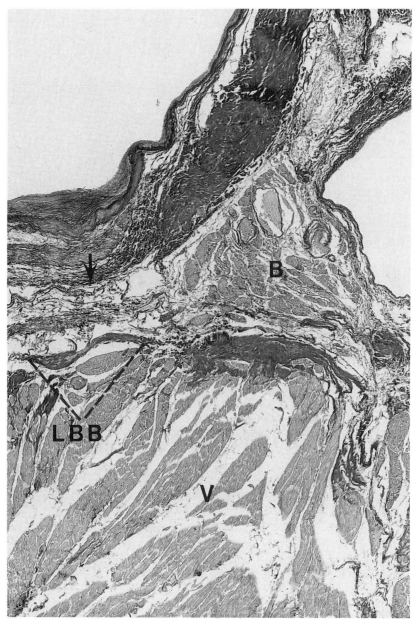

Figure 8-64: Fibroelastosis with replacement of the connection between the left bundle branch and the branching portion of the AV bundle. Weigert-van Gieson stain ×39. V = ventricular septum; B = branching bundle; LBB = left bundle branch. The arrow points to replaced LBB fibers.

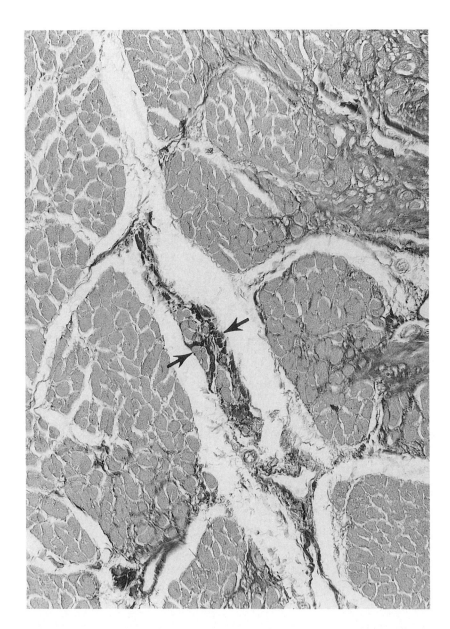

Figure 8-65: Fibroelastosis of the second portion of the right bundle branch. Weigert-van Gieson stain ×130. The arrows point to the right bundle branch.

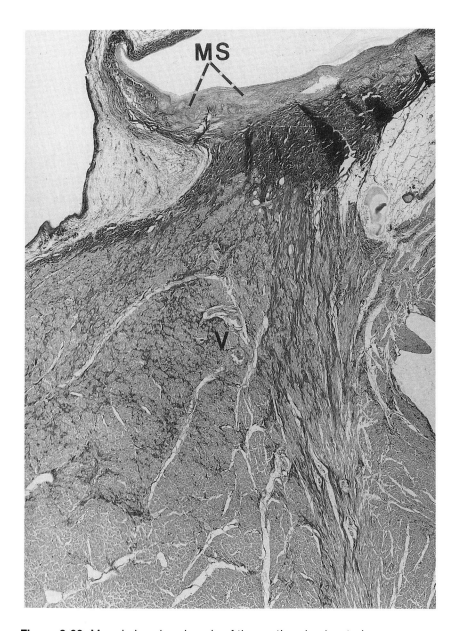

Figure 8-66: Monckeberg's sclerosis of the aortic valve (posterior noncoronary cusp). Note the fibrosis of the summit of the ventricular septum. Weigert-van Gieson stain ×22.5. MS = Monckeberg's sclerosis in sinus of Valsalva; V = ventricular septum. (Reprinted with permission from Rosen KM, Rahimtoola SH, Gunnar RM, Lev M: Site of heart block as defined by His bundle recording. *Circulation* 1972; 45:965–987.)

Microscopic Examination: Positive Findings

Approaches to the SA Node

There was marked fibrosis and elastosis, arteriolosclerosis, and infiltration of mononuclear cells.

AV Bundle, Penetrating Portion

Moderate fatty infiltration was present.

Left Bundle Branch

The connection of the left bundle branch with the main bundle was narrowed and markedly disrupted by collagen and elastic tissue. The periphery of the anterior radiation showed fibrosis (Fig. 8-64).

Right Bundle Branch

The second part showed marked fibroelastosis (Fig. 8-65).

Summit of the Ventricular Septum

There was marked fibrosis, with arteriolosclerosis anteriorly. The aortic valve showed Monckeberg's sclerosis of the noncoronary (posterior) cusp (Fig. 8-66).

Discussion

This elderly patient with hypertension but no narrowing of the coronary arteries had Monckeberg's sclerosis of the posterior cusp of the aortic valve and sclerosis of the summit of the ventricular septum. He developed heart block. He then developed ventricular tachyarrhythmias and died suddenly.

The cause of the heart block was found to be marked fibrosis and destruction of both bundle branches. This is related to Monckeberg's sclerosis of the aortic valve and sclerosis of the left side of the cardiac skeleton. The cause of the tachyarrhythmias and sudden death may lie in (1) the heart block, (2) the fibroelastosis of the approaches to the SA node, (3) the sclerosis of the left side of the cardiac skeleton, and (4) the hypertensive heart disease.

CASE #27[178]

A 5-year-old male child who had a Mustard procedure for simple complete transposition at 3 years of age died suddenly while playing. He had seizures and lost consciousness three times in the last year before his sudden death.

ECG

Two months before death, there was junctional rhythm with a rate of 70 beats per minute alternating with sinus rhythm with an occasional premature ventricular contraction. There was also first-degree AV block with right

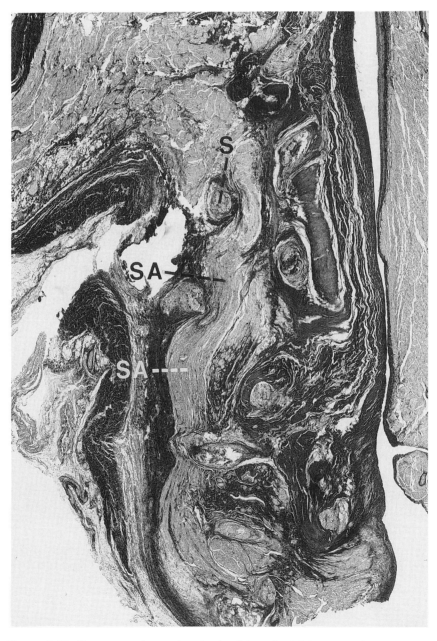

Figure 8-67: Sutures and reaction in the SA node. Weigert-van Gieson stain ×14.3. SA = SA node; S = suture.

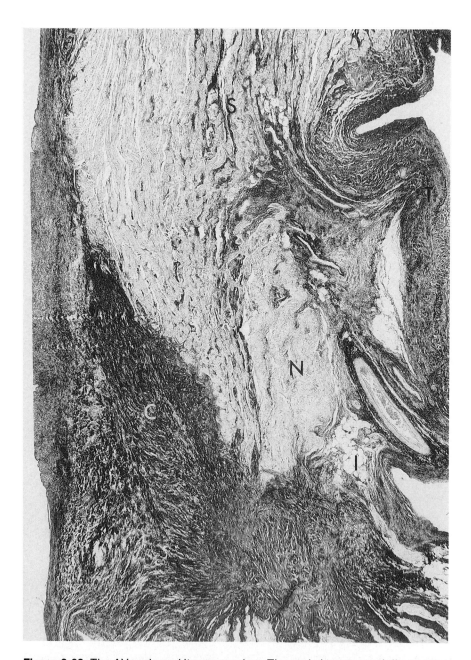

Figure 8-68: The AV node and its approaches. The node is seen partially encased in connective tissue with fibrotic separation from inferior and superior approaches. Weigert-van Gieson stain ×30. N = AV node; S = superior approaches; I = inferior approaches; C = central fibrous body; T = tricuspid valve. (Reprinted with permission from Bharati S, Molthan ME, Veasy G, Lev M: Conduction system in two cases of sudden death two years after the Mustard procedure. *J Thorac Cardiovasc Surg* 1979; 77:101–108.)

ventricular hypertrophy and strain and a suggestion of left atrial enlargement. Cardiac catheterization revealed normal pressures.

Pathology: Gross

The heart was enlarged and weighed 145 grams. After the Mustard procedure, the now-converted pulmonary venous atrium was hypertrophied and enlarged. There was no obstruction to the entry of the pulmonary veins. The right ventricle and the left atrium, now converted to the systemic venous atrium, were hypertrophied. There was no obstruction to the superior and inferior venae cavae or to the coronary sinus. The left ventricle was hypertrophied and enlarged.

Microscopic Examination: Positive Findings

SA Node

Sutures were present in the SA node. The node was compressed by the pericardial patch with fibrosis (Fig. 8-67).

Approaches to the SA Node

Sutures, fibrosis, and giant cell reaction compromised about 50% of the approaches.

Atrial Preferential Pathways

Only part of the superior preferential pathway remained, and it was interrupted in part by sutures.

Approaches to the AV Node

There was marked fibrosis and destruction of the inferior approaches, with slight to moderate fibrosis of the superior approaches (Fig. 8-68).

AV Node

Moderate fibrosis was present. It was partially encased in connective tissue (Fig. 8-68).

Discussion

This 5-year-old child had a Mustard procedure for transposition at 3 years of age. Junctional rhythm followed the procedure and he died suddenly.

The cause of the junctional rhythm was the sutures in the SA node and partial destruction of the node, the atrial preferential pathways, and the fibrosis and partial destruction of the superior approaches to the AV node. The sudden death was in some form or other related to the junctional rhythm.

CASE #28[178]

A 5-year-old male child had a Mustard procedure for simple complete transposition at 2½ years of age. He did well clinically and was completely asymptomatic until 2 months before death, when he had pneumonia. He recovered from this and was again asymptomatic. He was found unconscious and having a seizure at home and died suddenly.

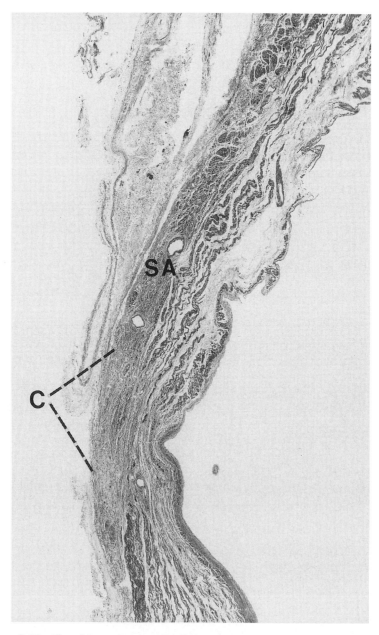

Figure 8-69: The SA node and its approaches. Gomori trichrome stain ×14.3. Part of the SA node and its approaches are almost completely replaced by connective tissue. SA = SA node; C = area of SA node almost completely replaced by connective tissue.

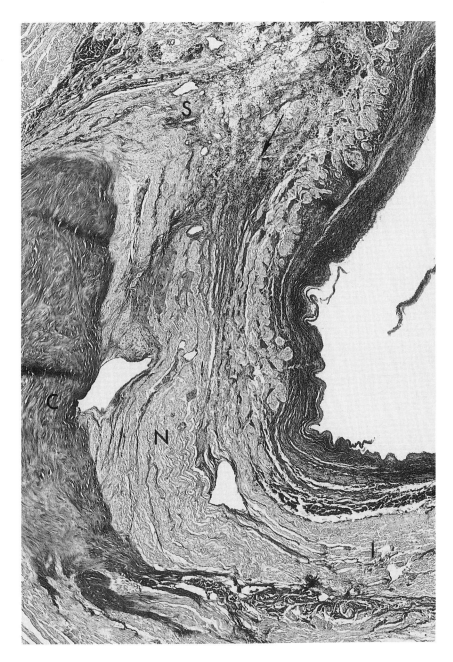

Figure 8-70: The AV node and its approaches. Weigert-van Gieson stain ×30. Considerable fibrosis is present in the superior approaches somewhat involving the node itself. The inferior approaches are intact. N = node; C = central fibrous body; I = inferior approaches; S = superior approaches. The arrow points to the fibrosis of the superior approaches. (Reprinted with permission Bharati S, Molthan ME, Veasy G, Lev M: *J Thorac Cardiovasc Surg* 1979; 77:101–108.)

ECG

Two months before death, an ECG revealed sinus rhythm changing to first-degree AV block and then to second-degree block with 2:1 conduction, varying with junctional rhythm with AV dissociation.

Pathology: Gross

The heart was enlarged and weighed 230 grams. The pulmonary venous atrium was greatly hypertrophied and enlarged. After the Mustard procedure, it received the coronary sinus and the pulmonary veins; however, the opening of the pulmonary veins was greatly restricted. The tricuspid orifice was greatly enlarged and the medial part of the anterior leaflet of the tricuspid valve was plastered against the septum; there was a closing ventricular septal defect. About 1 cm beneath the defect, there was a ridge of white thickening. There was no pulmonary stenosis.

Microscopic Examination: Positive Findings

SA Node

There was marked fibrosis (Fig. 8-69).

Approaches to the SA Node

Moderate to marked fibrosis (Fig. 8-69) was present.

Atrial Preferential Pathways

The superior and middle preferential pathways were replaced by fibrous tissue and the pericardial prosthesis. The inferior pathway had been removed by the surgeon.

Approaches to the AV Node

The superior approaches were markedly replaced by fibrous tissue. The inferior approaches were intact (Fig. 8-70).

Branching Bundle

This was markedly replaced by connective tissue with loss of about 80% of its parenchyma.

Bifurcation

This was partially replaced by fibrous connective tissue.

Left Bundle Branch

There was moderate fibrosis.

Lungs

There was focal acute pneumonitis.

Discussion

This 5-year-old child developed partial AV block about 2 years after the Mustard procedure for complete transposition and died suddenly and unexpectedly a few months later. The cause of the AV block was related to the fibrosis of the SA node and the approaches to the SA and AV nodes and the complete destruction of the atrial preferential pathways. This was further enhanced by the marked fibrosis of the branching bundle and moderate fibrosis of the left bundle branch. Both of the latter are related to the spontaneously closing ventricular septal defect. Whether the AV block itself or any of the pathological changes in the conduction system are related to the sudden death is speculative.

CASE #29[191]

A 17-year-old male had a Hancock heterograft valve placed from the right ventricle to the pulmonary trunk for tetralogy of Fallot with pulmonary atresia. Following surgery, he did very well and was totally asymptomatic. Three years prior to his death, a routine evaluation revealed that he had premature ventricular contractions on the electrocardiogram. He was found dead in bed 6 years after the surgery at the age of 23.

ECG

An ECG revealed normal sinus rhythm with no premature ventricular contractions. A 24-hour Holter electrocardiographic monitor revealed the presence of frequent premature ventricular contractions and a brief episode of supraventricular tachycardia.

Pathology: Gross

The heart was enlarged, weighing approximately 579 grams. All chambers were hypertrophied and enlarged. The tricuspid orifice was smaller than normal with a small accessory opening in the septal leaflet. The endocardium of the right atrium and ventricle and the left ventricle were diffusely thickened and whitened. The ventricular septum at its base presented a large defect which entered the right ventricle in the region of the arch. The defect had been closed by a prosthesis which was well endothelialized. The closure of the defect had resulted in a pouch-like formation between the aortic valve and the summit of the ventricular septum. The Hancock heterograft valve, although patent, revealed a considerable amount of calcification of the Dacron prosthesis. The outflow tract of the left ventricle was adequate in size. It was evident that the aorta emerged about 50% from the left ventricle and 50% from the right before closure of the defect. The aortic orifice was enlarged. Its valve was abnormally formed. Its cusps were distinctly thickened, irregular, and nodose. The coronary arteries were not narrowed.

Microscopic Examination: Positive Findings

Approaches to the SA and AV Nodes

Fibrosis and fatty infiltration with calcification were present. Fibrosis of nerves was also present.

AV Node

Marked edema was present.

Bundle, Penetrating

There was moderate lobulation.

AV Bundle, Branching

Fibrosis and fatty metamorphosis were evident (Fig. 8-71).

Left Bundle Branch

Marked fibrosis with fatty metamorphosis was seen (Fig. 8-71).

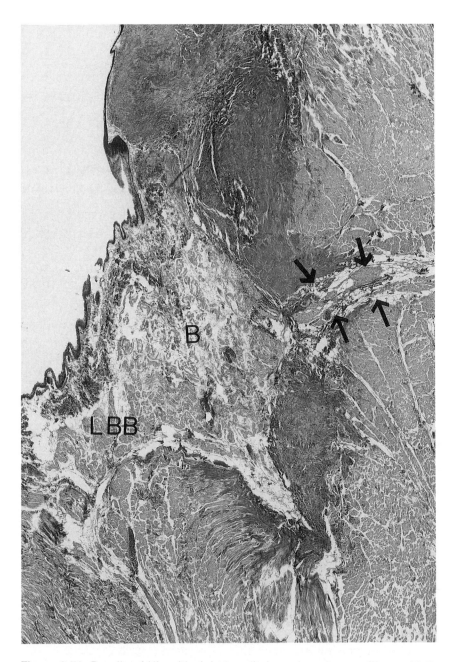

Figure 8-71: Bundle of His with right bundle branch and some fibers of left bundle branch being given off. Note the fatty metamorphosis of the right bundle branch, bundle, and left bundle branch. B = bundle; LBB = some fibers of the left bundle branch. The arrows point to right bundle branch. (Reprinted with permission from Bharati S, Lev M: Conduction system in cases of sudden death in congenital heart disease many years after surgical correction. *Chest* 1986; 90:861–868.)

Right Bundle Branch

Fatty metamorphosis and fibrosis were present (Fig. 8-71).

Summit of the Ventricular Septum

There was marked fibrosis with arteriosclerosis and arteriolosclerosis.

Discussion

The sudden death of this 23-year-old 6 years after repair of tetralogy of Fallot may be related to (1) the fibrosis and fatty metamorphosis of the approaches to the SA and AV nodes, and/or (2) the fibrosis and fatty metamorphosis of the bundle and bundle branches. Both of these may be related to the previous surgery.

CASE #30[191]

A male child had a Senning procedure at 6 months of age. At 15 months of age, he died suddenly during a swimming lesson. A few weeks before death, he was diagnosed as having juvenile rheumatoid arthritis. An electro-cardiogram before surgery showed sinus rhythm and right atrial hypertrophy and enlargement. Following the Senning procedure, the electrocardiogram showed ectopic atrial pacemaker and right ventricular hypertrophy, which converted to sinus rhythm 3 weeks later. The last ECG, done 2 months before death,

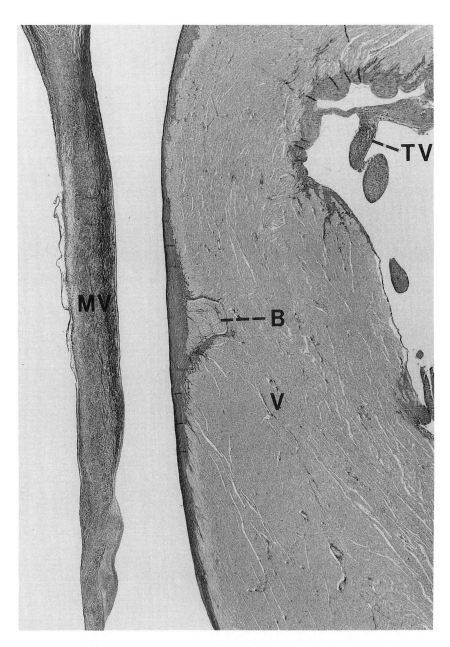

Figure 8-72: Left-sided AV bundle. V = ventricular myocardium; MV = mitral valve; B = bundle; TV = tricuspid valve.

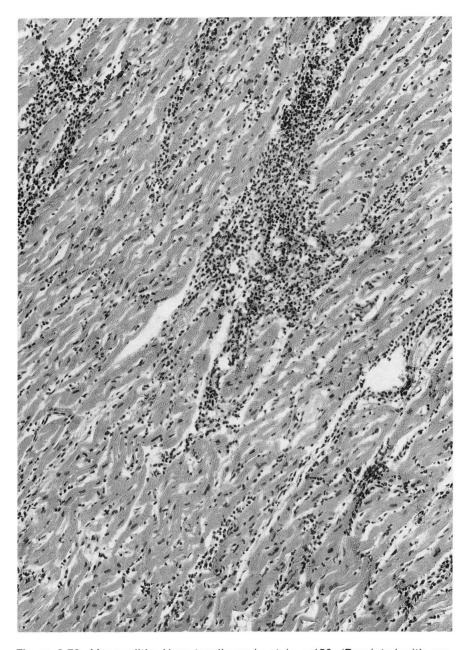

Figure 8-73: Myocarditis. Hematoxylin-eosin stain ×150. (Reprinted with permission from Bharati S, Lev M: Conduction system in cases of sudden death in congenital heart disease many years after surgical correction. *Chest* 1986; 90:861−868.)

revealed sinus rhythm, right axis deviation, and right ventricular hypertrophy.

Pathology: Gross

The heart was enlarged, weighing approximately 122 grams. All chambers were hypertrophied and enlarged. The tricuspid orifice was enlarged. The medial leaflet was divided into two well-developed segments. The endocardium of both atria was thickened and whitened.

Microscopic Examination: Positive Findings

Atrial Preferential Pathways

Marked fibroelastosis with replacement of muscle was present with chronic inflammation and atherosclerosis.

Approaches to the AV Node

Chronic inflammation was present.

AV Node

Marked fibrosis was present. There was an accessory AV node.

AV Bundle

This was distinctly on the left side (Fig. 8-72).

Myocardium

There was a diffuse distinct myocarditis (Fig. 8-73) in the atria and ventricles that was more concentrated in the infundibulum of the right ventricle.

Discussion

This child who had a Senning operation at 6 months of age died suddenly at 21 months. The cause of sudden death was a myocarditis, which is known to cause sudden death. The left-sided bundle, which has been compressed by the hypertrophied ventricular septal musculature, may be a contributing factor.

CASE #31[191]

An asymptomatic female died suddenly at the age of 30. Seventeen years earlier, at the age of 13, she had an ostium primum defect closed surgically. Although she had a loud persistent blowing apical systolic murmur of mitral regurgitation, she did extremely well and became a sports enthusiast and finished college. She was totally asymptomatic until her sudden death.

ECG

Before surgery, there was first-degree AV block with a P-R ranging from 0.16 to 0.2 and left axis deviation with biventricular enlargement. After surgery, there was left axis deviation, sinus rhythm notched P-waves interpreted as left atrial enlargement, and inversion of T-waves from $V_{3R}-V_6$.

Pathology: Gross

The heart was enlarged, weighing 472 grams in the fixed state. All chambers were hypertrophied and enlarged. The region of the patch closure of the primum defect revealed an area of calcification. The mitral orifice was somewhat enlarged. Both atria showed diffuse fibroelastosis.

Microscopic Examination: Positive Findings

Approaches to the SA Node

There was marked fatty metamorphosis. The nerves showed fibrosis.

Atrial Preferential Pathways

Marked fatty metamorphosis was noted.

Approaches to the AV Node

Marked fatty metamorphosis was present. The nerves showed fibrosis. Thickening of ramus septi fibrosi was noted.

AV Node

A sclerotic narrowed artery compressed the node (Fig. 8-74), which was partially embedded in the central fibrous body. There was partial separation of the node from the approaches.

AV Bundle, Penetrating and Branching

This showed marked fibrosis and fatty metamorphosis (Fig. 8-75).

Left Bundle Branch

Fibrosis of the left bundle branch.

Right Bundle Branch

Marked fibrosis was present.

Right Ventricle

This showed fatty metamorphosis.

Summit of the Ventricular Septum

This showed marked fibrosis (Fig. 8-76).

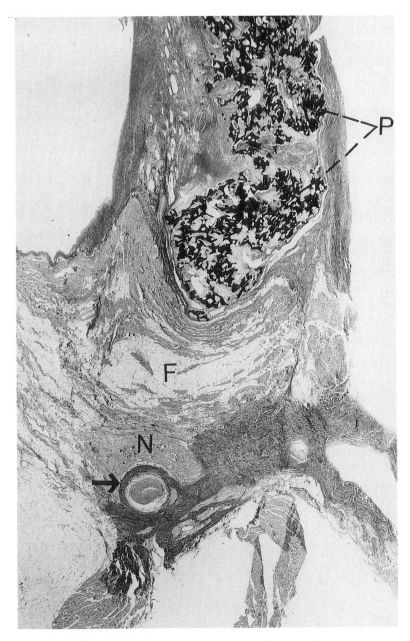

Figure 8-74: A sclerotic artery indenting AV node. N = AV node; F = fatty metamorphosis; Weigert-van Gieson stain ×10. P = atrial prosthesis. The arrow points to the sclerotic artery.

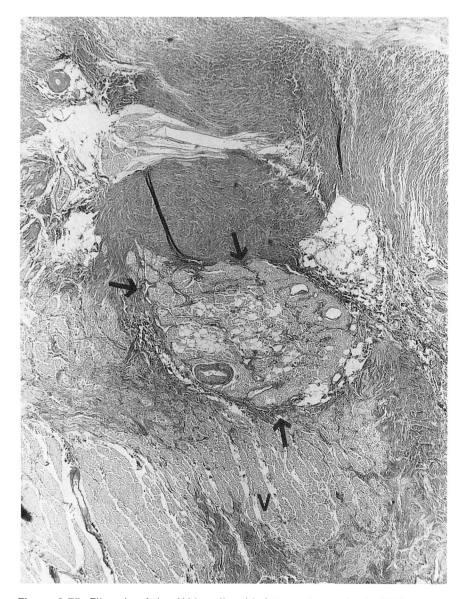

Figure 8-75: Fibrosis of the AV bundle with fatty metamorphosis. Weigert-van Gieson stain ×45. V = ventricular septum. The arrows point to the AV bundle.

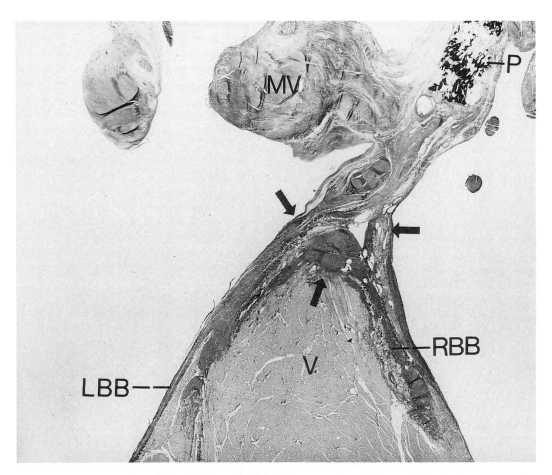

Figure 8-76: The summit of the ventricular septum showing marked fibrosis. Weigert-van Gieson stain ×10. MV = mitral valve; P = atrial prosthesis; RBB = right bundle branch showing marked fibrosis; LBB = left bundle branch; V = ventricular septum. The arrows point to the fibrosis of the summit of the ventricular septum. (Reprinted with permission from Bharati S, Lev M: Conduction system in cases of sudden death in congenital heart disease many years after surgical correction. *Chest* 1986; 90:861–868.)

Discussion

The cause of sudden death in this 30-year-old woman 17 years after the closure of a primum defect may lie in numerous findings. First the heart was enlarged as are so many hearts after cardiac surgery. Then the conduction system shows changes in the approaches to the SA and AV nodes, the AV node, the ramus septi fibrosi, the bundle of His, and both bundle branches. In addition, the summit of the ventricular septum showed fibrosis and the right ventricle showed fatty metamorphosis. It is thus difficult to assign an area as the cause of sudden death, if indeed the cause of death is cardiac.

CASE #32[191]

A 9-year-old male child died suddenly 4 years after a patch closure of a ventricular septal defect and insertion of a Hancock prosthesis from the right ventricle to the pulmonary artery for double outlet left ventricle. The patient did extremely well and was totally asymptomatic. All pressures were normal postoperatively and an angiocardiogram revealed an excellent repair. A treadmill electrocardiogram and 24-hour Holter monitoring revealed occasional premature atrial contractions and rare ventricular premature

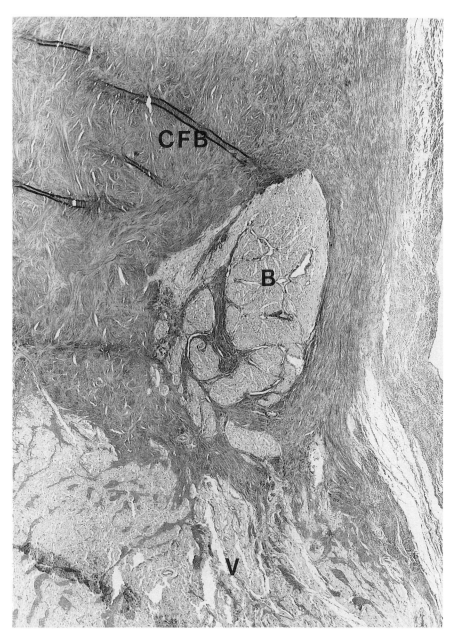

Figure 8-77: Fibrosis with lobulation of bundle. Weigert-van Gieson stain ×45. CFB = central fibrous body; B = bundle; V = ventricular septum.

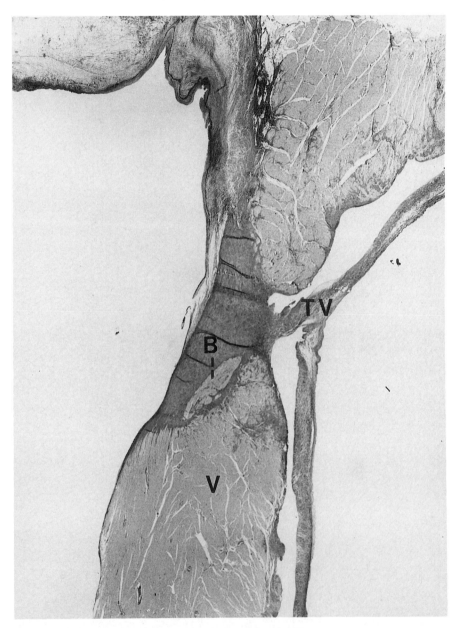

Figure 8-78: Fibrosis of the summit of the ventricular septum, especially on the right side. Weigert-van Gieson stain ×9.7. B = bundle; V = ventricular septum; TV = tricuspid valve.

contractions. The patient died suddenly while playing outside the house.

Pathology: Gross

The heart was enlarged, weighing 327 grams. All chambers were hypertrophied and enlarged. The tricuspid valve was smaller than normal and the leaflet structure was divided into several segments. The Hancock prosthesis revealed a considerable amount of calcification of the conduit. The porcine valve leaflets revealed some calcification. Originally, the ventricular septum presented a large defect in its anterior part, which did not involve the membranous septum. It entered the right ventricle in the region of the arch. The defect had been closed by means of a prosthesis and revealed calcification. Originally the aorta emerged overriding the defect. The pulmonary trunk originally emerged from the morphologically left ventricle situated between the mitral and the aortic valves. The main pulmonary trunk had been tied off by the surgeon.

Microscopic Examination: Positive Findings

Approaches to the SA Node

Chronic inflammation was noted.

Atrial Preferential Pathways

Marked fibrosis and fibroelastosis were evident.

AV Node

Fatty metamorphosis was present with partial separation of the node.

AV Bundle, Penetrating

Moderate fibrosis and lobulation were seen (Fig. 8-77).

AV Bundle, Branching

The bundle was left-sided (Fig. 8-78).

Summit of the Ventricular Septum

This showed an increase in fibrosis (Fig. 8-78), especially on the right side.

Myocardium

Myocarditis was present in the right ventricle and the ventricular septum.

Discussion

This 9-year-old boy died suddenly 4 years after insertion of a Hancock prosthesis from the right ventricle to the pulmonary artery and closure of a ventricular septal defect for double outlet left ventricle. The cause of sudden death may be related to (1) fibrosis and lobulation of the penetrating bundle, (2) myocarditis of the right ventricle and septum, and (3) partial separation of the AV node from the atrial septum by fat. In all of these surgical cases, the deformation of the central fibrous body and pars membranacea may be a factor.

CASE #33[198]

A 25-year-old previously healthy man was stabbed in the anterior chest, which resulted in a ventricular septal defect and complete atrioventricular block. A permanent pacemaker was inserted because of persistent congestive heart failure and bradycardia due to AV block. The patient subsequently became asymptomatic. Three and one-half years later, he died suddenly.

ECG

This showed complete AV block with QRS of the right bundle branch block pattern.

EPS

This showed AV disassociation with split His potentials. The escape QRS shifted from right to left bundle branch block with H potentials still preceding each QRS interval with an H2-V interval of 40 ms.

Pathology: Gross

The heart was greatly enlarged, weighing 680 grams. There was hypertrophy and enlargement of all chambers. The tricuspid valve was enlarged, and it presented a defect in the septal and anterior leaflets close to the annulus (Fig. 8-79). The mitral valve was greatly

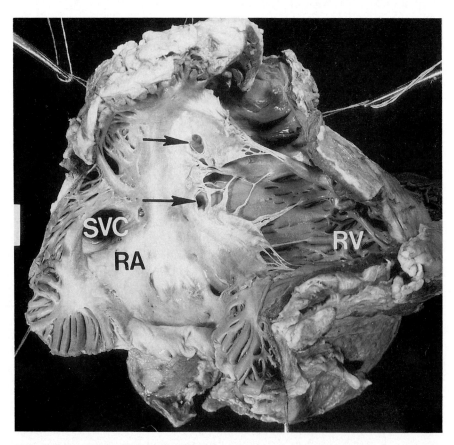

Figure 8-79: Right atrial and right ventricular view of the heart. RA = right atrium; RV = right ventricle; SVC = superior vena cava. The arrows point to the openings in the anterior and medial tricuspid leaflets produced by the knife.

enlarged and there was a circular defect in the anterior leaflet (Fig. 8-80). At the base of the ventricular septum, there was a defect measuring 0.5 × 0.4 cm (Fig. 8-80). This was situated beneath the junction of the posterior and right aortic cusps in the region of the lower part of the pars membranacea, partly involving the muscular portion of the septum. The coronary arteries were normal.

Microscopic Examination: Positive Findings

AV Bundle

Marked fibrosis was present until only a rim remained (Fig. 8-81). The bifurcation was destroyed.

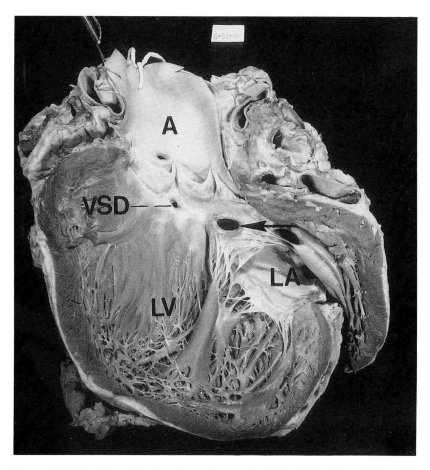

Figure 8-80: Left ventricular view. A = aorta; LA = left atrium; LV = left ventricle; VSD = ventricular septal defect produced by the knife. The arrow points to the opening in the anterior leaflet of the mitral valve produced by the knife. Note the thickening of the endocardium around the ventricular septal defect.

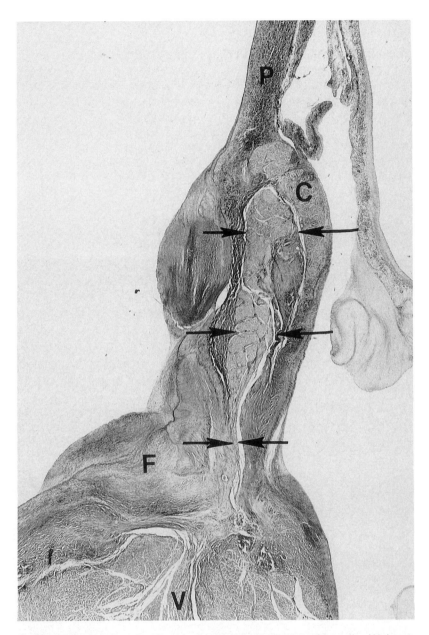

Figure 8-81: The proximal part of branching portion of bundle. Weigert-van Gieson stain ×17. C = conal musculature; F = fibroelastosis; P = pars membranacea; V = ventricular septum. The arrows point to the bundle and the beginning of the obliterated posterior fibers of the main left bundle branch. (Reprinted with permission from Bharati S, Towne WD, Patel R, Lev M, Rahmtoola SN, Rosen KM: Pathologic correlations in the case of complete heart block with split His potentials resulting from stab wound of the heart. *Am J Cardiol* 1976; 38:388–393.)

Bundle Branches

Most proximal portions of both bundle branches were absent, replaced by fibroelastosis.

Summit of the Ventricular Septum

There was marked fibrosis and fibroelastosis.

Discussion

This 25-year-old healthy man was stabbed in the chest, resulting in a ventricular septal defect and complete AV block. The block was the result of destruction of the branching bundle and the beginning of both bundle branches. The pacemaker was functioning normally. Thus, the cause of sudden death is difficult to explain, as it is in most cases of AV block.

CASE #34[189]

A 19-year-old girl with mild to moderate pulmonary stenosis and prolonged QT interval had had syncopal episodes lasting 5 to 10 minutes during which she was unresponsive. During her last attack, she was found to have no pulse or respiration. On resuscitation, her

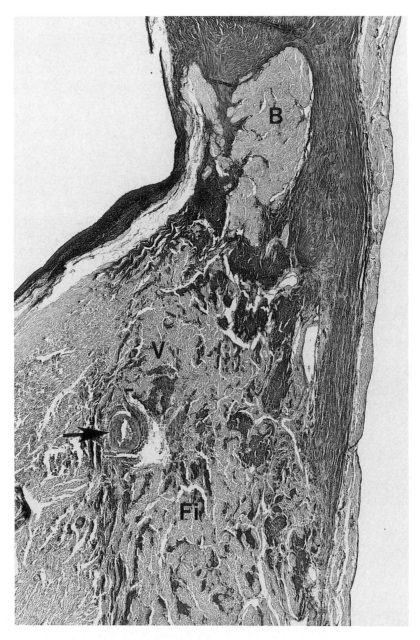

Figure 8-82: Lobulated atrioventricular bundle and fibrosis of the summit of the ventricular septum. Weigert-van Gieson stain ×22. B = bundle; V = ventricular septum; Fi = fibrosis of right side of summit of ventricular septum. The arrow points to arteriolosclerosis. (Reprinted with permission from Bharati S, Dreifus L, Bucheleres G, Molthan M, Covitz W, Isenberg NS, Lev M: The conduction system in patients with a prolonged QT interval. *J Am Coll Cardiol* 1985; 6:1110–1119.)

electrocardiogram showed asystole, subsequently ventricular fibrillation, idioventricular rhythm, and then sinus tachycardia. She became comatose and died 10 days later. She had no hearing problem. An electrocardiogram showed prolonged QT interval.

Pathology: Gross

The heart was enlarged. All chambers were hypertrophied and enlarged. There was an atrial septal defect of the fossa ovalis type. The tricuspid orifice was somewhat smaller than normal. The pulmonary orifice was smaller than normal and the pulmonary valve was abnormal. Although there were three cusps, the commissures and valvular tissue were markedly thickened and whitened.

Microscopic Examination: Positive Findings

SA Node

This was divided into two segments, one in normal position and the other in the roof of the right atrium.

Atrial Preferential Pathways and Approaches to the AV Node

Marked fatty infiltration was in evidence.

AV Node

This showed fatty infiltration and fibrosis and moderate mononuclear cell infiltration. This was partially present in the central fibrous body.

AV Bundle, Penetrating

This was lobulated (Fig. 8-82).

AV Bundle, Branching

There was moderate fibrosis.

Bundle Branches

Moderate fibrosis was in evidence.

Summit of the Ventricular Septum

The right side showed marked fibrosis with arteriolosclerosis (Fig. 8-82).

Discussion

Although this 19-year-old girl died 10 days after a seizure, we are including this under the category of sudden death since she was comatose during this period. The patient had pulmonary stenosis with an atrial septal defect of the fossa ovalis type and a prolonged QT interval.

The prolonged QT interval may be related to (1) fatty infiltration of the approaches to the SA node and the atrial preferential pathways and the approaches to the AV node, (2) fatty infiltration and fibrosis of the AV node, (3) the lobulated AV bundle, and (4) the fibrosis of the bundle branches. We cannot overlook the massive fibrosis of the right side of the summit of the ventricular septum with arteriolosclerosis. Is this the cause of changes in the bundle and bundle branches?

CASE #35[189]

A 9-month-old female child had documented QT prolongation since birth. She had normal growth and development. At 9 months of age, she had a seizure and cardiopulmonary resuscitation was performed. She continued to have multiple cardiac arrests associated with recurrent ventricular tachycardia of which she died. The hearing was normal.

ECG

Prolonged QT with a corrected QT interval of 0.65 sec was present. The ventricular rate was 64 per minute with a 2:1 ventricular response with every P-wave occurring before the T-wave.

Pathology: Gross

All chambers were hypertrophied and enlarged. The posterior crest region was abnormal, with several muscles demarcating off the atrial appendage from the atrium. The left ventricle showed fibroelastosis.

Microscopic Examination: Positive Findings

Atrial Preferential Pathways

There was distinct mononuclear cell infiltration and hemorrhage.

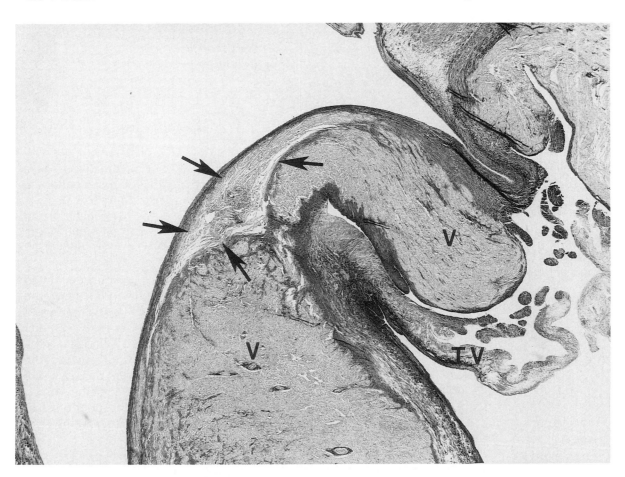

Figure 8-83: The atrioventricular bundle on the left side of the ventricular septum showing fibrosis. Weigert-van Gieson stain ×22. V = ventricular septum; TV = tricuspid valve. The arrows point to the bundle.

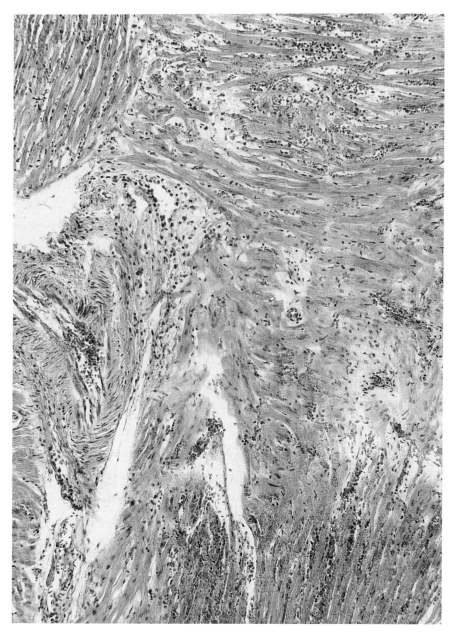

Figure 8-84: Myocarditis of the ventricular septum. Hematoxylin-eosin stain ×150. (Reprinted with permission from Bharati S, Dreifus L, Bucheleres G, Molthan M, Covitz W, Isenberg HS, Lev M: The conduction system in patients with a prolonged QT interval. *J Am Coll Cardiol* 1985; 6:1110–1119.)

Approaches to the AV Node

An infiltration of mononuclear cells and red cells with fibrosis and fatty infiltration was noted.

AV Node

This showed distinct mononuclear cell infiltration.

AV Bundle, Branching

This was distinctly on the left side and showed fibrosis and an infiltration of mononuclear cells (Fig. 8-83).

Bundle Branches

Both showed fibrosis.

Summit of the Ventricular Septum

This showed a myocarditis (Fig. 8-84) with fibrosis on the left side and hemorrhages.

Myocardium

A myocarditis and hemorrhage were present on both sides (Fig. 8-84).

Discussion

This 9-month-old child had documented QT prolongation since birth. She died in ventricular fibrillation at 9 months of age. The ventricular fibrillation was due to a myocarditis of the atria and ventricles and of the conduction system. Since the child had a QT prolongation since birth, it is unlikely that this was due to the myocarditis. This could be related to the left-sided bundle with fibrosis of the bundle branches.

CASE #36[189]

A 15-month-old black infant (an identical twin) was found not breathing in the playpen and was taken to the hospital. He could not be resuscitated. His identical twin brother is known to have had prolonged QT interval (0.47 sec, corrected).

Pathology: Gross

The heart was somewhat enlarged. The left atrium and ventricle were hypertrophied and enlarged. The limbus was distinctly accentuated as it reached the tubercle of Lower. The limbus bifurcated into two portions distally, producing a small pouch. Distinct fibroelastosis was present in the bundle, the tubercle of Lower, and the mouth of the inferior vena cava.

Microscopic Examination: Positive Findings

Approaches to the AV Node

There was marked fatty metamorphosis.

AV Node

This was partly embedded in the central fibrous body.

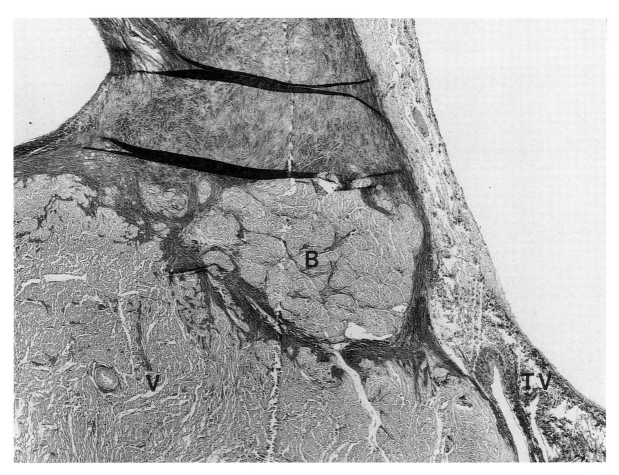

Figure 8-85: Penetrating bundle, showing slight to moderate fibrosis with lobulation. Weigert-van Gieson stain ×45. B = bundle; TV = tricuspid valve; V = ventricular septum.

AV Bundle, Penetrating and Branching

There was slight to moderate fibrosis with lobulation (Fig. 8-85).

Bundle Branches

These were larger than normal for his age.

Discussion

This 15-month-old child whose identical twin had QT prolongation had findings in the conduction system that may be related to arrhythmia and sudden death. They are: (1) fatty metamorphosis in the approaches to the AV node; (2) the AV node was partly embedded in the central fibrous body; (3) the AV bundle showed slight to moderate fibrosis and lobulation; and (4) the bundle branches were larger than normal for his age.

CASE #37[189]

A 2-year-old black boy was the identical twin of the previous case. The patient had cardiac arrest 1½ weeks before the death of his twin brother. He was documented to have had prolonged QT and was given propranolol. His hearing was normal. As he was eating, he began choking and collapsed. In the hospital, he was stabilized. He subsequently had a second cardiac arrest, then developed ventricular tachycardia, followed by bradycardia, arrhyth-

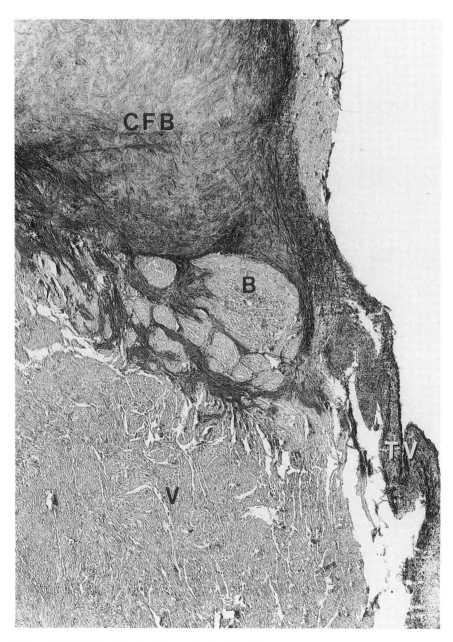

Figure 8-86: Lobulated atrioventricular bundle. Weigert-van Gieson stain ×45. B = bundle; CFB = central fibrous body; V = ventricular septum; TV = tricuspid valve.

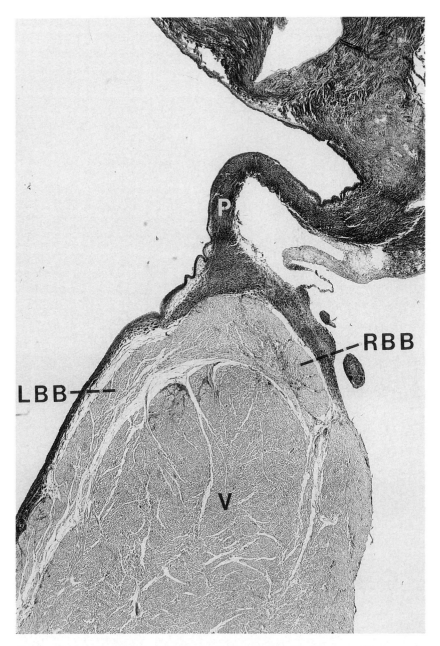

Figure 8-87: Large right and left bundle branches. Weigert-van Gieson stain ×30. RBB = right bundle branch; LBB = left bundle branch; P = pars membranacea; V = ventricular septum. (Reprinted with permission from Bharati S, Dreifus L, Bucheleres G, Molthan M, Covitz W, Isenberg HS, Lev M: *J Am Coll Cardiol* 1985; 6:1110–1119.)

mias, multiple arrests, and died 4 hours after admission.

Pathology: Gross

The heart was slightly enlarged. The left ventricle was hypertrophied and enlarged. The endocardium of the right atrium was thickened and whitened, especially in the region of the atrial preferential pathways. That of the left ventricle was distinctly thickened and whitened at the base and throughout the left bundle branch.

Microscopic Examination: Positive Findings

Approaches to the AV Node

There was marked fatty metamorphosis.

AV Node

This was partly embedded in the central fibrous body.

AV Bundle, Penetrating

This was lobulated with slight fibrosis (Fig. 8-86).

Bundle and Bundle Branches

Slight to moderate fibrosis was present. Both bundle branches were large for the age of the patient (Fig. 8-87).

Discussion

This 2-year-old boy was known to have prolonged QT syndrome. He died suddenly. The prolonged QT syndrome may be related to the lobulated bundle of His and the fibrosis of the bundle branches. The sudden death may be related to the fatty metamorphosis of the approaches to the AV node. The role of the large bundle branches in this case cannot be ascertained. The QT prolongation and sudden death in the identical twins suggests the possibility of genetically abnormally formed conduction system or tendency for arrhythmias in an abnormal conduction system.

CASE #38[199]

A 13-year-old boy had a 6-year history of documented recurrent ventricular tachycardia and died suddenly. The episodes of ventricular tachycardia were short and well tolerated, but several lasted many hours and recurred despite treatment with combinations of procainamide, quinidine, digoxin, propranolol, and diphenylhydantoin. Cardiac catheterization was normal, except for mildly elevated pulmonary artery and right ventricular systolic pressures.

ECG

During sinus rhythm, it showed a PR interval of 0.16 sec and narrow QRS complexes with normal morphology except for Q-waves in lead III and left ventricular hypertrophy by voltage criteria. Ventricular tachycardia was characterized by rates of 150 to 220 beats per minute, left bundle branch block QRS morphology, and AV dissociation with capture and fusion beats. Some rhythm strips demonstrated intermittent nonsustained bursts of ventricular tachycardia.

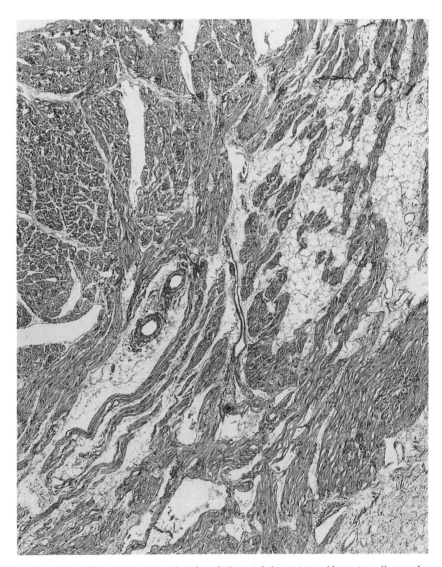

Figure 8-88: Fatty metamorphosis of the atrial septum. Hematoxylin-eosin stain × 45.

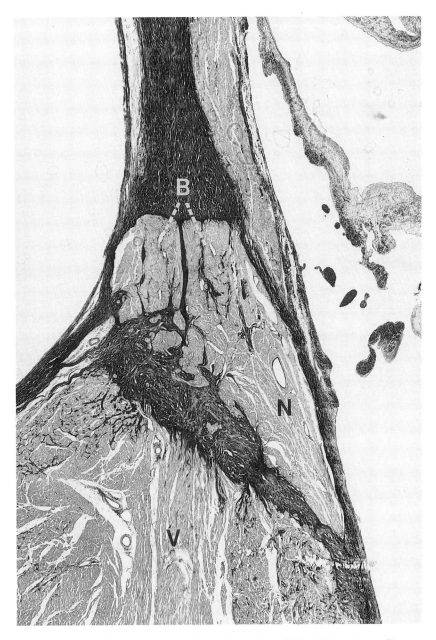

Figure 8-89: Atrioventricular node and bundle of His. Weigert-van Gieson stain × 30. There is no sharp line of differentiation between the node, partly engulfed in the central fibrous body, and the markedly septated bundle of His. N = AV node; B = bundle of His; V = ventricular septum. (Reprinted with permission from Bharati S, Bauernfiend R, Scheinman M, Massie B, Cheitlin M, Denes P, Wu D, Lev M, Rosen KM: Congenital abnormalities of the conduction system in two patients with tachyarrhythmias. *Circulation* 1979; 59:593–606.)

EPS

There were normal PA and AH intervals, with prolonged HV intervals, with normal AV nodal function determined by rapid atrial pacing and extrastimulus testing. Only short bursts of ventricular tachycardia were recorded. The tachycardia could not be initiated with right ventricular incremental pacing or extrastimulus testing.

Pathology: Gross

The heart was enlarged, weighing 357 grams. All chambers were hypertrophied and enlarged. A rete Chiari was present in the right atrium.

Microscopic Examination: Positive Findings

Atrial Preferential Pathways

Fatty metamorphosis was present (Fig. 8-88).

AV Node

This was partly engulfed in the central fibrous body.

Penetrating Bundle

It was septated (Fig. 8-89).

Branching Bundle

This showed moderate fibrosis.

Bundle Branches

Fibrosis was noted.

Summit of the Ventricular Septum

There was an increase in loose connective tissue.

Myocardium

There was fatty infiltration of the right ventricle.

Discussion

This 13-year-old boy had recurrent ventricular tachycardia and died suddenly. The tachycardia may be related to the fatty metamorphosis of the atrial preferential pathways, the markedly septated bundle, and the fibrosis of the bundle branches.

CASE #39[203]

A 59-year-old woman with recurrent atrial fibrillation, refractory to treatment with digoxin, beta blockers, verapamil, quinidine, procainamide, and amiodarone, had atrioventricular junctional ablation by means of 500 joules (2 shocks) which produced complete AV block. Despite the insertion of a permanent pacemaker, she died suddenly in ventricular fibrillation 6 weeks later.

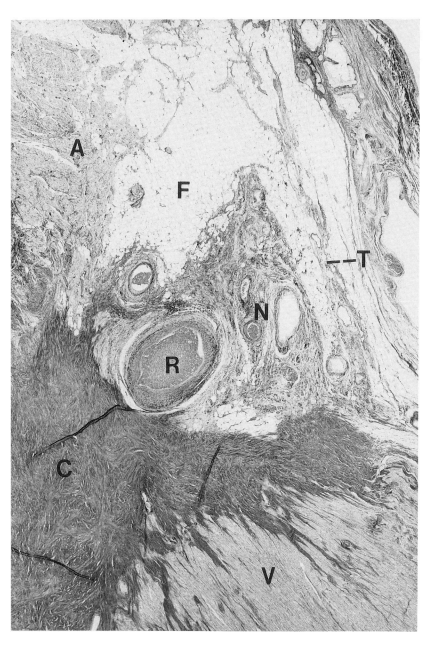

Figure 8-90: AV node showing marked fibroelastosis, with replacement of the approaches by fat. Weigert-van Gieson stain ×24. C = central fibrous body; R = ramus septi fibrosi; N = AV node; F = fat tissue; A = atrial muscle; V = ventricular septum; T = trace of muscle in approaches.

ECG

Atrial fibrillation with rapid ventricular rate (170–220 beats per minute) were present. A 24-hour Holter recording and exercise tolerance test performed 4 weeks after the ablative procedure showed complete AV block with a ventricular paced rate of 72 per minute, with occasional ventricular premature complexes. Two weeks later, the electrocardiogram revealed complete AV block with 100% capture and no ventricular ectopic complexes.

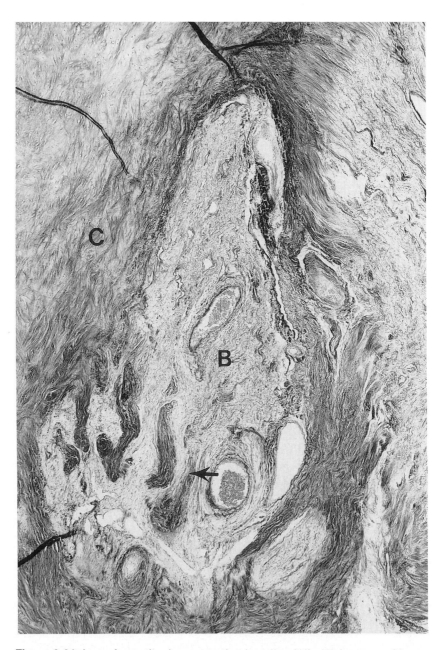

Figure 8-91: Loop formation in penetrating bundle of His. Weigert-van Gieson stain ×45. B = bundle of His; C = central fibrous body; The arrow points to the loop formation.

Fifteen minutes after the check-up, she collapsed in a rest room.

Pathology: Gross

The heart was somewhat enlarged and weighed 434 grams in the fixed state. Both atria were hypertrophied and enlarged, especially the left, and the left ventricle was hypertrophied. The endocardium was thickened and whitened throughout the left atrium and over the junction of the eustachian valve with the septum. The pacemaker was well endothelialized.

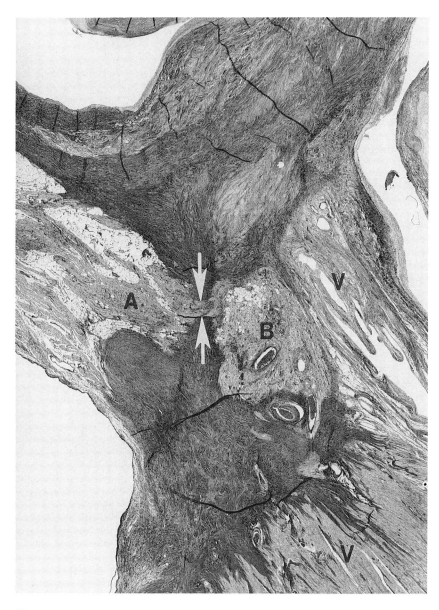

Figure 8-92: Atrio-Hisian connection. Weigert-van Gieson stain ×17. A = atrial septum; B = bundle of His; V = ventricular septum. The arrows point to the atrio-Hisian connection.

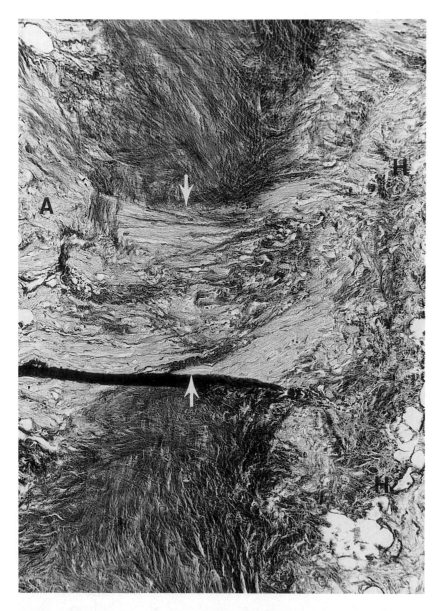

Figure 8-93: Higher power view of Figure 8-92. Weigert-van Gieson stain ×150. A = atrial septum; H = bundle of His. The arrows point to atrio-Hisian connection.

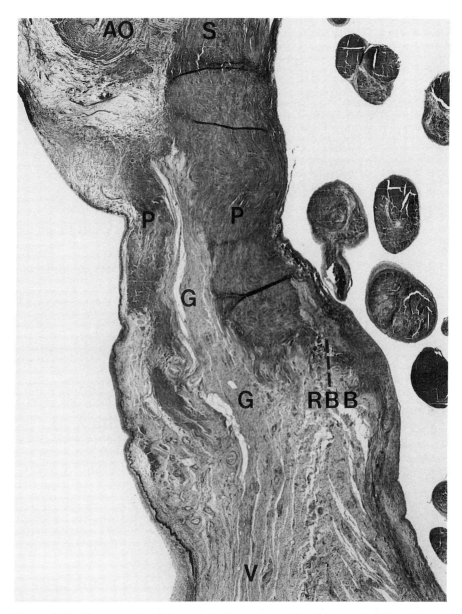

Figure 8-94: The summit of the ventricular septum showing marked fibrosis and thickening of the pars membranacea. Weigert-van Gieson stain ×15. V = ventricular septum; P = thickened pars membranacea; S = scar beneath aorta meeting pars membranacea; AO = base of aorta at sinus of Valsalva; G = granulation tissue; RBB = right bundle branch. (Reprinted with permission from Bharati S, Scheinman MM, Morady F, Hess DS, Lev M: Sudden death after catheter-induced atrioventricular junctional ablation. *Chest* 1985; 89:883–889.)

Microscopic Examination: Positive Findings

SA Node and Its Approaches, the Atrial Preferential Pathways, and Approaches to the AV Node

Fatty infiltration was present in all these regions with neuritis. A thick fibrous scar extended from the endocardium of the right atrium to the base of the aorta. The elastic tissue of the aorta in this region was almost replaced by connective tissue. Only a tenuous connection remained between the atrial musculature and the AV node (Fig. 8-90).

AV Node

This showed marked fibroelastosis (Fig. 8-90) with a moderate infiltration of mononuclear cells.

AV Bundle, Penetrating

This showed marked fibrosis and elastosis, fatty metamorphosis with a moderate infiltration of mononuclear cells, and loop formation (Fig. 8-91). An atrio-Hisian tract was noted (Figs. 8-92, 8-93).

AV Bundle, Branching

Marked fibroelastosis was seen.

Right Bundle Branch

The first portion showed marked fibroelastosis (Fig. 8-94) and was infiltrated with mononuclear cells and neutrophils.

Left Bundle Branch

The beginning of the left bundle branch revealed focal destruction of fibers, hemorrhage, and marked elastosis.

Summit of the Ventricular Septum

There was marked fibrosis (Fig. 8-94) with chronic inflammation.

Discussion

The cause of sudden death in this patient may be related to several of the following factors. The atrio-Hisian tract, although scarred, may have permitted re-entry. The marked fatty metamorphosis of the atrial septum may be associated with arrhythmia leading to sudden death. Loop formation in the bundle may also be incriminated. Furthermore, the chronic inflammatory changes of the ventricular septum with fibrosis following the ablative procedure might form a milieu for arrhythmogenicity and sudden death.

CASE #40[201]

A 26-year-old male, with a history of paroxysmal tachycardia and Wolff-Parkinson-White syndrome, diagnosed 7 years previously, died suddenly at home. Two years before death, he was readmitted for paroxysmal tachycardia. An electrocardiogram at that time revealed typical pre-excitation with a PR interval of 0.10 sec, a QRS duration of 0.16 sec, and initial slurring of the QRS pattern (delta wave). The 20-ms vector was positive in leads I, II, AVL, and AVF, suggesting a right free wall or anteroseptal anomalous pathway. Cardiac catheterization 2 years before death revealed congestive cardiomyopathy with mild mitral regurgitation and moderate pulmonary hypertension.

EPS

A bidirectional conducting anomalous pathway with short refractoriness was seen, with an easily inducible re-entrant paroxysmal supraventricular tachycardia.

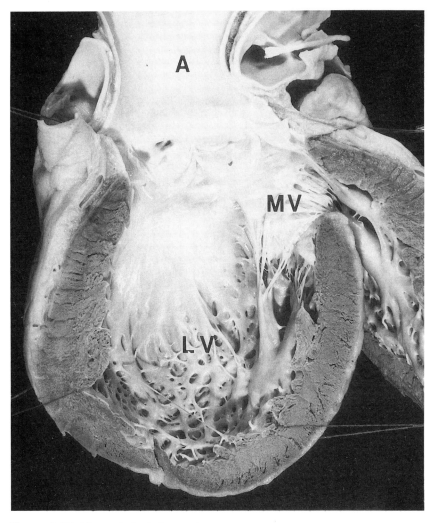

Figure 8-95: View of the left ventricle showing the outflow tract with endocardial fibroelastosis. A = aorta; LV = left ventricle; MV = mitral valve.

Pathology: Gross

The heart was enlarged, weighing 640 grams. There was hypertrophy and enlargement of the left atrium and left ventricle and hypertrophy of the right atrium and right ventricle. The right posterior aortic sinus of Valsalva gave off both coronary arteries. There was diffuse fibroelastosis of the left ventricle (Fig. 8-95).

Microscopic Examination: Positive Findings

SA Node and Its Approaches and the Approaches to the AV Node

Moderate fatty infiltration was present.

AV Node

Copious Mahaim fibers were present.

AV Bundle, Penetrating

This was septated with loop formation and copious Mahaim fibers.

AV Bundle, Branching

This was septated with fatty infiltration and fibrosis at the bifurcation.

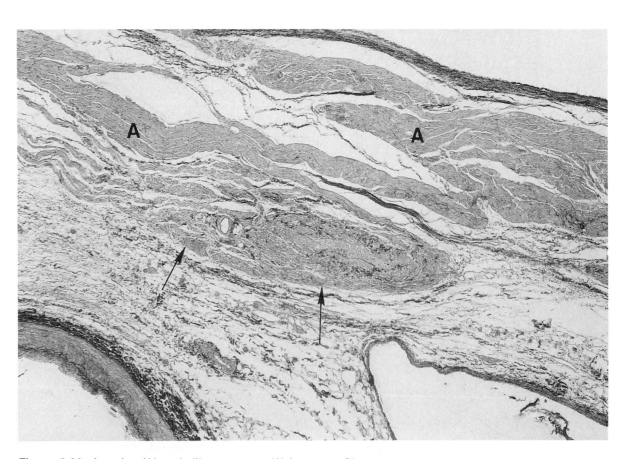

Figure 8-96: Anterior AV node-like structure. Weigert-van Gieson stain × 40. A = atrial musculature. The arrows point to the AV node-like structure.

Right Bundle Branch

There was moderate fibrosis in the first part.

Ventricular Septum

There was marked endothelial fibroelastosis.

Right AV Rim

There was a sizable accessory AV node situated in the anterior part of the right side of the atrial septum close to the roof of the right atrium (Fig. 8-96). This node connected with the atrial musculature, which joined the infundibular musculature of the right ventricle where the infundibular septum met the free wall of the right ventricle (Fig. 8-97).

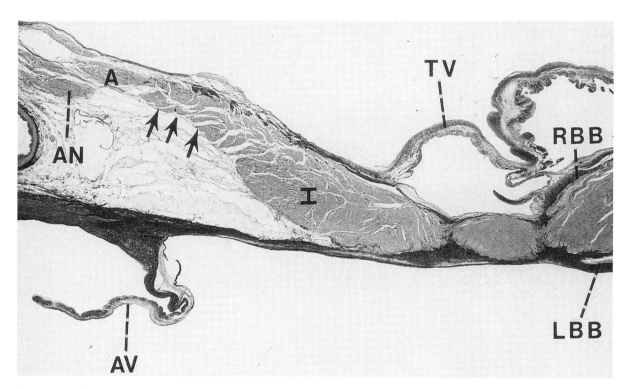

Figure 8-97: Bypass tract in anterior portion of the atrial septum and in the bulbar septum. Weigert-van Gieson stain ×30. A = atrial musculature; AN = anterior node-like structure; AV = aortic valve; TV = tricuspid valve; I = infundibular musculature; LBB = left bundle branch; RBB = right bundle branch. The arrows point to the area of interdigitation of atrial and infundibular fibers. (Reprinted with permission from Bharati S, Strasberg B, Bilitch M, Salibi H, Mandel W, Rosen KM, Lev M: Anatomic substrate for preexcitation in idiopathic myocardial hyperthrophy with fibroelastosis of the left ventricle. *Am J Cardiol* 1981; 48:47–58.)

Discussion

This 26-year-old man with Wolff-Parkinson-White syndrome and paroxysmal tachycardia died suddenly. The Wolff-Parkinson-White syndrome was related to a right AV connection. The paroxysmal tachycardia was due to re-entry in the anomalous pathway. The sudden death may be related to the following pathology in the conduction system: (1) fatty metamorphosis in the SA node and its approaches, and the approaches to the AV node, (2) a septated AV bundle with loop formation, (3) fibrosis of the right bundle branch, and (4) the anomalous pathway.

CASE #41[172]

A 46-year-old female was admitted several times in a 2-year period for syncopal episodes and mild convulsions due to intermittent complete AV block and Stokes-Adams syndrome. She died suddenly. Her past history revealed that she had had typhoid fever as a child.

ECG

This showed sinus rhythm, second-degree AV block with 3:1 conduction, and posterior hemiblock of the left bundle branch type, which progressed to intermittent complete AV block. She also showed on various occasions complete right bundle branch block pattern.

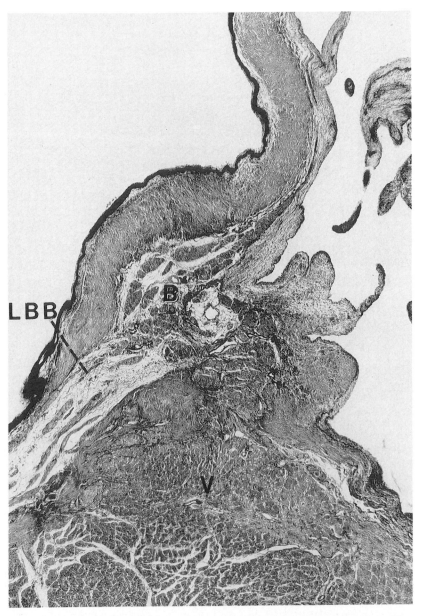

Figure 8-98: Destruction of part of the left bundle branch. Weigert-van Gieson stain ×40. B = bundle, branching portion; LBB = left bundle branch showing focal destruction; V = ventricular septum.

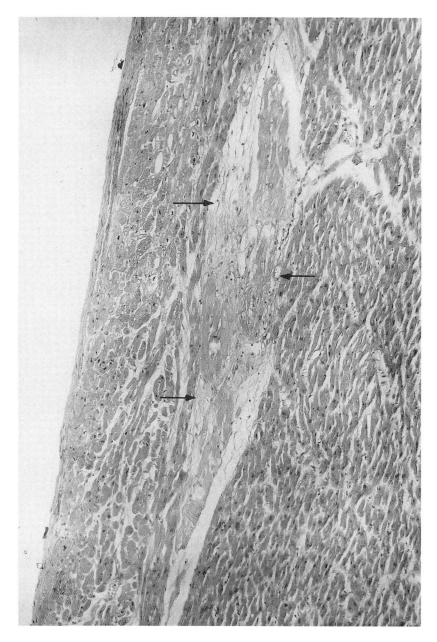

Figure 8-99: Distal part of the second part of right bundle branch showing necrosis of cells and an infiltration of mononuclear cells. Hematoxylin-eosin stain ×105. The arrows point to the right bundle branch.

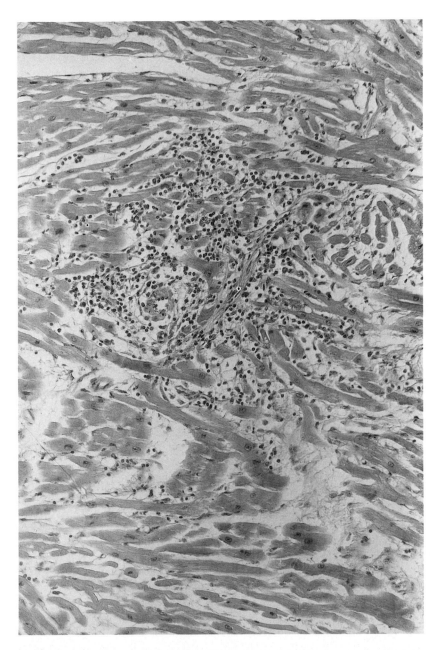

Figure 8-100: Myocardium showing myocarditis. Hematoxylin-eosin stain ×190. (Reprinted with permission from Harris R, Siew S, Lev M: Smoldering myocarditis with intermittent complete A-V block and Stokes-Adams syndrome: A histopathologic and electrocardiographic study of "trifascicular" bundle branch block. *Am J Cardiol* 1969; 24:880–889.)

Pathology: Gross

The heart weighed 270 grams. The chambers were normal in size and thickness. There were severe irregular areas of wrinkling of the endocardium of the left ventricle adjacent to the pars membranacea. The left coronary lay high above the sinus of Valsalva. The coronary arteries were patent.

Microscopic Examination: Positive Findings

Approaches to the SA Node

This showed a myocarditis.

Both Bundle Branches

Marked degeneration of both bundle branches (Fig. 8-98), especially the right (Fig. 8-99), with myocarditis was present.

Summit of the Ventricular Septum

Fibrosis was present.

Myocardium

Myocarditis was present throughout (Fig. 8-100).

Discussion

This 46-year-old woman developed a smoldering myocarditis with intermittent complete heart block. The cause of the heart block was complete destruction of both bundle branches. Sudden death in heart block is a common occurrence, with or without myocarditis. Likewise sudden death can occur in myocarditis, in the acute, chronic, or smoldering forms.

CASE #42[190]

A 24-year-old white male was found unconscious by his roommate. He gasped for breath, had a seizure, and rolled over onto his stomach. There was a history of recreational drug usage. He had used cocaine on the day before and marijuana on the day that he died.

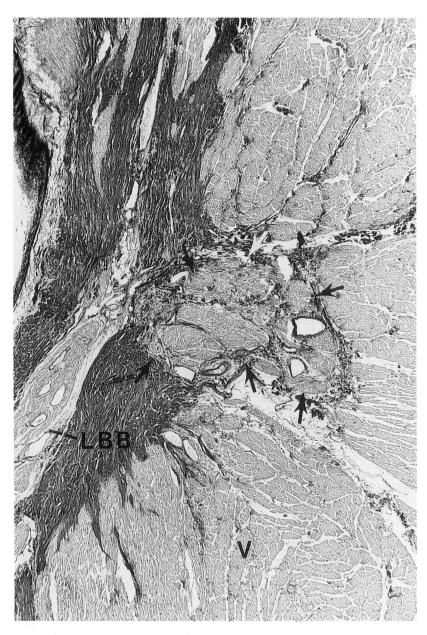

Figure 8-101: The right bundle branch showing fibrosis. Weigert-van Gieson stain ×45. LBB = left bundle branch; V = ventricular septum. The arrows point to the right bundle branch.

Pathology: Gross

The toxicologic examination did not show a toxic level of either marijuana or cocaine. The heart was not enlarged. The anterior leaflet of the tricuspid valve was divided into two segments. There were three coronary ostia for the right coronary artery. The arteries were patent throughout. The myocardium of the left ventricle showed areas of fat spreading from the epicardium.

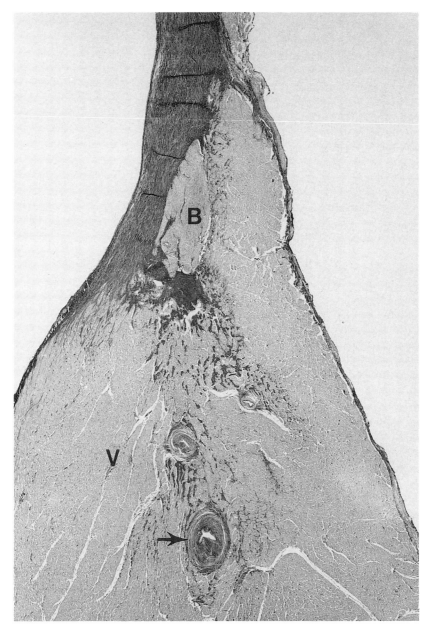

Figure 8-102: The summit of the ventricular septum showing fibrosis and arteriolosclerosis. Weigert-van Gieson stain ×17. B = bundle; V = ventricular septum. The arrow points to the sclerotic vessel.

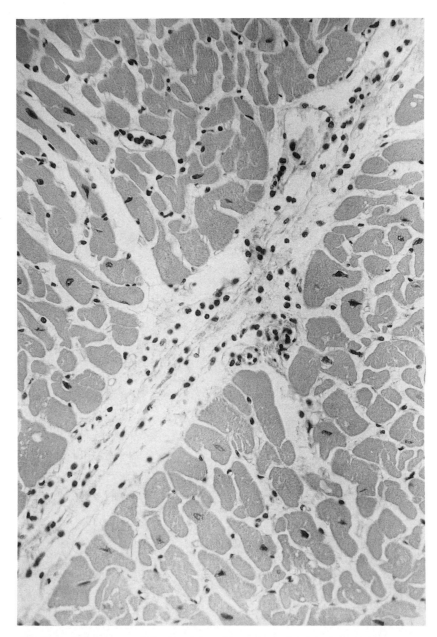

Figure 8-103: Myocarditis. Hematoxylin-eosin stain ×150. (Reprinted with permission from Bharati S, Lev M: Congenital abnormalities of the conduction system in sudden death in young adults. *J Am Coll Cardiol* 1986; 8:1096–1104.)

Microscopic Examination: Positive Findings

Approaches to the SA Node and the AV Node

There was fatty infiltration and neuritis.

AV Node

Thickening of the AV nodal artery was seen.

AV Bundle, Penetrating

This showed moderate lobulation and loop formation and moderate fatty metamorphosis.

AV Bundle, Branching

This was left-sided.

Right Bundle Branch

This showed marked fibrosis at the beginning (Fig. 8-101).

Left Bundle Branch

This revealed marked fibrosis.

Summit of the Ventricular Septum

This showed an increase in connective tissue and arteriolosclerosis mostly on the right side with myocarditis (Fig. 8-102).

Myocardium

This showed subacute and chronic myocarditis in left ventricle but not in the right (Fig. 8-103).

Discussion

This 24-year-old man who died suddenly was found to have a myocarditis of the left ventricle but not the right. Patients with myocarditis may die suddenly. Is this due, however, to the involvement of the conduction system? In this heart, we found: (1) fatty infiltration in the approaches to the SA and AV nodes, accompanied by neuritis; (2) thickening of the ramus septi fibrosi; (3) moderate lobulation and loop formation and fatty metamorphosis of AV bundle; (4) a left-sided branching bundle; (5) marked fibrosis of the right bundle branch; and (6) fibrosis and arteriolosclerosis of the summit of the ventricular septum. Thus, a possible thesis is that in myocarditis, the involvement of the conduction system, either localized or diffuse, may cause sudden death, or the sudden death in this case may not be due to the myocarditis but related to the many abnormalities in the conduction system. Or is there a tendency for the development of myocarditis where there are changes in the conduction system?

CASE #43

A 28-year-old white male was watching television and suddenly fell over, rolled off the sofa, stopped breathing, and died suddenly.

He was in good health until the morning of his death when he suffered a transient episode of difficulty in breathing and light-headedness from which he recovered almost immediately. He was fine for the rest of the day.

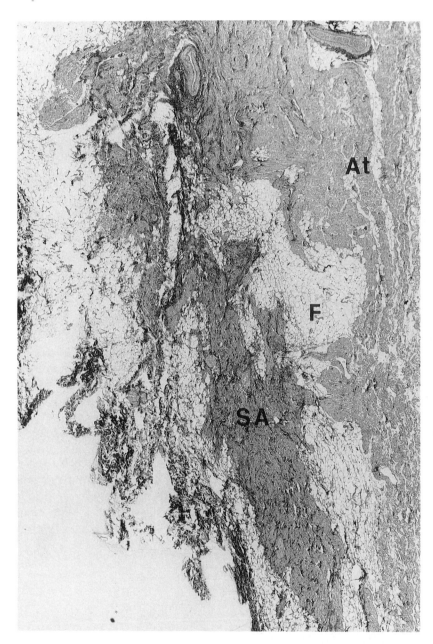

Figure 8-104: The SA node, almost completely isolated from atrial muscle by fat. Weigert-van Gieson stain ×21. SA = SA node; At = atrial muscle; F = fat tissue.

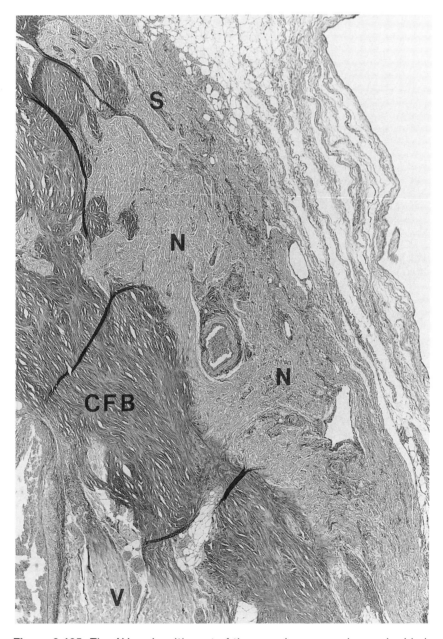

Figure 8-105: The AV node with part of the superior approaches embedded in the central fibrous body. Weigert-van Gieson stain ×45. S = superior approaches; N = AV node; CFB = central fibrous body; V = ventricular septum.

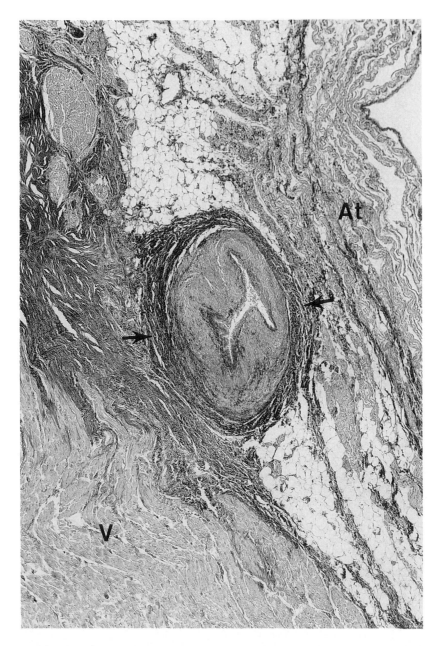

Figure 8-106: Thickening of the ramus septi fibrosi. Weigert-van Gieson stain ×45. At = atrial muscle; V = ventricular septum. The arrows point to the ramus septi fibrosi.

Pathology: Gross

The heart weighed 415 grams. Hypertrophy was evident and there was enlargement of all chambers. There was an aneurysm in the space of His and an abnormal formation of the atrial septum.

Microscopic Examination: Positive Findings

SA Node

The node was partially isolated from the atrium by fat (Fig. 8-104).

Approaches to the SA Node, Atrial Preferential Pathways, and Approaches to the AV Node

There was marked fatty metamorphosis. The superior approaches to the AV node were entrapped within the central fibrous body, still retaining the characteristics of atrial cells (Fig. 8-105).

AV Node

This was partly embedded in the central fibrous body. The AV nodal artery was thickened (Fig. 8-106).

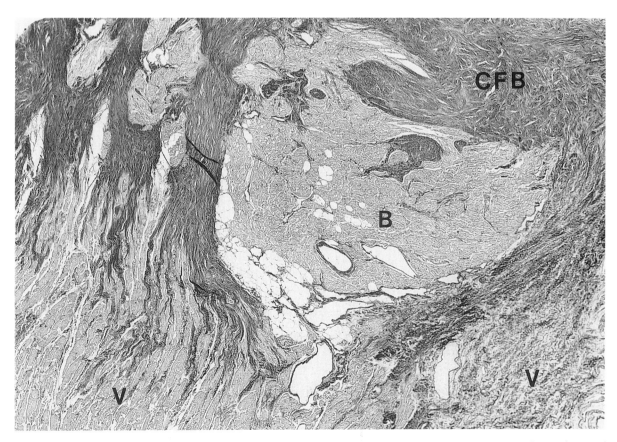

Figure 8-107: Bundle of His. Weigert-van Gieson stain ×45. B = bundle of His showing loop formation and fatty metamorphosis; V = ventricular septum; CFB = central fibrous body.

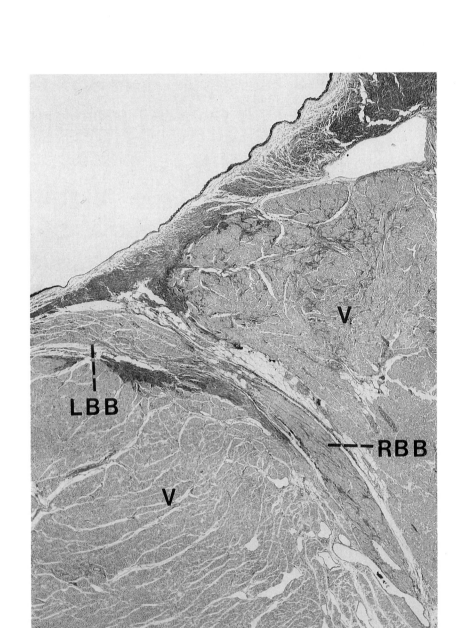

Figure 8-108: Bifurcation with right bundle branch showing fibrosis. Weigert-van Gieson stain ×30. RBB = right bundle branch; LBB = left bundle branch; V = ventricular septum.

AV Bundle, Penetrating

This showed loop formation and fatty infiltration (Fig. 8-107).

AV Bundle, Branching

This was left-sided with moderate fibrosis.

AV Bundle, Bifurcating

This showed fibrosis of both the right and the left side (Fig. 8-108).

Right Bundle Branch

This showed moderate fibrosis in the beginning (Fig. 8-108).

Left Bundle Branch

There were foci of linear degeneration in the beginning.

Summit of the Ventricular Septum

There was marked fatty metamorphosis mostly on the right side with arteriolosclerosis.

Ventricular Myocardium

Moderate fatty metamorphosis was present in the left ventricle and marked fatty metamorphosis in the right ventricle.

Discussion

This 28-year-old allegedly healthy man who died suddenly had a generally hypertrophied heart and numerous abnormalities in the conduction system. The SA node was partially isolated from the atria by fat, and there was fatty metamorphosis of the approaches to the SA node, the atrial preferential pathways, and the approaches to the AV node. The superior approaches to the AV node were in part entrapped in the central fibrous body, as was part of the node itself. The ramus septi fibrosi was thickened and narrowed. The penetrating bundle showed loop formation and fatty metamorphosis. The branching bundle was left-sided. The right bundle branch showed moderate fibrosis in the beginning, and foci of linear degeneration were seen in the beginning of the left bundle branch. The summit of the ventricular septum showed marked fatty metamorphosis, mostly on the right side, with arteriolosclerosis. The left ventricle showed fatty metamorphosis and there was marked fatty metamorphosis in the right ventricle.

Thus, the fatty metamorphosis so widely distributed stands out as a possible cause of rhythm disturbances and sudden death. However, the numerous abnormalities present in the conduction system may have played some role in the death of this individual.

CASE #44[173]

A 16-year-old female had frequent episodes of alternating bidirectional ventricular tachycardia and died during attempted suppressive therapy. At age 6, an irregular heart beat was noted. She had no clinical evidence of heart disease until 2 weeks before her death. Two weeks before admission, she experienced pleuritic substernal pain associated with dyspnea and numbness of the left arm after an episode of strenuous exertion. She was transferred to the California School of Medicine.

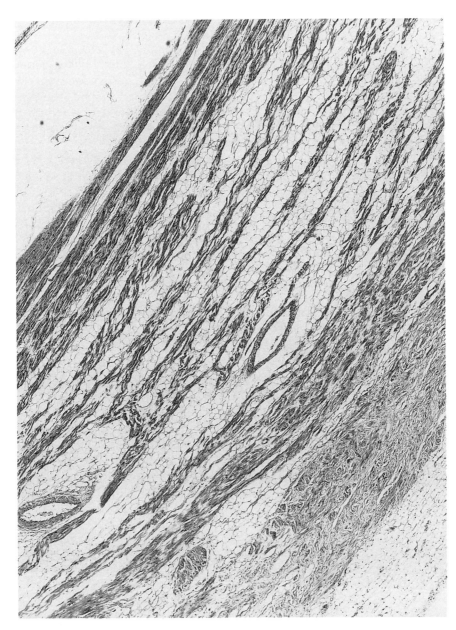

Figure 8-109: Approaches to SA node showing fatty metamorphosis. Hematoxylin-eosin stain ×39.

ECG

At this time, she showed paroxysmal bidirectional tachycardia with alternating left anterior and posterior hemiblock in the presence of right bundle branch block with a number of fusion beats. During the arrhythmia, AV dissociation was present, usually with a slow sinus rhythm. The PR interval and QT intervals were normal. An attempt was made to establish a satisfactory suppressive drug routine in combination with atrial pacing, with overdrive suppression.

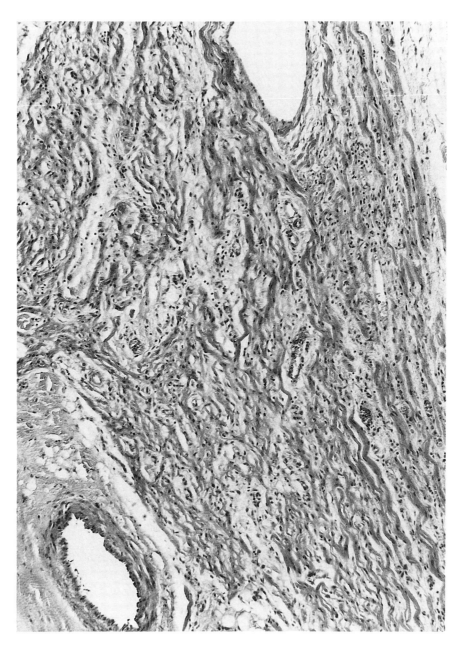

Figure 8-110: AV node showing proliferation of mononuclear cells and interstitial cells. Hematoxylin-eosin stain ×104.

Course

The patient had numerous bouts of ventricular tachycardia with a QRS configuration different from that of the previous tachycardia.

The tachycardia degenerated into ventricular fibrillation, and defibrillation was performed approximately 50 times. The patient became comatose and died 2 weeks after the onset of her illness.

Her family history documented a similar

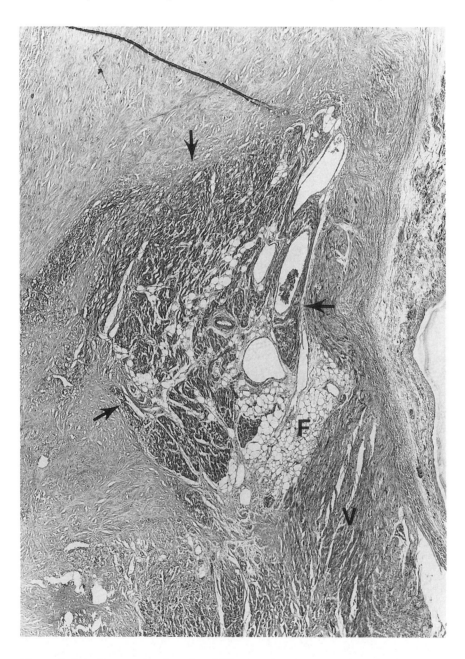

Figure 8-111: Penetrating bundle of His showing fatty metamorphosis. Hematoxylin-eosin stain ×39. V = ventricular septum; F = fatty tissue. The arrows delineate the bundle.

arrhythmia in an 18-year-old sister who died suddenly 9 months after discovery of arrhythmia. Conduction system studies were not done on this case. A brother 21 years old and a mother aged 45 also revealed ventricular bi-geminal rhythm, and a maternal uncle and grandmother died suddenly, the latter with a knowledge of an irregular heart beat. There was no QT prolongation. Auditory defects were not present.

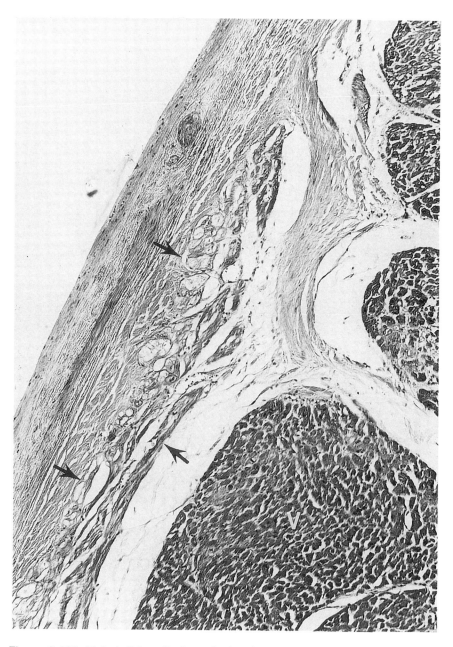

Figure 8-112: Main left bundle branch showing vacuolar degeneration. Hematoxylin-eosin stain ×104. The arrows point to the left bundle branch.

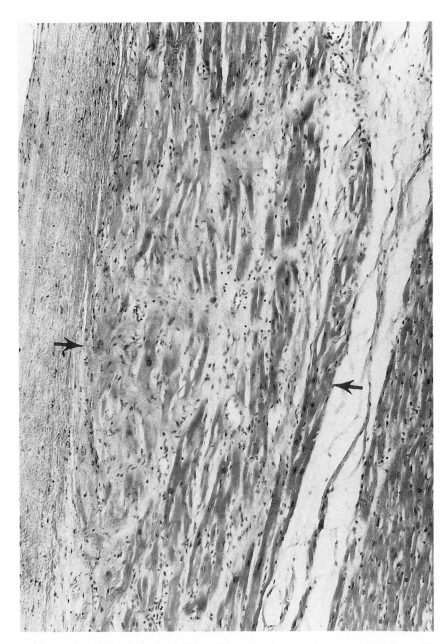

Figure 8-113: Fasciculi of posterior radiation showing irregular staining with infiltration of mononuclear cells. Hematoxylin-eosin stain ×104. The arrows point to the left bundle branch. (Reprinted with permission from Gault JH, Cantwell J, Lev M, Braunwald E: Fatal familial cardiac arrhythmias. *Am J Cardiol* 1972; 29:548–553.)

Pathology: Gross

The heart was enlarged and weighed 370 grams. The right atrium and right ventricle were hypertrophied and enlarged. The left atrium and ventricle were hypertrophied. The left ventricular endocardium was thickened. The coronary arteries were not restricted.

Microscopic Examination: Positive Findings

Approaches to the SA and the AV Nodes

There was fatty infiltration in these areas (Fig. 8-109) with a neuritis. The ramus septi fibrosi was thickened.

AV Node

This showed a myocarditis (Fig. 8-110) with proliferation of sheath cells.

AV Bundle, Penetrating

Fatty metamorphosis was present (Fig. 8-111) with an infiltration of mononuclear cells.

AV Bundle, Branching

There was an infiltration of mononuclear cells.

Left Bundle Branch

The main left bundle branch (Fig. 8-112), its radiations, and the peripheral Purkinje cells showed distinct vacuolar degeneration (Fig. 8-112) with an infiltration of mononuclear cells (Fig. 8-113).

Summit of the Ventricular Septum

This showed an infiltration of mononuclear cells with fibrosis and arteriolosclerosis.

Myocardium

Fatty infiltration was present in both ventricles with fibroelastic proliferation.

Discussion

This 16-year-old girl had frequent episodes of bidirectional ventricular tachycardia and died 2 weeks after an attack during suppressive therapy. This is not a case of sudden death, but a case of bidirectional ventricular tachycardia leading to death. Thus, the findings and death are related to the arrhythmia and possibly to the suppressive therapy. These findings are: (1) fatty metamorphosis in the approaches to the SA and AV nodes and in the bundle of His and both ventricles; (2) a myocarditis in the AV node, the bundle of His, and left bundle branch, with an associated neuritis; and (3) slight thickening and narrowing of the ramus septi fibrosi. Since the patient had a long history of the tachycardia, it is difficult to ascribe this to the myocarditis. One would, therefore, prefer to think that the fatty changes in the approaches to the SA and AV nodes and in the bundle of His are related to the arrhythmia. We do not know what is the cause and what is the effect.

It is interesting that she belongs to a family in which arrhythmias were present and sudden death had occurred. One, therefore, speculates that the fatty changes in the conduction system here is a family trait, or that there is a genetic tendency in the formation of the conduction system which makes it vulnerable for myocarditis to involve only the conduction system and not involve the surrounding myocardium. One also speculates that the myocarditis is secondary to the arrhythmia, and that the arrhythmia has a tendency to produce myocarditis.

CASE #45[181]

A 25-year-old white female had idiopathic hypertrophic subaortic stenosis proved by catheterization. She had dizzy and near-syncopal episodes for which a permanent pacemaker was inserted. One week later she died suddenly.

An ECG showed left bundle branch block pattern. An EPS revealed normal PA and AH intervals, but a prolonged H-V interval. A clear reproducible split His potential was demonstrated with atrial extrastimulus technique.

Pathology: Gross

The heart was enlarged, weighing 408 grams (Fig. 8-114). The left atrium and ventricle were hypertrophied and enlarged. The septal surface of the left ventricle was sigmoid (Fig. 8-114) with a bulge in its midportion. It was coarsely trabeculated. At the top of the septum, there was a 1.2-cm indentation surrounded by a thickened endocardium. The parietal wall was also covered by thickened trabeculae with numerous areas of thickened endocardium. The lumen of the left ventricle was

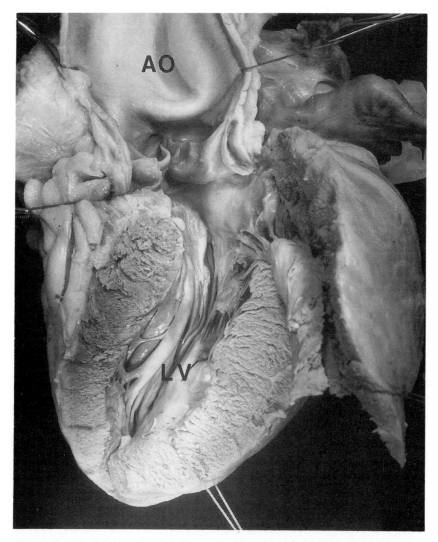

Figure 8-114: Outflow tract of the left ventricle. LV = left ventricle; AO = aorta.

relatively restricted. The coronary arteries were not restricted. The thickening of the anterior and posterior walls of the left ventricle and of the septum were increased without trabeculation. The septum measured 1.8 cm and the anterior and posterior walls measured 1.4 cm.

Microscopic Examination: Positive Findings

Approaches to the SA Node

Some large arterioles were thickened and narrowed.

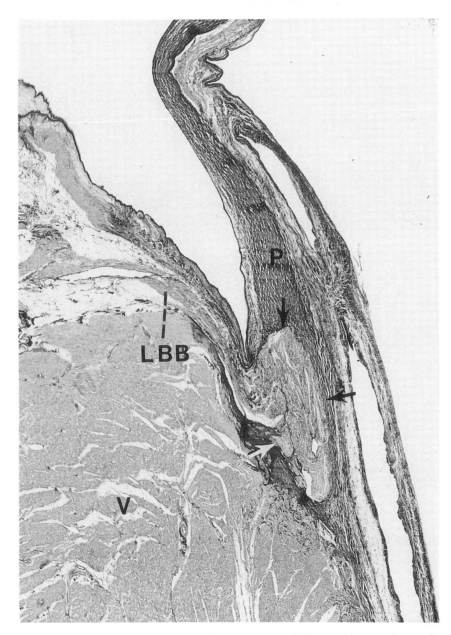

Figure 8-115: Branching portion of the bundle of His showing moderate fibrosis of the bundle with marked fibrosis of the beginning of the left bundle branch. Weigert-van Gieson stain ×22. V = ventricular septum; P = pars membranacea; LBB = left bundle branch.

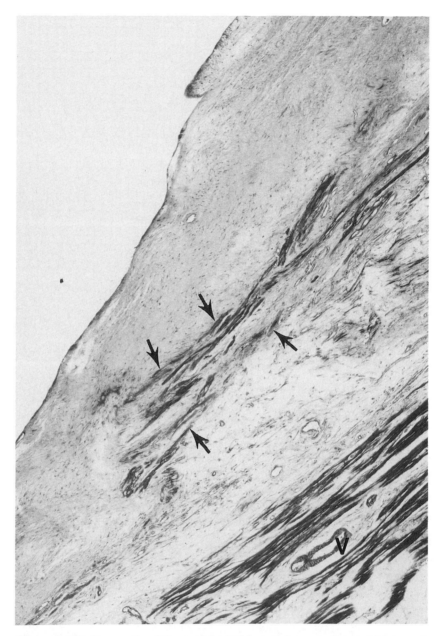

Figure 8-116: Remnants of fibers of the left bundle branch. Gomori trichromic stain ×45. V = ventricular septum. The arrows point to fibers of the left bundle branch.

Approaches to the AV Node

There was moderate thickening and narrowing of the ramus septi fibrosi.

AV Node

This was flattened in a vertical direction.

AV Bundle, Penetrating and Branching

This showed moderate fibrosis (Fig. 8-115).

Left Bundle Branch

This went over a bulge in the summit of the ventricular septum to get to the left side (Fig. 8-115). It showed marked fibrosis with an infiltration of neutrophils and mononuclear cells (Figs. 8-115, 8-116). More peripherally, only remnants of the bundle were in evidence (Fig. 8-116).

Right Bundle Branch

In the first part, there was moderate fibrosis.

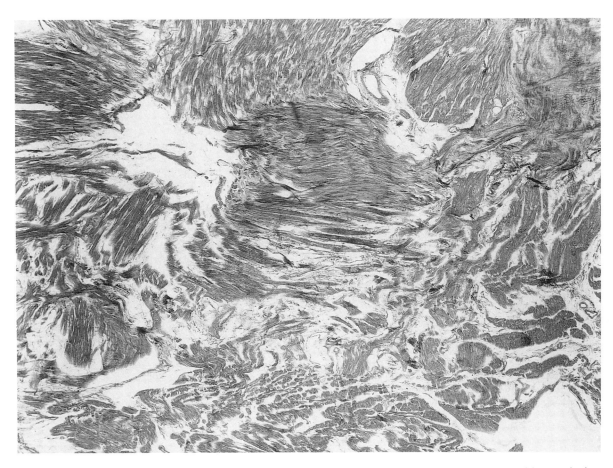

Figure 8-117: Ventricular septum showing disarray. Hematoxylin-eosin stain × 45. (Reprinted with permission from Bharati S, McAnulty JH, Lev M, Rahmitoola SH: *Circulation* 1980; 62:1373–1380.)

Summit of the Ventricular Septum

The architecture was altered by thick trabeculation on the left side. There was a proliferation of recent and older connective tissue. Large and small arterioles were thickened and narrowed. Areas of disarray were in evidence (Fig. 8-117).

Myocardium

Arteriolosclerosis was in evidence in the left ventricle.

Discussion

This 25-year-old woman had idiopathic hypertrophic subaortic stenosis and she died suddenly. She had had left bundle branch block and shortly before death had split His potentials. The left bundle branch block was explained by the marked fibrosis of the left bundle branch. The split His bundle potentials may have been due to the fibrosis of the bundle of His.

It is well known that people with split His potentials die suddenly. The cause in this case may be due to: (1) the narrowing of the ramus septi fibrosi, (2) the fibrosis of the bundle of His, left bundle branch, and right bundle branch, and (3) the arteriolosclerosis or sudden left ventricular outflow tract obstruction.

CASE #46²⁰²

A 36-year-old female was diagnosed as having myotonia dystrophica at age 30. She had a history of nonsustained bursts of polymorphic ventricular tachycardia a year before she died suddenly in ventricular fibrillation. Her father and brother were also found to have myotonia dystrophica. She had brief episodes of paroxysmal palpitations at the age of 32.

ECG

At age 32, an ECG revealed right bundle branch block, left anterior fascicular block, first-degree AV block, and atrial and ventric-

ular premature beats. At age 35, ECG monitoring revealed intermittent Mobitz type II 2:1 and complete AV block as well as nonsustained bursts of polymorphic ventricular ejection fraction of 36% with inferolateral akinesia and septal hypokinesia.

An echocardiogram showed pansystolic mitral valve prolapse.

EPS

Studies revealed block distal to His with episodes of polymorphic ventricular tachycardia. Ten months later, she developed left-sided pleuritic chest pain. Six hours later, she developed ventricular fibrillation and died.

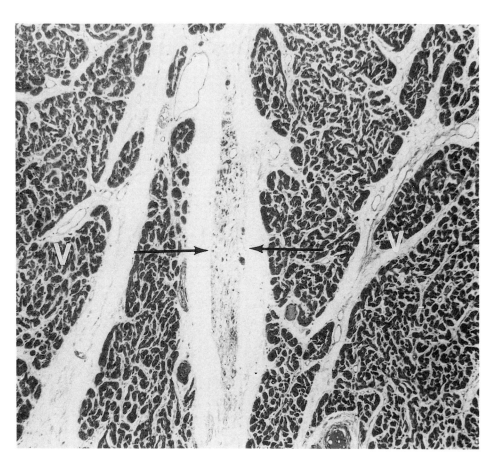

Figure 8-118: The second portion of the right bundle branch showing almost complete disruption. Gomori trichrome stain ×45. V = ventricular septum. The arrows point to the right bundle branch.

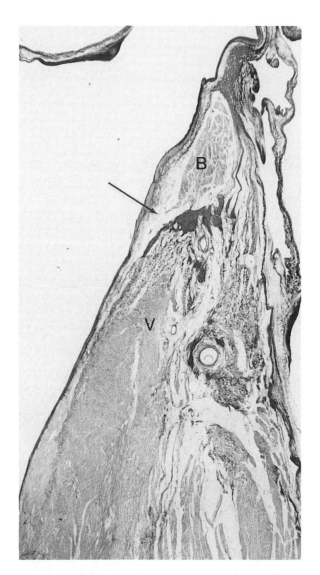

Figure 8-119: Beginning of left bundle branch. Weigert-van Gieson stain ×45. B = bundle of His; V = ventricular septum. The arrow points to the disruption of the beginning of the left bundle branch. (Reprinted with permission from Bharati S, Bump T, Bauernfeind R, Lev M: Dystrophica myotonia: correlative, electrocardiographic, electrophysiologic, and conduction system study. *Chest* 1984; 86:444–450.)

Pathology: Gross

The heart was enlarged, weighing about 414 grams. The left ventricle was distinctly hypertrophied. There were recent thrombi in the oblique branches of the left coronary artery. A thrombus was present in the main pulmonary trunk. The inferior cusp of the mitral valve was somewhat enlarged and thickened.

Microscopic Examination: Positive Findings

Atrial Preferential Pathways and the Approaches to the AV Node

These showed marked fatty metamorphosis.

Penetrating Bundle

This showed some lobulation in the beginning.

Right and Left Bundle Branches

These showed marked fibrosis and disruption (Figs. 8-118, 8-119).

Summit of the Ventricular Septum

Marked fibrosis was present on both sides, but mostly on the right.

Remainder of the Myocardium

The difference in diameter of myocardial fibers was in evidence throughout, with atrophy of cells, vacuolization of cytoplasm, and loss of myofibrils in the center. This was associated with slight mononuclear cell infiltration. Zones of fibrosis were also noted through the atria and ventricles. Marked fatty infiltration was present in the right ventricle and in areas of the left ventricle. Some ganglion cells showed fibrosis.

Striated Muscle

The fat and fibrous content was increased and the number and size of muscle cells were decreased.

Discussion

This 36-year-old female with familial myotonia dystrophica gradually developed AV block. This was due to fibrosis of both bundle branches. However, she also had bursts of polymorphic ventricular tachycardia. This could be due to the degeneration of the myocardial cells, which is part of myotonia, or could possibly be secondarily related to the fatty metamorphosis of the approaches to the SA and AV nodes and the atrial septum. The familial nature of the disease also suggests a genetic abnormality in the formation of the myocardium including the conduction system, and the susceptability for arrhythmias and sudden death.

CASE #47[204]

This patient was a 36-year-old Caucasian male diagnosed as having Kearns-Sayre syndrome and bifascicular block. A permanent pacemaker was inserted because of marked prolongation of the HV interval, and the patient felt well for 1 year. Ten days before death, he was treated for pulmonary edema. On the tenth day of hospitalization, he developed ventricular tachycardia, which degenerated into ventricular fibrillation, and he died.

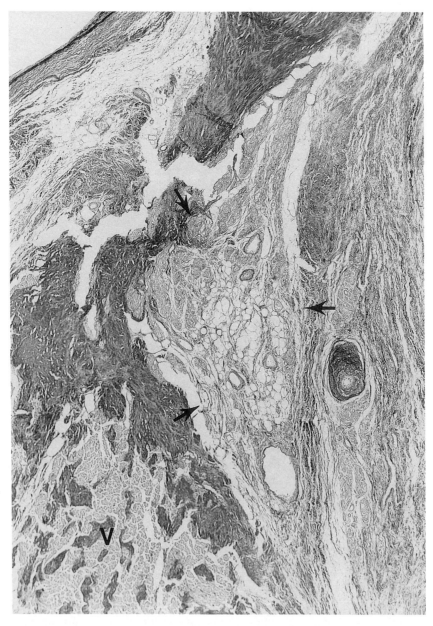

Figure 8-120: Bundle of His showing fatty metamorphosis. Weigert-van Gieson stain ×45. V = ventricular septum. The arrows point to the penetrating bundle.

ECG

Sinus rhythm, right bundle branch block with left anterior hemiblock, and possible inferior wall myocardial infarction of undetermined age were present. The treadmill test was normal. A chest x-ray showed cardiomegaly.

Cardiac catheterization showed normal coronaries with decreased ejection fraction of 42%. Hypokinesia of the inferior and anterior apical walls was present. Left ventricular volumes were increased and left ventricular end-diastolic pressure was elevated to 16 mm.

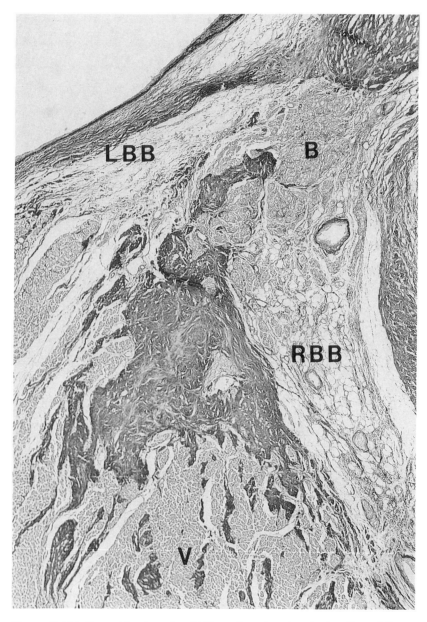

Figure 8-121: Branching bundle at bifurcation showing destruction of fibers of the left bundle branch and fatty metamorphosis of the right bundle branch. Weigert-van Gieson stain ×45. B = branching bundle; LBB = left bundle branch; RBB = right bundle branch; V = ventricular septum.

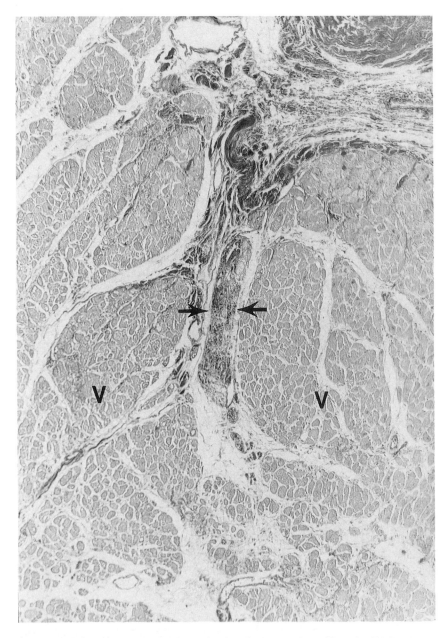

Figure 8-122: Right bundle branch showing complete fibrosis. Weigert-van Gieson stain ×90. V = ventricular septum. The arrows point to the right bundle branch. (Reprinted with permission from Gallastequi J, Hariman RJ, Handler B, Lev M, Bharati S: Cardiac involvement in the Kearns-Sayre syndrome. *Am J Cardiol* 1987; 89:385–388.)

EPS

Prolonged HV of 80 ms, dual AV nodal conduction curves, and inducible sustained supraventricular tachycardia was possible.

Pathology: Gross

Aside from the findings in the heart, there was pulmonary embolism bilaterally. The heart was enlarged, weighing 720 grams. All four chambers were hypertrophied and enlarged. There was considerable fatty infiltration of the anterior wall of the right ventricle. The mitral valve revealed thickening and nodularity from the line of closure to the edge. The coronary arteries were widely patent.

Microscopic Examination: Positive Findings

Atrial Preferential Pathways and Approaches to the AV Node

Marked fatty metamorphosis was present. The nerves showed fibrosis.

Bundle of His, Penetrating Portion

Fatty metamorphosis was present (Fig. 8-120).

Bundle of His, Branching Portion

The bifurcation showed destruction of fibers of the left bundle branch and fatty metamorphosis of the right bundle branch (Fig. 8-121).

Left Bundle Branch

The beginning of the posterior radiation was replaced by linear formations. Peripherally, there was marked fibrosis.

Right Bundle Branch

Fatty metamorphosis was present at the beginning. The third part was completely replaced by connective tissue (Fig. 8-122).

Summit of the Ventricular Septum

Marked fibrosis and fatty infiltration on the right side were seen. In addition, the nerves showed fibrosis.

Left Ventricle

There was marked fibrosis throughout.

Right Ventricle

Marked fatty infiltration was present.

Discussion

This 36-year-old man had Kearns-Sayre syndrome. The cause of the AV block was marked fibrosis of both bundle branches. The patient suddenly developed ventricular tachycardia, which degenerated into fibrillation, and he died suddenly. Of course, we know that patients with AV block may develop fibrillation and may die suddenly. However, in addition to this, the patient had fatty metamorphosis in the atrial preferential pathways, in the approaches to the AV node, and in the AV bundle. Are these changes associated with sudden death? Of course, the bilateral pulmonary embolism might have caused the sudden death and/or triggered an arrhythmic event.

CASE #48[183]

A 20-year-old female died suddenly after having had recurrent ventricular tachycardia for 5 years. She had had 17 hospitalizations for episodes of ventricular tachycardia during which time she had palpitations, dizziness, light-headedness, and chest pain. Some episodes ended spontaneously, but most required cardioversion with either intravenous lidocaine or direct current cardioversion. The ventricular tachycardias were refractory to antiarrhythmic drugs including propranolol, quinidine, procainamide, and phenytoin, and

to pacing. The patient was fully ambulatory and felt well between hospitalizations.

Cardiac catheterization showed normal right and left ventricle pressures, with a slight decrease in cardiac index. Right ventricular angiography suggested a thin-walled, enlarged, and abnormally contracting right ventricle. Selective coronary arteriogram showed a dominant left system without abnormalities.

Electrocardiogram during sinus rhythm showed a normal PR interval varying from 0.14 to 0.18 sec. The mean frontal plane QRS axis was −60 with a Q-wave in lead 1 and RS complexes in leads 2 and 3. Augmented lead aVF

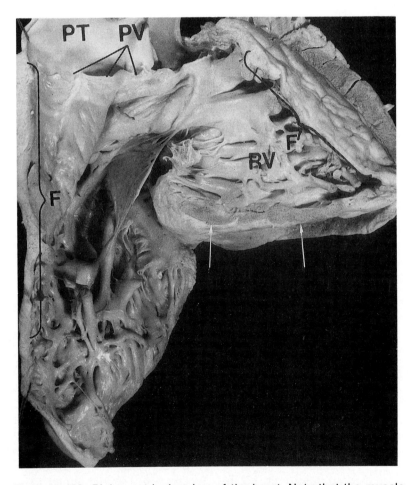

Figure 8-123: Right ventricular view of the heart. Note that the muscle in the inferior wall is intact. The remainder of the wall is replaced by fat. However, trabeculation is intact. RV = right ventricle; PT = pulmonary trunk; F = fat tissue; PV = quadricuspid pulmonary valve. The arrows point to the inferior wall.

suggested the presence of left anterior fascicular block. R-wave progression was poor and S-waves were noted in chest lead V_6. In addition, voltage criteria for left ventricular hypertrophy was noted in several ECGs. During ventricular tachycardia, the rate was 120 to 220 beats per minute. These tachycardias had distinct QRS morphology. One was characterized by left bundle branch block pattern with normal axis and the other by left bundle branch block pattern with left axis. Both ventricular tachycardias occurred as sustained and nonsustained arrhythmias. Atrioventricular dissociation, captures, and fusion beats were frequently noted during episodes of ventricular tachycardia.

Pathology: Gross

The heart was dilated and weighed 290 grams. The right ventricle was tremendously enlarged and the muscular portion of the wall was extremely thin. Most of the wall was replaced by fat (Figs. 8-123, 8-124, and 8-125), with the exception of the papillary muscles. The parietal band was abnormal in configuration and consisted of several short muscles. The endocardium of the right ventricle was focally whitened. The pulmonic valve was quadricuspid. (Fig. 8-123). The right coronary artery was hypoplastic, terminating on the anterior wall of the right ventricle, while the left coronary artery formed the posterior descending.

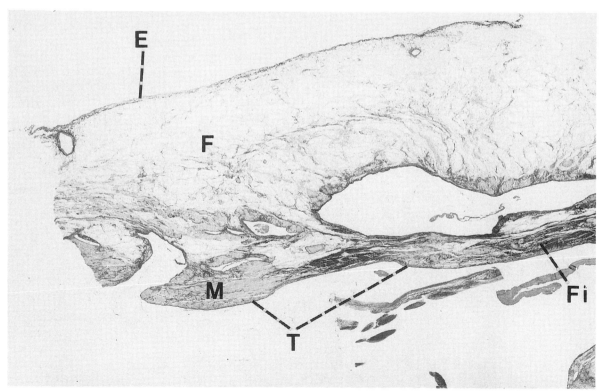

Figure 8-124: Right ventricular myocardium, anterior wall, sinus area. Weigert-van Gieson stain ×16. E = epicardium; F = fat tissue; T = trabeculation showing muscle; M = muscle; Fi = fibrosis.

Microscopic Examination: Positive Findings

Approaches to the AV Node

Fatty metamorphosis was noted.

AV Bundle, Penetrating

The bundle was septated with moderate fibrosis (Fig. 8-126).

AV Bundle, Branching

Moderate fibrosis was present. The bundle was left-sided.

Right Bundle Branch

Marked fibrosis was present.

Left Bundle Branch

Moderately severe vacuolization of cells with zones of fibrosis was noted. Peripherally, fatty metamorphosis and focal necrosis of cells were present.

Summit of the Ventricular Septum

Large and small areas of necrosis were in evidence. The right side of the septum showed necrosis of muscle and severe fatty metamorphosis and fibrosis. Arteriolosclerosis was also noted.

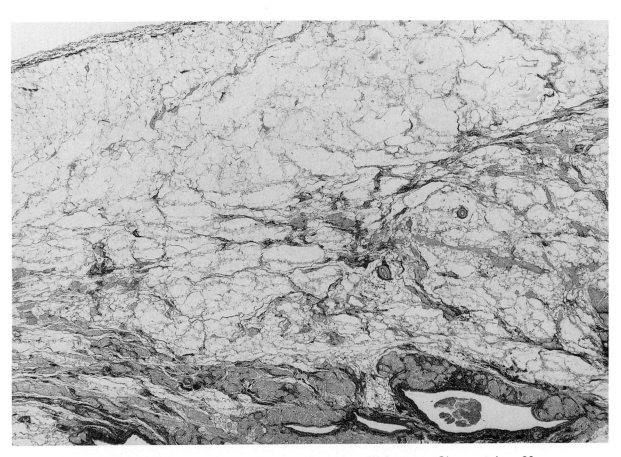

Figure 8-125: Higher power of the previous view. Weigert-van Gieson stain ×30.

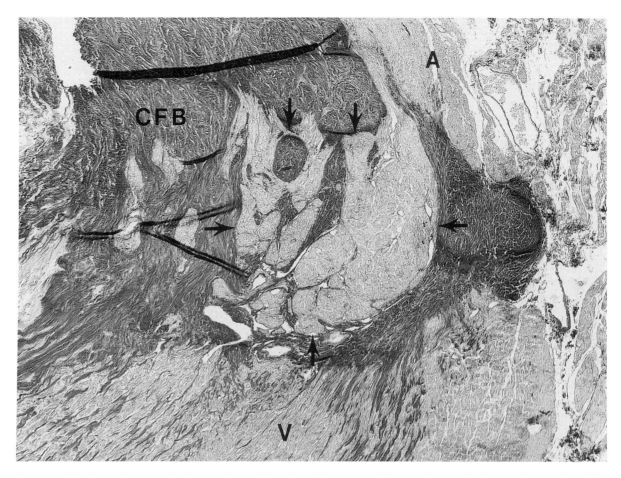

Figure 8-126: Septated penetrating portion of bundle. Weigert-van Gieson stain ×45. A = atrial septum; V = ventricular septum; CFB = central fibrous body. The arrows point to bundle. (Reprinted with permission from S Bharati, AW Feld, R Bauernfeind, A Kattus, M Lev: Hypoplasia of the right ventricular myocardium with ventricular tachycardia. *Arch Pathol Lab Med* 1983; 107:249–253.)

Right Ventricle

Anterior wall: The myocardium was mostly replaced by fat, except in the trabecular area.

Posterior wall: There was severe fatty metamorphosis. Degenerative changes were present in the muscle cells.

Left Ventricle

Focal areas of necrosis, fibrosis with an infiltration of mononuclear cells, and neutrophils were noted.

Discussion

This 20-year-old female died suddenly after having recurrent ventricular tachycardia for 5 years. Pathologically she was found to have Uhl's disease with replacement of most of the right ventricle by fat. The tachycardia characterized by left bundle branch block may have originated in the right ventricle. Another cause of the tachycardia may be the septated bundle or the fibrosis of the left and right bundle branches. The role of the hypoplastic right coronary in the genesis of arrhythias and/or Uhl's anomaly is not understood at present.

CASE #49[194]

A 47-year-old female with systemic hypertension (166/97) died suddenly 2½ months after surgical closure of an atrial septal defect of fossa ovalis type. She was asymptomatic before surgery. An electrocardiogram 4 months before surgery showed atrial flutter. This was converted to normal sinus rhythm after digitalis, quinidine, and cardioversion, with first-degree AV block and ST-T wave changes. An ECG after surgery showed incomplete right bundle branch block, first-degree AV block, and ST-T wave changes.

Pathology: Gross

The heart was hypertrophied and enlarged in all chambers. No further changes were in evidence.

Microscopic Examination: Positive Findings

SA Node and Its Approaches

Sutures with marked fibrosis and foreign body granulomas were in evidence. Neuritis was present.

Atrial Preferential Pathways

These revealed marked fatty infiltration with fibroelastosis of muscle and fibrosis and perifibrosis of nerves.

Approaches to the AV Node

Here again sutures were in evidence with foreign body reaction and fatty metamorphosis.

AV Node

Fatty metamorphosis and fibroelastosis were noted.

Penetrating and Branching Bundle

These showed fatty metamorphosis (Fig. 8-127). The branching bundle occupied a considerable part of the membranous septum.

Left Bundle Branch

This was partially destroyed (Fig. 8-128).

Right Bundle Branch

The first part lay at the base of the tricuspid valve and showed fibrosis.

Summit of the Ventricular Septum

There was marked increase in fibrosis, especially on the left side (Fig. 8-127).

Myocardium

Fibrosis was present in both ventricles, but was more marked on the right.

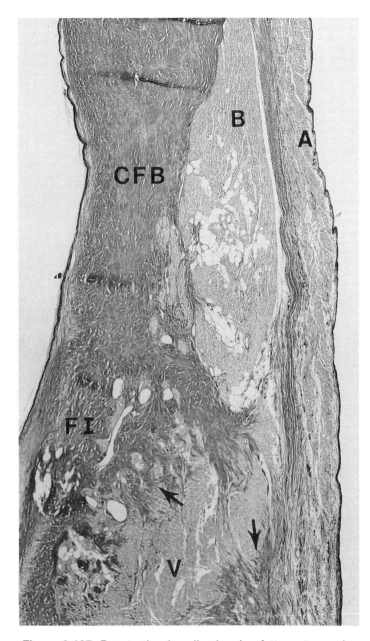

Figure 8-127: Penetrating bundle showing fatty metamorphosis. Note the marked fibrosis of the left and right sides of the summit of the ventricular septum. Weigert-van Gieson stain ×30. B = bundle; V = ventricular septum; CFB = central fibrous body; A = atrial muscle; FI = fibrosis of the left side of summit. The arrows point to the fibrosis of the left and right side of the summit of the ventricular septum.

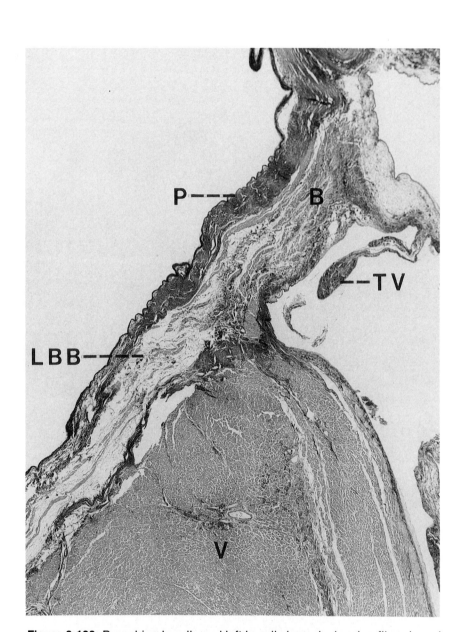

Figure 8-128: Branching bundle and left bundle branch showing fibrosis and space formation in both. Note that the bundle occupies a considerable part of the pars membranacea. Weigert-van Gieson stain ×30. B = bundle; LBB = left bundle branch; P = pars membranacea; V = ventricular septum; TV = tricuspid valve. (Reprinted with permission from S Bharati, M Lev: Conduction system in sudden unexpected death a considerable time after repair of atrial septal defect. *Chest* 1988; 94:142–148.)

Discussion

This 47-year-old woman died suddenly 2½ months after surgical repair of an atrial septal defect. Here we are confronted with the cause of sudden death after surgical repair of a congenitally abnormal heart. Since this was 2½ months after surgery, it may be too soon for the heart to return to normal.

The abnormalities in the conduction system were: (1) sutures in the SA node and its approaches and in the approaches to the AV node with foreign body reaction and neuritis; (2) fatty metamorphosis of the AV bundle; (3) partial destruction of the left bundle branch and fibrosis of the right bundle branch; (4) marked fibrosis of the summit of the ventricular septum; and (5) fibrosis of both ventricles. We do not know which of these or whether all of these are related to her sudden death.

CASE #50[188]

The Conduction System in Sudden Infant Death Syndrome (SIDS)

The cause of sudden unexpected death in infants is today unknown. The conduction systems of 23 hearts were examined without knowing which individual hearts belonged to the sudden infant death group and which ones belonged to the control group. There were 15 hearts from the SIDS group and eight from the control group. All hearts were submitted by Dr. Krongrad from the Medical Examiner's Office, New York City, New York. The AV node was situated in part within the central fibrous body in some cases. The branching portion of the His bundle was located on the left side in eight cases out of 15 and only in two cases out of eight in the control group. We hypothesize that a left-sided His bundle may be prone to or vulnerable to arrhythmia during the transition from the relative predominance of the right ventricle at term to the relative predominance of the left ventricle at 2–4 months of age. The increase in left ventricular pressure may influence the His bundle which is in the subendocardial region in some infants and may be responsible for arrhythmia and sudden death. The effect of the presence of the AV node in part in the central fibrous body, the fragmentation of the His bundle, and the presence of a neuritis in the atria cannot be evaluated.

Pathology: Microscopic Examination — Positive Findings

Conduction System

AV Node: This was partly embedded in the central fibrous body. Fibrosis was noted.
AV Bundle, Penetrating: Fibrosis was present with fragmentation.
AV Bundle, Branching: This was left-sided and showed fibrosis (Fig. 8-129).
Left Bundle Branch: Fibrosis was noted.

Nerves

Neuritis was noted throughout.

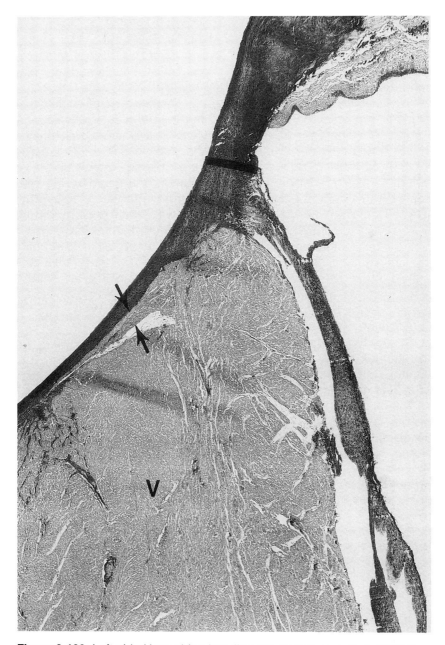

Figure 8-129: Left-sided branching bundle seen more frequently in SIDS than in the normal heart. Weigert-van Gieson stain ×30. V = ventricular septum. The arrows point to the left-sided bundle. (Reprinted with permission from Bharati S, Krongrad E, Lev M: Study of the conduction system in a population of patients with sudden infant death syndrome. *Pediatr Cardiol* 1985; 6:20–40.)

Discussion

The fundamental finding in the hearts appeared to be the left-sidedness of the bundle of His. We speculate that between 2 and 4 months, when the right-sidedness of the fetal circulation is changed to the left-sidedness of the adult circulation, that this change may effect a left-sided bundle to produce SIDS.

CASE #51

A 32-year-old Japanese-American male collapsed suddenly while skiing and died. The patient was thought to have familial type 2 hyperlipoproteinemia. His cholesterol levels varied from 313 mg to 341 mg while triglycerides varied from 48 mg to 275 mg. Over a 3-year period, he was treated intermittently with chlofibrate and para-amino cylic acid. He did not take the medications regularly, nor did he attend the clinic regularly. Six months before he died suddenly, he became a father of twins and began to take his hypercholesterolemia seriously. He took bile acid binding resin, 24 mg, every day. On this regimen, his serum cholesterol fell to a low of 246 mg % and averaged 267 on four determinations throughout the year. This was a 21% reduction from levels prior to initiating Questran therapy. His triglyceride levels on this therapy were higher than before, averaging 126 mg %. He went skiing with his friend, going from sea level to an altitude of 8,000 feet overnight. He slept at that altitude, and the following morning skied on slopes varying from 1,000 to 10,000 feet. The patient finished a vigorous downhill run, joked about fatigue, went to lay down, and stopped breathing. Despite all resuscitative attempts, he could not be resuscitated.

His two aunts, both with myocardial infarctions in their mid-forties, have xanthomas and elevated blood cholesterol. His uncle, who died of coronary atherosclerosis at age 47, had xanthomatosis, with cholesterol in the range of 360 to 420 mg %. A number of his other relatives are being treated for similar conditions.

ECG

His electrocardiogram revealed first-degree AV block, sinus bradycardia, and intraventricular conduction defect.

Pathology: Gross

Severe coronary arteriosclerosis and generalized atherosclerosis with xanthomas in the Achilles tendon were present.

The heart weighed 300 grams. The aortic-mitral annulus revealed atherosclerotic plaques and there was distinct fenestration and calcification of the aortic valve. There were marked atherosclerotic plaques in the ascending aorta involving the ostia of both coronary arteries extending to the sinuses of Valsalva. Extensive atherosclerosis was seen throughout the aorta.

The anatomical diagnosis was familial xanthomatosis with severe atherosclerotic coronary artery disease with type 2 hyperlipoproteinemia.

Microscopic Examination: Positive Findings

SA Node and Its Approaches

Marked fatty infiltration of the approaches to the SA node was present. The SA node showed an increase in fibrosis.

AV Node and Its Approaches

The AV nodal artery was thickened and narrowed. Marked fatty infiltration of the AV node was present. The AV node was partly in the central fibrous body (Fig. 8-130).

AV Bundle, Penetrating

Fatty infiltration was present (Fig. 8-131).

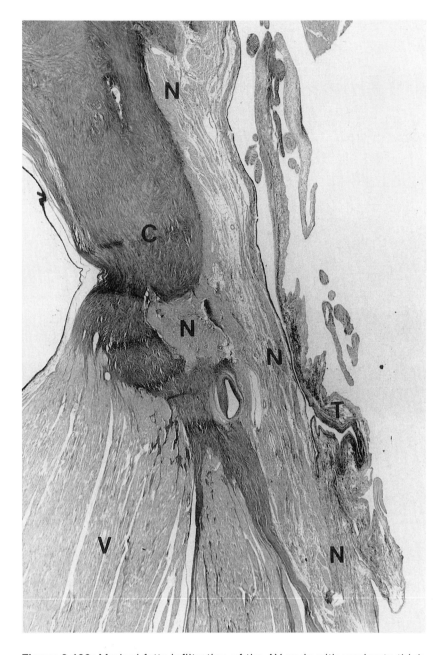

Figure 8-130: Marked fatty infiltration of the AV node with moderate thickening of the AV nodal artery. The node is in part in the central fibrous body. Weigert-van Gieson stain ×16.5. N = AV node; V = ventricular septum; C = central fibrous body; T = tricuspid valve.

AV Bundle, Branching

There was fine fibrosis, with marked space formation.

Left Bundle Branch

Fibrosis was noted with marked space formation (Fig. 8-132).

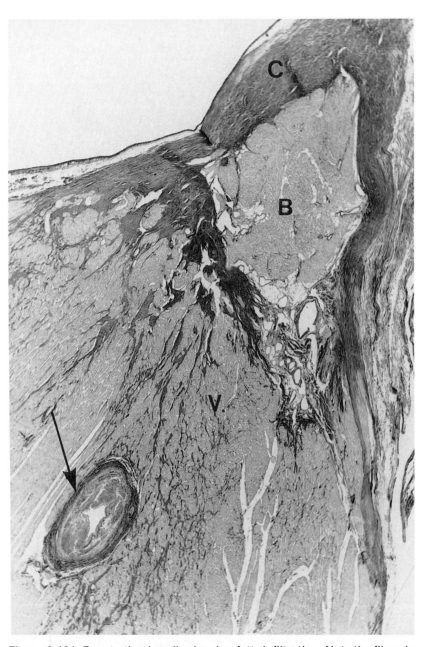

Figure 8-131: Penetrating bundle showing fatty infiltration. Note the fibrosis of the septum and arteriolosclerosos. Weigert-van Gieson stain ×30. B = penetrating bundle; V = ventricular septum; C = central fibrous body; The arrow points to the arteriole.

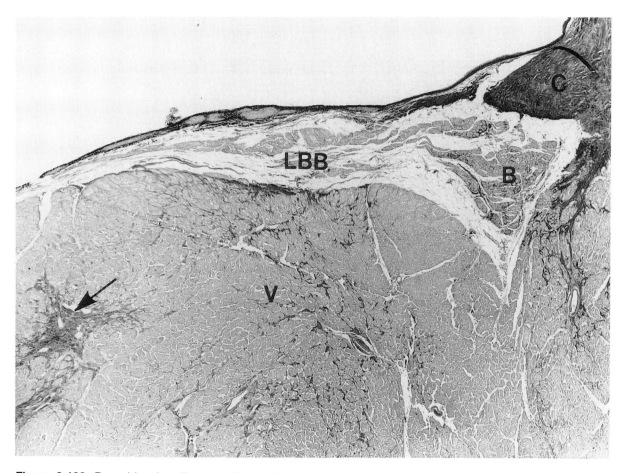

Figure 8-132: Branching bundle and left bundle branch showing space formation. Note the fibrosis of the septum. Weigert-van Gieson stain ×45. B = branching bundle; LBB = left bundle branch; V = ventricular septum; C = central fibrous body. The arrow points to the fibrosis.

Right Bundle Branch

The first and second parts were intramyocardial. Mild fibrosis was present in the first part.

Summit of the Ventricular Septum

Marked arteriolosclerosis was in evidence with moderate fibrosis (Fig. 8-132).

Discussion

The sudden death of this patient is in some way related to his hyperlipoproteinemia. From the morphological standpoint, the fatty infiltration of the AV node and the penetrating bundle, the presence of the node in the central fibrous body, the fibrosis and arteriolosclerosis of the summit of the ventricular septum, the marked space formation in the branching bundle and left bundle branch all stand out as contributing factors.

CASE #52

A 64-year-old hypertensive, diabetic male developed atrioventricular block. He was doc-umented as having a large sinus venosus type of atrial septal defect and had a pacemaker inserted for syncopal episodes. Despite the pacemaker, he suddenly went into ventricular tachycardia, fibrillation, and he died.

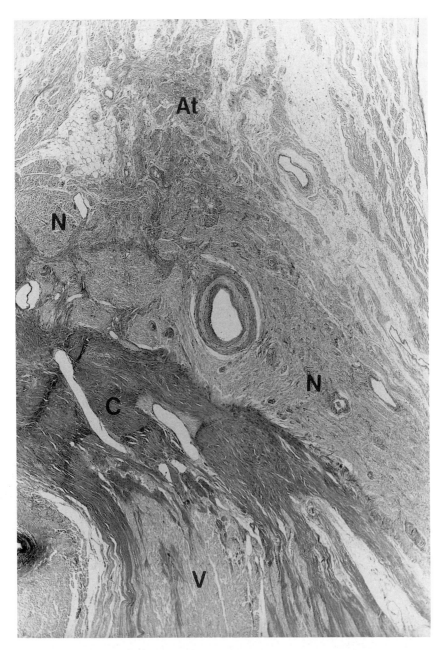

Figure 8-133: The AV node showing marked fibrosis. Weigert-van Gieson stain ×45. N = AV node; C = central fibrous body; V = ventricular muscle; At = atrial muscle.

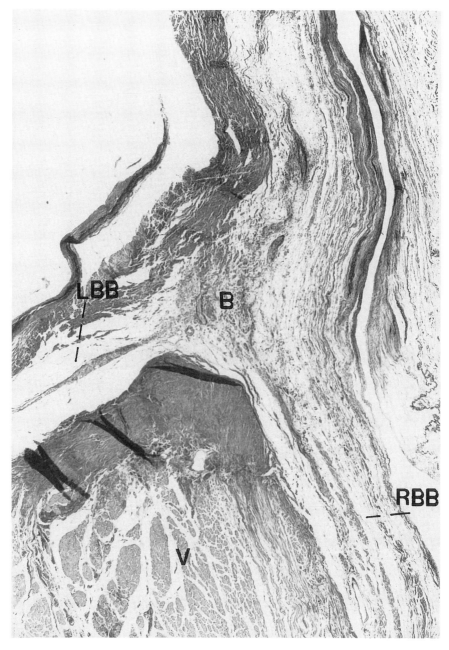

Figure 8-134: Branching bundle and left bundle branch showing complete fibrosis, and right bundle branch showing almost complete fibrosis. Weigert-van Gieson stain ×30. B = branching bundle; LBB = left bundle branch; RBB = right bundle branch; V = ventricular septal muscle.

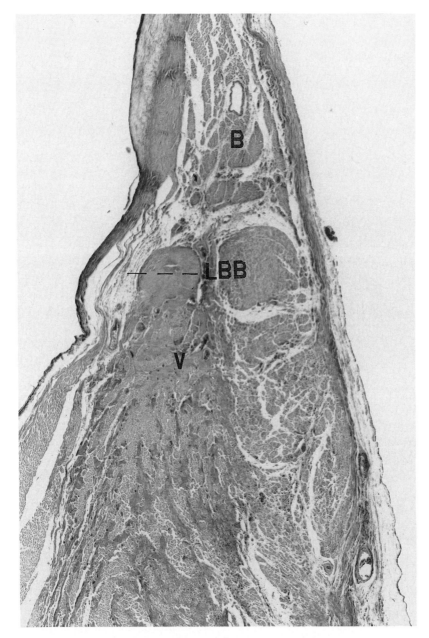

Figure 8-135: Branching bundle and left bundle branch, and summit of the ventricular septum showing fibrosis. Weigert-van Gieson stain ×30. B = branching bundle; LBB = left bundle branch; V = ventricular septal muscle.

EPS

His bundle studies revealed second-degree block distal to the His bundle recording site. He developed recurrent congestive heart failure and the block progressed to third-degree AV block in the last 5 years.

Pathology: Gross

Generalized atherosclerosis, arteriolosclerosis, arteriolo-nephrosclerosis, and atrophy of the right kidney were present. Pulmonary emphysema, acute ulcers in larynx and trachea, bronchopneumonia, pleural adhesions, and cerebral arteriolosclerosis with infarcts of the cerebrum, cerebellum, focal demyelination of the spinal cord, ectopic adrenal gland in the celiac area, and fat necrosis of the pancreas (mild) were present.

The heart was enlarged, weighing 600 grams. There was a sinus venosus type of a large atrial septal defect measuring about 1.5 to 2 cm in greatest dimension. The superior vena cava straddled the defect, emerging in part from the right atrium and in part from the left atrium. The right two pulmonary veins entered the right atrium directly. There was a localized narrowing of the left circumflex and the anterior descending coronary arteries.

Microscopic Examination: Positive Findings

SA Node and Its Approaches

There was partial separation of the SA node by fat with fibroelastosis of the node.

AV Node, Bundle, and Bundle Branches

Marked fibrosis was present in these structures (Fig. 8-133) with obliteration of the branching bundle (Fig. 8-134) and almost all of the left bundle branch (Fig. 8-135).

Summit of the Ventricular Septum

Marked fibrosis of the summit was evident.

Discussion

The AV block in this case was related to the destruction of the branching bundle and both bundle branches. Sudden death in complete AV block is common.

CASE #53

A 23-year-old white female, while shopping in a convenience store with her daughter, suddenly fell to the floor and collapsed. A phy-sician who was near by started immediate re-suscitative efforts but she could not be resus-citated.

According to the mother of the deceased, her daughter had complained of numbness, radiating to the left shoulder and left fingertips

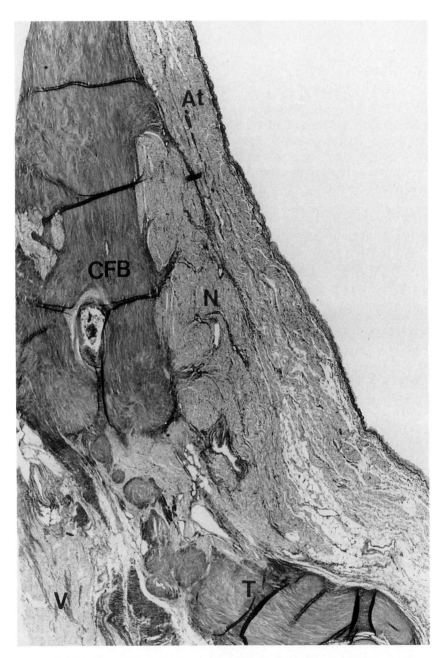

Figure 8-136: The AV node in the central fibrous body showing segmentation. Weigert-van Gieson stain ×32. N = AV node; At = atrial musculature; CFB = central fibrous body; V = ventricular septal muscle; T = tricuspid prong.

lasting 1 to 2 hours, and she felt that her heart was "jelly" in her chest. That sensation lasted for 10 to 15 minutes and it occurred every month. She was noted to have said that her heart had stopped and that she felt faint and that she was going to die. None of these symptoms were related to exercise. The mother also stated that her daughter had a fear of cats and that there were three cats present in the store at the time she died.

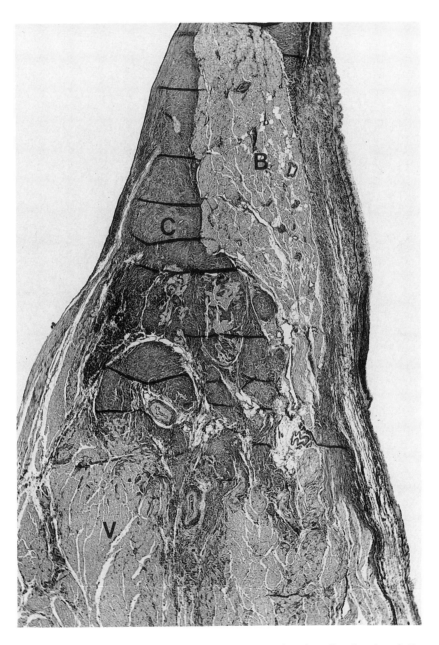

Figure 8-137: The proximal part of the penetrating bundle showing fatty metamorphosis. Note the fibrosis of the ventricular septum. Weigert-van Gieson stain ×30. B = penetrating bundle; C = central fibrous body; V = ventricular septal musculature.

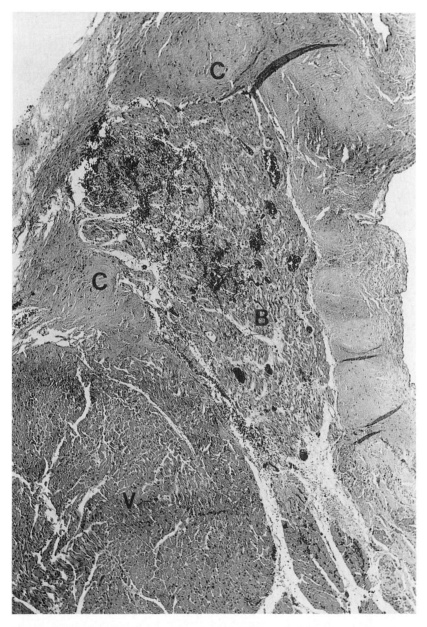

Figure 8-138: Massive hemorrhage in the distal part of the penetrating bundle. Weigert-van Gieson stain ×52.5. B = AV bundle; V = ventricular septal muscle; C = central fibrous body.

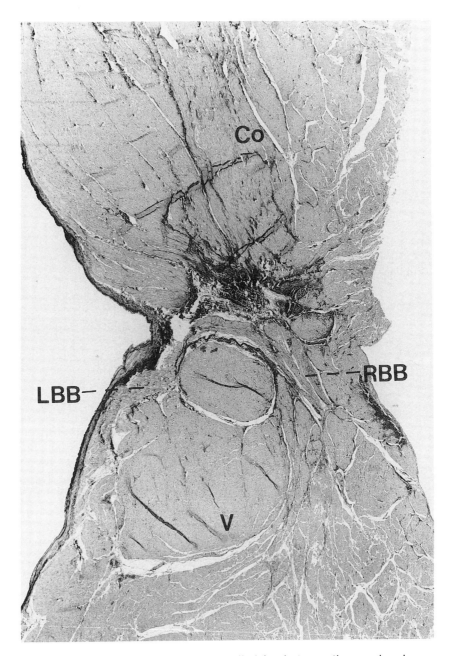

Figure 8-139: Bifurcation of the AV bundle lying between the conal and ventricular septal musculature. Weigert-van Gieson stain ×21. LBB = left bundle branch; RBB = right bundle branch; V = ventricular septal muscle; Co = conal muscle.

Pathology: Gross

The heart weighed 265 grams. The coronary sinus did not enter the right atrium; instead it entered the left atrium. In addition, the left coronary originated between the aorta and the pulmonary trunk.

Microscopic Examination: Positive Findings

AV Node and Its Approaches

Marked fatty metamorphosis was present. The AV node was segmented and was in part within the central fibrous body (Fig. 8-136). It lay directly adjacent to the aorta.

AV Bundle, Penetrating

In the beginning (Fig. 8-137), fat was noted within the bundle. Massive hemorrhage was evident in the distal part (Fig. 8-138).

AV Bundle, Branching

This lay within the muscular part of the ventricular septum, unrelated to the aortic valve and membranous septum (Fig. 8-139). The bundle was located about 1.5 cm beneath the aortic valve, within the muscle.

Left Bundle Branch

This revealed hemorrhage in the beginning. Peripherally, there was an infiltration of mononuclear cells.

Right Bundle Branch

The first and second parts of the right bundle branch were intramyocardial and showed slight fibrosis. The third part was infiltrated with mononuclear cells.

Summit of the Ventricular Septum

This showed marked fibrosis on the left side with arteriolosclerosis. The fibrosis appeared to originate from the aorta going down.

Central Fibrous Body

This was abnormally formed. It basically consisted of the aortic prong meeting the ventricular septum. The tricuspid prong occurred later.

Discussion

This is a remarkable case. The central fibrous body was abnormally formed, mostly by the aorta and the fibrous tissue of the ventricular septum. The bulbus was abnormally absorbed into the ventricles, so that there were two well-developed coni, and the bifurcation of the branching bundle was sandwiched in between the conal and ventricular muscles. The coronary sinus entered the left atrium. The left coronary passed between the aorta and the pulmonary trunk and was therefore compressed. Massive hemorrhage was noted in the bundle. All of the above abnormalities are probably related to the sudden death in this case.

CASE #54[207]

A 4½-year-old boy, diagnosed as having mucocutaneous lymph node syndrome (Kawasaki disease), had an unexpected cardiac arrest on the 13th day of his illness and died suddenly. He had no symptoms of heart failure and the electrogram revealed no evidence of any arrhythmia, but did show some nonspecific ST-T wave changes and rsr' pattern in V1. An echocardiogram 3 days before death revealed large right and left coronaries with some enlargement of the left ventricle, with a moderately good ejection fraction of about 67%.

Pathology: Gross

The heart was enlarged, weighing 123 grams (normal 73 to 88 grams). There were aneurysms of coronary arteries but no rupture.

Microscopic Examination: Positive Findings

Myocarditis of the entire conduction system with chronic subendocardial inflammation was evident. In addition, the conduction system showed diffuse periarteritis and neu-

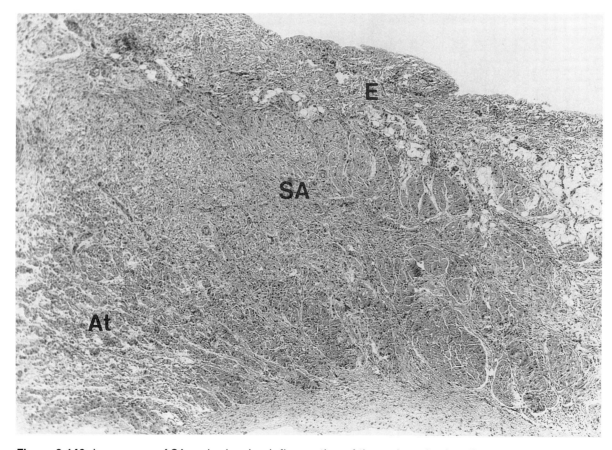

Figure 8-140: Low power of SA node showing inflammation of the node and epicardium. Hematoxylin-eosin stain ×60. SA = SA node; At = atrial musculature; E = epicardium.

ritis. The above findings were present throughout the heart. In summary, the sudden death occurred in the early phase of the illness of Kawasaki disease, unrelated to coronary aneurysm but as a lethal arrhythmia secondary to myocarditis.

Entire Conduction System (Figs. 8-140– 8-148)

The entire conduction system showed myocarditis. In addition, there was diffuse neuritis and perineuritis.

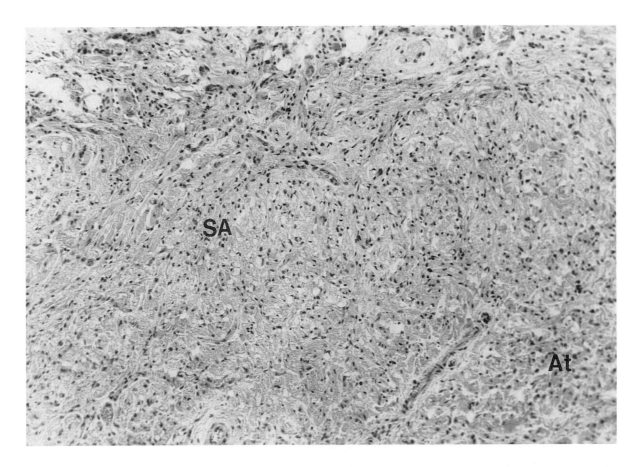

Figure 8-141: Higher power view of Figure 8-140. Hematoxylin-eosin stain ×120. SA = SA node; At = atrial musculature.

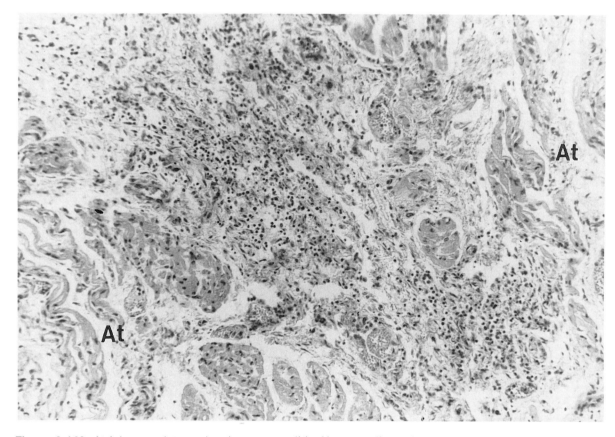

Figure 8-142: Atrial musculature showing myocarditis. Hematoxylin-eosin stain ×150. At = atrial musculature.

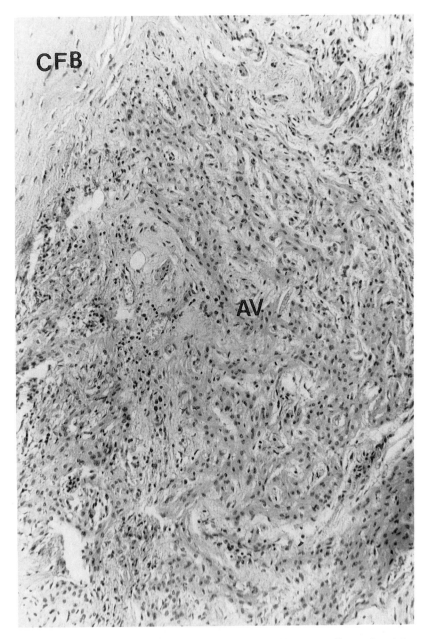

Figure 8-143: AV node showing inflammation. Hematoxylin-eosin stain ×120. AV = AV node; CFB = central fibrous body.

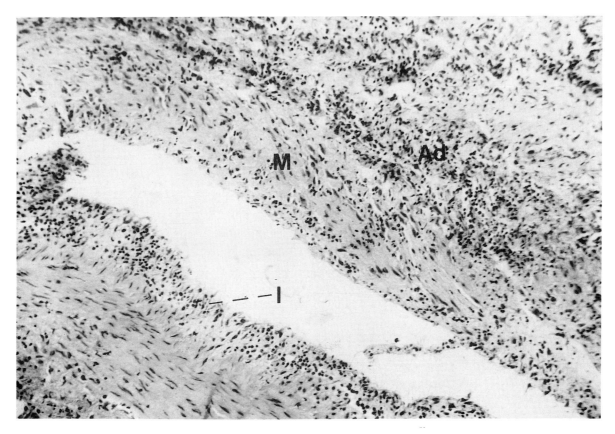

Figure 8-144: Artery showing inflammation mostly in intima and adventitia. Hematoxylin-eosin stain ×150. I = intima; M = media; Ad = adventitia.

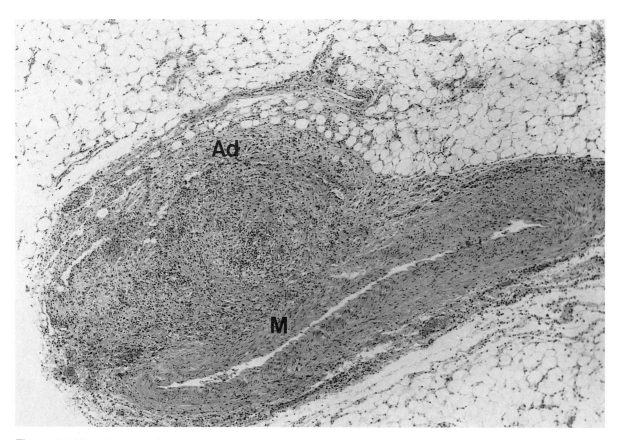

Figure 8-145: Artery showing marked inflammation in adventitia. Hematoxylin-eosin stain ×60. M = media; Ad = adventitia.

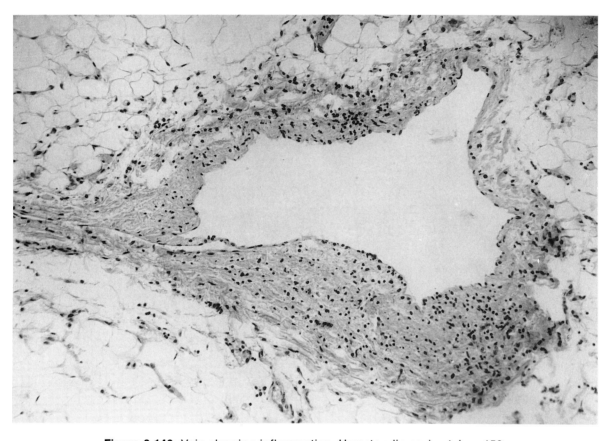

Figure 8-146: Vein showing inflammation. Hematoxylin-eosin stain ×150.

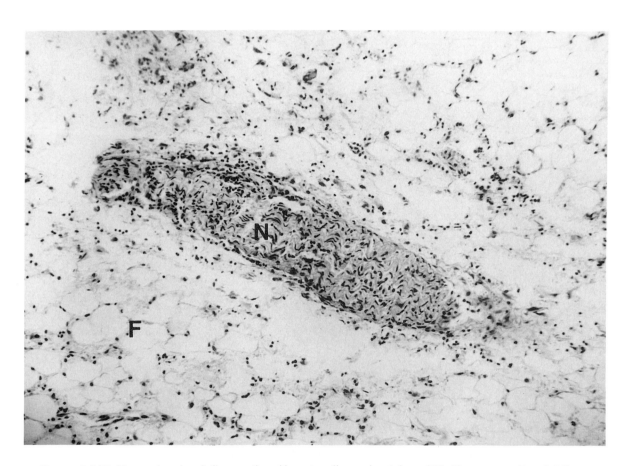

Figure 8-147: Nerve showing inflammation. Hematoxylin-eosin stain ×150. N = nerve; F = fat tissue.

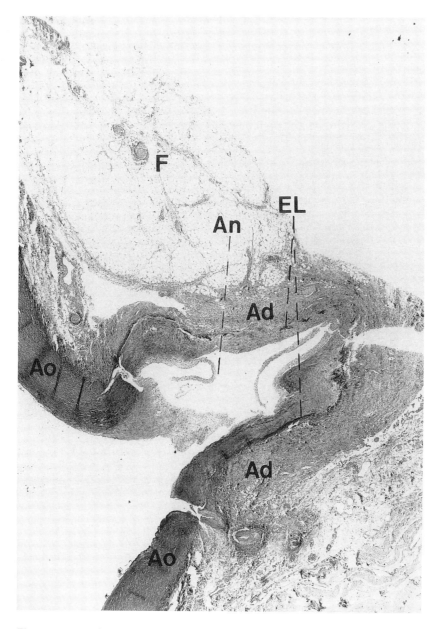

Figure 8-148: Origin of coronary artery from aorta showing inflammatory changes. Hematoxylin-eosin stain ×16.5. Ao = aorta; F = fat tissue; EL = elastic tissue showing disruption; Ad = adventitia; An = aneurysm formation. (Reprinted with permission from Bharati S, Engle MA, Fatica NS, et al: The heart and conduction system in acute Kawasaki disease. Report of fraternal cases: one lethal, one relapsing. *Am Heart J* 1990; 120:359–365.)

Discussion

Sudden death occurs in Kawasaki disease in less than 2% of cases. However, sudden death in early phase of the illness is rare. Death is usually related to myocarditis, cardiac failure, ischemic heart disease, rupture of the coronary aneurysm, or cardiac arrhythmia.

This case is one of significance in that this was an acute fatal case of fraternal Kawasaki disease, with panvasculitis, and severe pancarditis with involvement of all parts of the conduction system including neuritis. The exact mechanism of an arrhythmic episode is probably related to an altered metabolic state of the myocardium with neuritis.

It is of interest that the brother of this child, born 1 year later, survived relapsing Kawasaki disease and is asymptomatic at the present time. He was treated early with intravenous gamma globulin during each relapse.

CASE #55

A 1-month-old infant was diagnosed as having truncus arteriosus communis persistens. He died suddenly at home. He was diagnosed as having gastroenteritis 3 weeks before he died.

Pathology: Gross

The infant was found to have DiGeorge syndrome with the following: (1) hypertensive pulmonary vascular disease grade 3; (2) hyperplasia and hypertrophy of the islets of the pancreas; and (3) moderate diffuse swelling of cerebral hemispheres and the cerebellum.

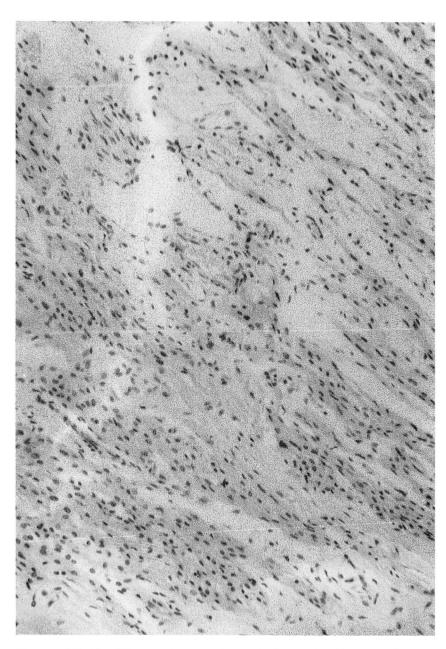

Figure 8-149: The AV node showing chronic inflammation. Hematoxylin-eosin ×225.

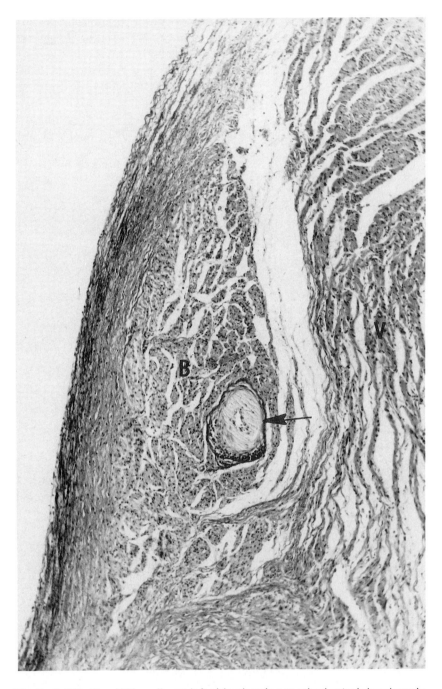

Figure 8-150: The AV bundle on left side showing marked arteriolosclerosis. Weigert-van Gieson stain ×82.5.

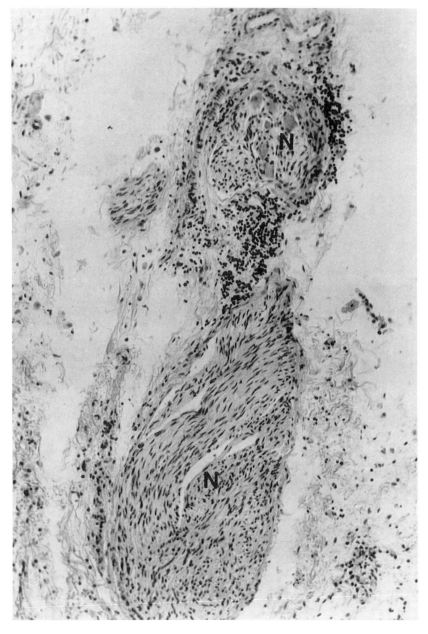

Figure 8-151: The Nerve showing chronic inflammation. Hematoxylin-eosin stain ×82.5. N = nerve.

The heart was enlarged. Truncus arteriosus was present with right aortic arch: (1) incomplete cortriatriatum dexter, and (2) bicuspid dysplastic truncal valve.

Microscopic Examination: Positive Findings

Chronic inflammation of the AV node was present (Fig. 8-149). Marked arteriolosclerosis of the AV bundle was noted (Fig. 8-150). Chronic inflammation of the nerves adjacent to the truncus was seen (Fig. 8-151), and epicarditis was evident.

Discussion

This was a case of myocarditis in a case of truncus arteriosus in an infant. It is well known that in myocarditis of any etiology, either in the acute or during the chronic phase of the illness, arrhythmias may be generated which may end fatally.

The mechanisms for the development of arrhythmias in myocarditis are unknown today. One may hypothesize that various disturbances in the metabolic level which result in abnormal physiological states of the myocardial tissue may play a role in provoking arrhythmias in myocarditis.

CASE #56[210]

A 74-year-old male physician was admitted for dizziness and syncope and died suddenly while being investigated. An asymptomatic enlarging abdominal aneurysm was replaced by means of a Dacron prosthesis 4 years earlier. During the ensuing years, his mental status deteriorated severely and he was in a nursing home. An electrocardiogram revealed paroxysmal atrial fibrillation followed by atrial arrest and depression of atrioventricular junctional pacemaker. In addition, an electrocardiogram revealed recent ischemia of the anterolateral and posterior walls superimposed on a pattern of left ventricular hypertrophy.

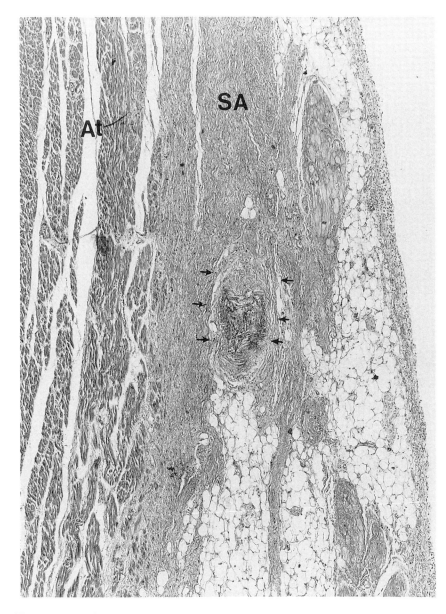

Figure 8-152: SA node showing sclerotic vessel. Hematoxylin-eosin stain ×45. SA = SA node, At = atrial muscle. The arrows point to the sclerotic artery.

Pathology Gross

The findings included arterial and arteriolar nephrosclerosis, pulmonary edema, saccular aneurysm of the descending aorta with a large mural thrombus, adenocarcinoma of the ascending colon with metastases to the liver, and massive hemopericardium.

The heart weighed 416 grams. The right, the main left, and the anterior descending arteries showed atherosclerosis but no distinct narrowing. However, the circumflex 2 cm distal to its origin was markedly narrowed by atherosclerosis and completely occluded by a recent thrombus. In addition, there was a huge recent infarct of the proximal two-thirds of the

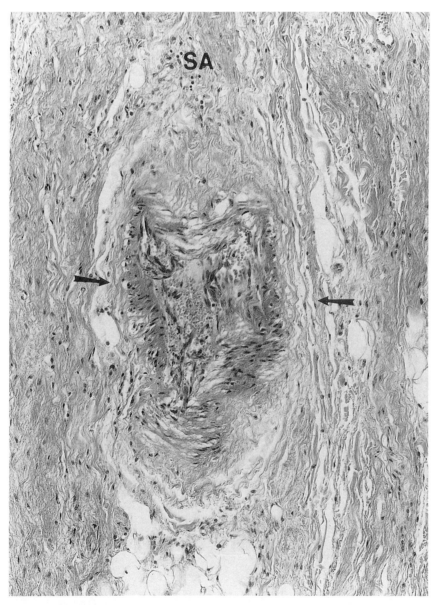

Figure 8-153: Enlargement of Figure 8-152. Hematoxylin-eosin stain ×150. SA = SA node showing sclerotic artery. The arrows point to the sclerotic vessel.

posterior ventricular septum. The posterior and lateral walls had ruptured.

Microscopic Examination: Positive Findings

SA Node

This showed degeneration, early necrosis, and arteriolosclerosis (Figs. 8-152, 8-153).

Approaches to the SA Node

There was considerable fibrosis, elastosis, chronic pericarditis, and arteriolonecrosis.

Approaches to AV Node

This showed fat, chronic inflammation, and arteriolosclerosis. Acute degenerative changes of the AV nodal artery was also seen.

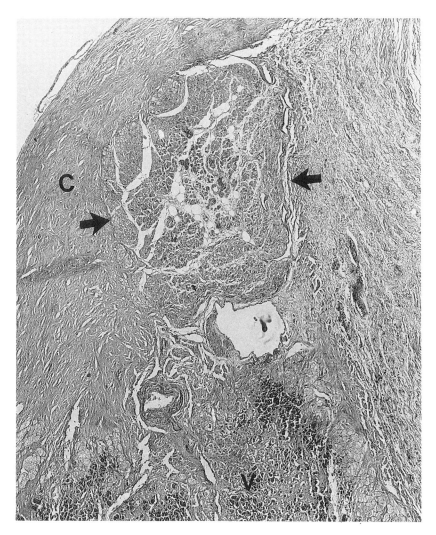

Figure 8-154: Penetrating portion of the bundle showing degenerative changes in the bundle. Hematoxylin-eosin stain ×45. C = central fibrous body; V = ventricular septal muscle. The arrows point to the bundle.

AV Node

Chronic inflammation with proliferation of sheath cells and fibrosis was noted.

AV Bundle, Penetrating

Degenerative changes were seen focally in some of the cells (Figs. 8-154, 8-155).

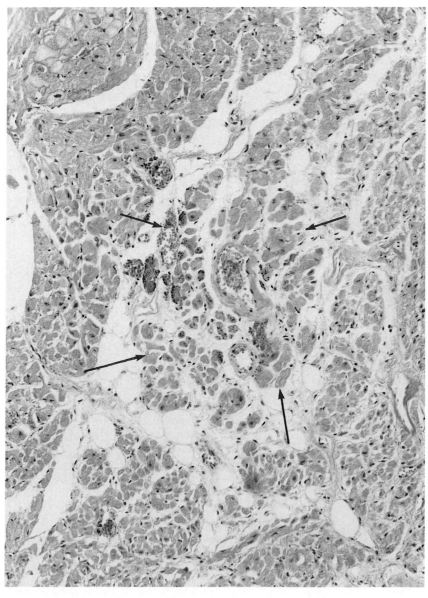

Figure 8-155: Enlargement of Figure 8-154. Hematoxylin-eosin stain ×150. The arrows point to the degenerating cells.

AV Bundle, Bifurcating

There was marked fibrosis, falling out of cells and space formation (Fig. 8-156).

Right Bundle Branch

Marked fibrosis with space formation was evident (Fig. 8-157).

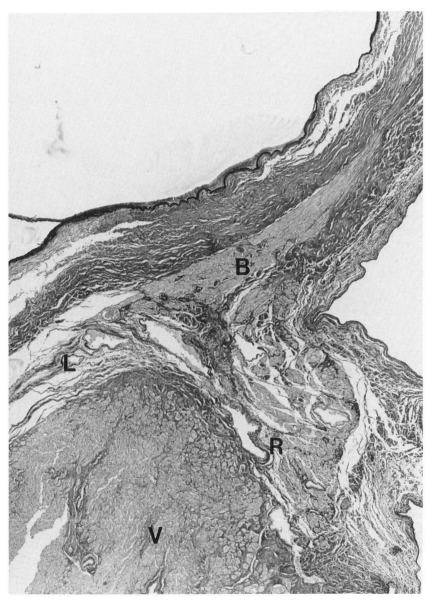

Figure 8-156: Bifurcating bundle showing space formation and fibrosis of the left and right sides. Weigert-van Gieson stain × 45. B = branching bundle; L = left side of bifurcation; R = right side of bifurcation; V = ventricular septal muscle.

Left Bundle Branch

Marked fibrosis was present (Fig. 8-158).

Myocardium

There was recent infarct 24–48 hours old.

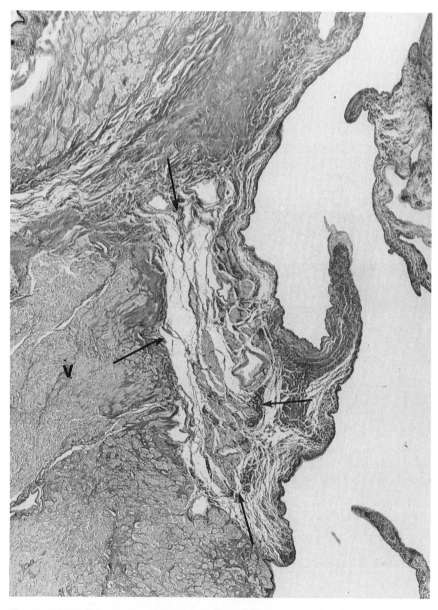

Figure 8-157: The first part of the right bundle branch showing fibrosis and space formation. Weigert-van Gieson stain ×45. V = ventricular septal muscle. The arrows point to the right bundle branch.

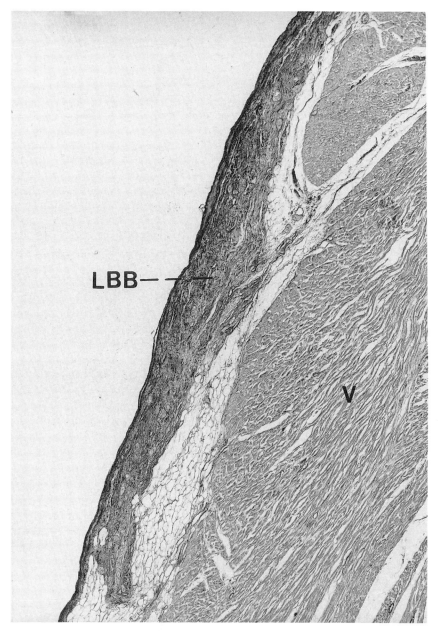

Figure 8-158: Left bundle branch showing marked fibrosis. Weigert-van Gieson stain ×120. LBB = left bundle branch; V = ventricular septal muscle.

Discussion

In addition to the infarct of the myocardium, the vessels of the conduction system showed marked sclerotic changes with parenchymal changes in the SA node, the AV node, the bundle of His, and the bundle branches. All of these changes certainly can be related to the sudden death of the individual, with sick sinus syndrome.

CASE #57[206]

This case was a 6-month-old white female born full-term following a normal pregnancy, who weighed 3150 grams. Approximately 36 hours postdelivery, the baby was noted to have a heart rate of 160–180/min. The rate pro-

gressed to greater than 250 beats/min, although there was no evidence of congestive heart failure or respiratory compromise. A diagnosis of junctional ectopic tachycardia was made and the patient was digitalized.

A 2D echocardiogram revealed no evidence of structural heart disease. Her admis-

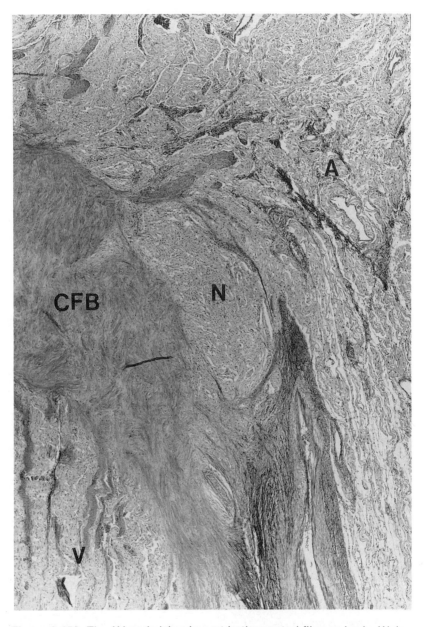

Figure 8-159: The AV node lying in part in the central fibrous body. Weigert-van Gieson stain ×45. CFB = central fibrous body; N = AV node; A = atrial musculature, V = ventricular musculature.

sion was complicated by staph scalded skin syndrome and an allergic reaction to procainamide. She was discharged on digoxin, quinidine, and Dicloxacillin. She was admitted 6 months later for a trial of amiodarone. Approximately 6 hours after the dose of amio-

darone (25 mg) she became tachypnic with an irregular heart rate of 190 and cyanosis. She developed seizures and a temperature of 105.8° and she grew increasingly acidotic. A 2D echocardiogram revealed a grossly dilated noncontractile heart with dyskinesis. She de-

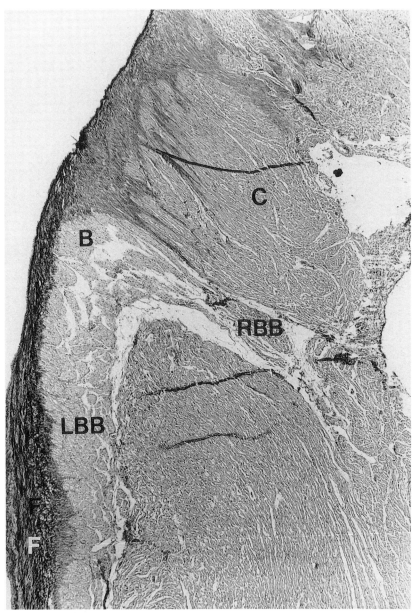

Figure 8-160: Left-sided bundle showing slight fibrosis. Weigert-van Gieson stain ×45. F = subendocardial fibroelastosis of the left ventricle; LBB = left bundle branch; B = bundle; RBB = right bundle branch; C = conal muscle above the bundle.

veloped a gallop with premature ventricular contractions and episodes of bradycardia. Despite medical management, she went into acute renal failure, thrombocytopenia, developed ventricular tachycardia, and despite defibrillation, died.

Pathology Gross

Congestion of all the organs was present with pleural effusion and ascites.

The heart was enlarged, weighing 80 grams. There was diffuse fibroelastosis of the

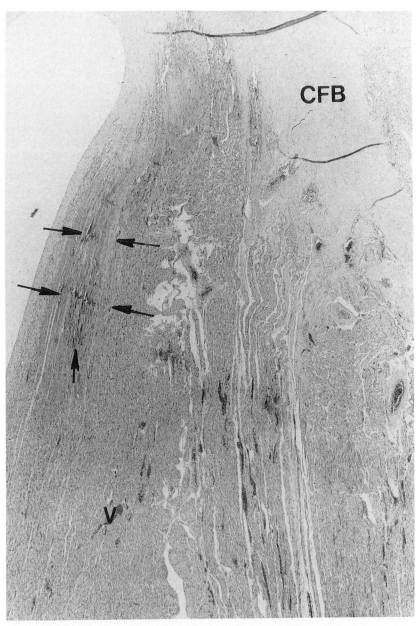

Figure 8-161: Subendocardial necrosis of the myocardium of the ventricular septum. Hematoxylin-eosin stain ×30. V = ventricular septal muscle; CFB = central fibrous body. The arrows point to the zone of necrosis.

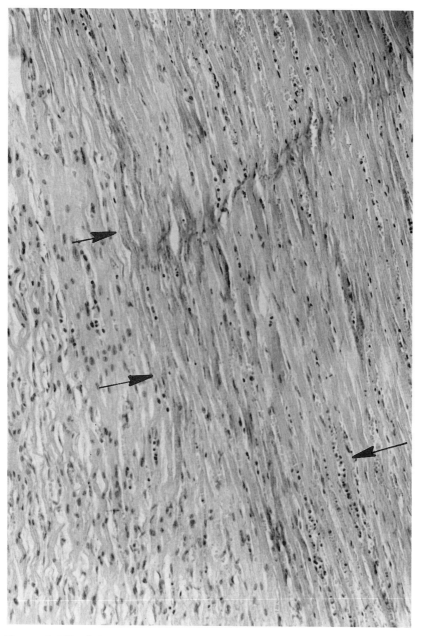

Figure 8-162: Subendocardial necrosis of the ventricular septum. Hematoxylin-eosin stain ×180. The arrows point to the necrosis and infiltration of mononuclear cells.

left ventricle with fibrosis of the papillary muscles and the anteroseptal wall of the left ventricle.

Microscopic Examination: Positive Findings

Atrioventricular Node

This was in part within the central fibrous body (Fig. 8-159).

Bundle of His

This was left-sided with slight fibrosis (Fig. 8-160).

Left Bundle Branch

Marked fibrosis was present, including the peripheral Purkinje nets (Fig. 8-160).

Right Bundle Branch

This was sandwiched between muscle layers (Fig. 8-160).

Summit of the Ventricular Septum and Myocardium

There was generalized focal necrosis and degeneration of the myocardium, with chronic organizing epicarditis (Figs. 8-161, 8-162).

Discussion

The presence of the AV node in part within the central fibrous body, we believe, might cause re-entry phenomenon or fractionization of impulse generation. In addition, there was a left-sided bundle and focal necrosis of the myocardium. These pathological findings could have triggered an arrhythmia and sudden death.

CASE #58[206]

A 5-month-old infant, with a long history of tachycardia, went into ventricular fibrillation during cardiac catheterization and despite defibrillation, died.

He had a long history of tachycardia managed on digoxin and propranolol. His heart rate was 206/min. There were no murmurs. An electrocardiogram revealed a junctional tachycardia. The patient's hospital course was complicated by viral infection and small bowel intussusception, which apparently reduced spontaneously during general anesthesia.

Propranolol was changed to flecainide over a period of several days.

Pathology: Gross

This was limited to the chest and abdomen. There was congestion of the abdominal organs with ectopic pancreas and mild dilatation of the small bowel.

The heart was enlarged, weighing 60 grams. There was diffuse fibroelastosis of the left ventricle, and the coronary sinus was displaced close to the central fibrous body with absent eustachian and thebesian valves (Fig. 8-163).

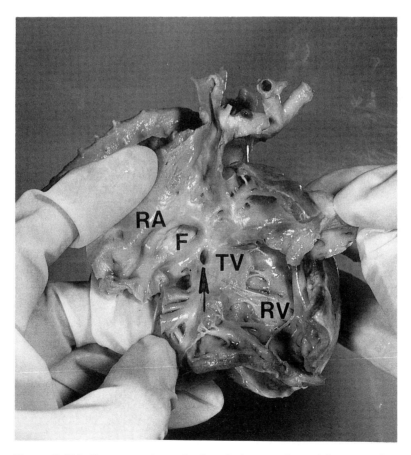

Figure 8-163: Coronary sinus displaced close to the atrial septum. RA = right atrium; F = fossa ovalis; TV = tricuspid valve; RV = right ventricle. The arrow points to the displaced coronary sinus.

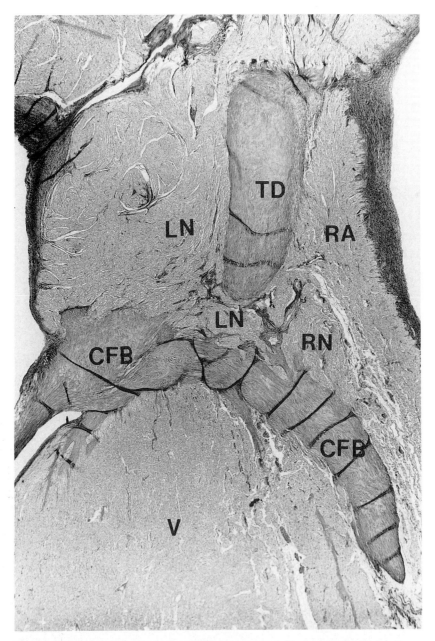

Figure 8-164: Double AV node within the central fibrous body. Weigert-van Gieson stain ×19.5. RN = right-sided AV node; LN = left-sided AV node; RA = right atrium; TD = tendon of Todaro; V = ventricular septum; CFB = central fibrous body.

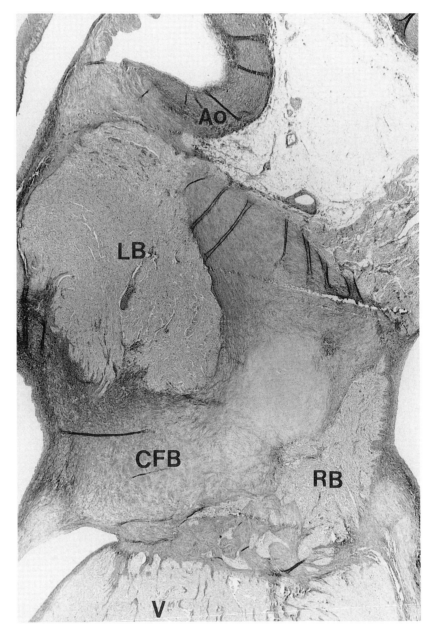

Figure 8-165: Two His bundles within the central fibrous body. Weigert-van Gieson stain ×19.5. CFB = central fibrous body; RB = small right-sided bundle; LB = large left-sided bundle; V = summit of the ventricular septum.

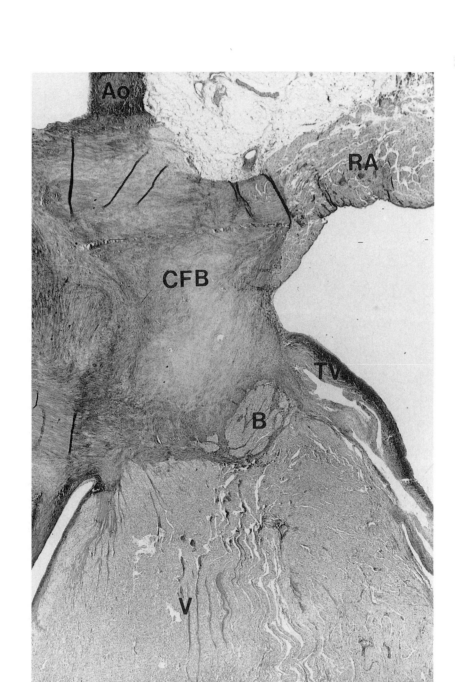

Figure 8-166: Small right-sided septated bundle. Weigert-van Gieson stain ×19.5. CFB = central fibrous body; RA = right atrium; B = small right-sided bundle; Ao = Aorta; V = summit of ventricular septum; TV = tricuspid valve.

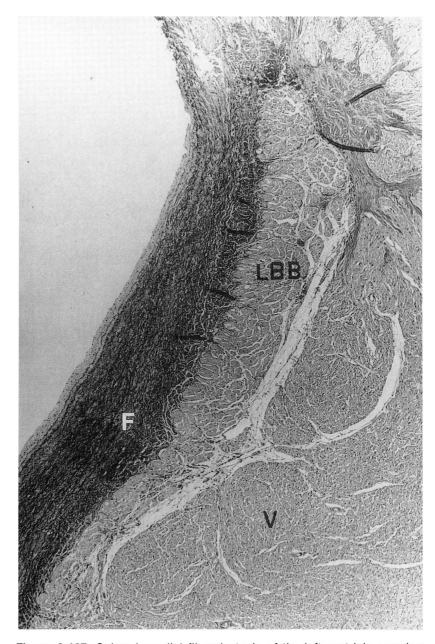

Figure 8-167: Subendocardial fibroelastosis of the left ventricle pressing on the discrete large left bundle branch. Weigert-van Gieson stain ×54. F = fibroelastosis; V = left ventricle; LBB = left bundle branch.

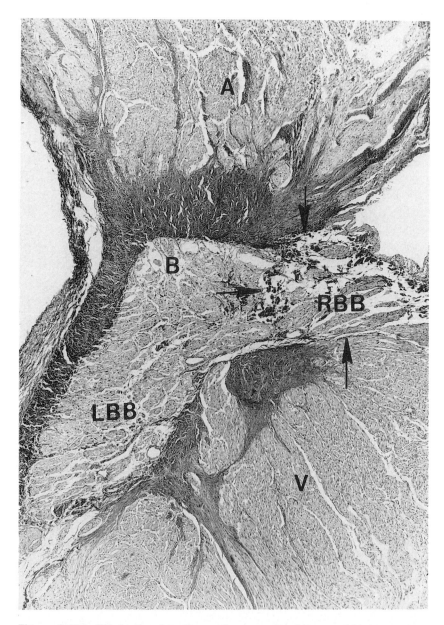

Figure 8-168: Bifurcating bundle on the summit of the ventricular septum. Weigert-van Gieson stain ×54. B = bundle; LBB = left bundle branch; RBB = right bundle branch; V = ventricular septal musculature; A = atrial muscle. The arrows point to the fibrosis of the right bundle branch.

Microscopic Examination: Positive Findings

SA Node

Arteriolosclerosis was present.

Approaches to SA Node

Mononuclear cells were present in the approaches.

AV Node and Bundle of His

The central fibrous body was divided into several segments. The atrioventricular node was present within one of the segments. It was situated on either side of the tendon of Todaro. Thus, part of the node was on the right side and part was on the left side (Fig. 8-164). The left-sided node was quite large. In addition, the central fibrous body had masses of normal atrial tissue. The left-sided node became a left-sided bundle (Fig. 8-165). In the beginning, it was quite large. The right-sided node became a right-sided bundle and was quite small (Fig 8-165). Both bundles showed marked fibrosis. The right-sided bundle was very small and markedly septated, with fibrosis (Fig 8-166). Eventually, this became the branching bundle.

Left Bundle Branch

This showed fibrosis and was pressed on by the fiberoelastosis of the left ventricle (Fig. 8-167).

Bifurcating Bundle

This was on the summit of the ventricular septum. (Fig. 8-168)

Discussion

In this fascinating case, the heart had two AV nodes and two bundles. The left-sided AV node and the bundle were quite large. It was therefore conceivable that impulses could have reached both nodes and the bundles which might be responsible for re-entry phenomenon and junctional tachycardia. The other abnormal findings, such as the markedly septated right-sided bundle, could have contributed to the arrhythmia and sudden death.

CASE #59[206]

A 22-year-old white female nurse died suddenly at work. She was diagnosed as hav-

ing intractable junctional tachycardia with intervening normal sinus rhythm since the age of 10 weeks. She experienced syncope at age 13 and was diagnosed as having sick sinus syndrome. A VVI pacemaker was inserted.

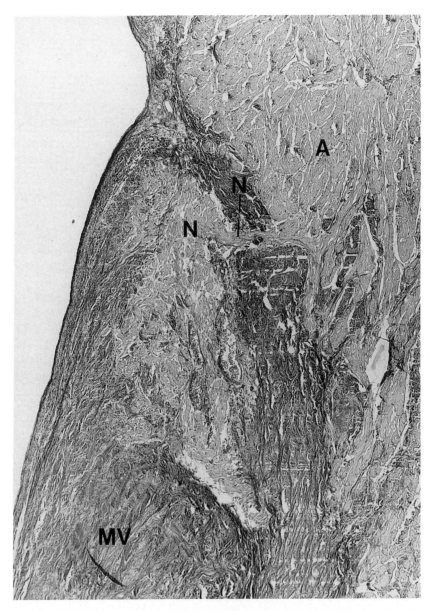

Figure 8-169: Node-like cells from the mitral valve, joining the atrial muscle. Weigert-van Gieson stain ×60. MV = annulus of mitral valve; N = node-like cells; A = atrial muscle.

ECG

At age 19, an intranodal re-entry pathway was documented for her supraventricular tachycardia. There were no bypass tracts. The supraventricular tachycardia proved to be unresponsive to verapamil, digoxin, Pronestyl, quinidine, Inderal, and amiodarone.

Cardiac Catheterization

The coronaries were normal and the left ventricular ejection fraction was 25%. A myocardial biopsy at that time was negative. The supraventricular tachycardia was interrupted by pacing at electrophysiological studies. A Holter monitor at that time revealed 5,000 premature ventricular contractions and 180 runs of supraventricular tachycardia and sinus pauses of up to 18 seconds. Amiodarone was started and she was asymptomatic. She was admitted 2 years later for catheter ablation of the AV node.

ECG

Supraventricular tachycardia at the rate of 120/min with inverted T-waves in leads 2, 3, and aVF was present.

Catheter AV node ablation was attempted twice with 200 watt seconds. This resulted in transient complete heart block after each event. The patient then developed normal sinus rhythm with first-degree block and Mobitz type I block after the first ablation, and then normal sinus rhythm with first-degree AV block past the second ablation. The supraventricular tachycardia redeveloped. The patient underwent repeat AV nodal ablation with temporary production of complete heart block which eventually resulted in slow supraventricular tachycardia with the right bundle branch block pattern at the rate of 120/min. Flecainide was begun with the hope that the partially ablated AV node would have greater effects on suppressing the supraventricular tachycardia. Four months later, she still had palpitations but was otherwise asymptomatic.

The first cryoprobic ablation of the AV node resulted in complete heart block and the area was surgically dissected. It became apparent that intermittent retrograde conduction was persisting, thereby mandating a deeper dissection. Ventricular pacing was performed while both atria were mapped, and it was determined that the earliest activation was in the low mid-septal atrium, just above the AV node. This was consistent with a retrograde fiber of the AV node rather than a bypass tract. She recovered uneventfully from the surgical ablation of the AV node and went back to her standard nursing duties, including lifting of patients. Seven months later, her DDD unipolar Medtronic pacemaker was checked and was found to be functioning normally. Eight days later, she suddenly collapsed and was found to be in ventricular fibrillation and could not be resuscitated.

Pathology: Gross

The heart was enlarged.

Microscopic Examination: Positive Findings

AV Node and Its Approaches

The AV node was surgically ablated with marked fibrosis, fatty infiltration, and chronic inflammatory cells in the right atrium and atrial septum. Node-like cells from the mitral valve annulus jointed the atrial muscle (Fig. 8-169).

AV Bundle, Penetrating

A small piece of penetrating bundle first appeared within the central fibrous body and showed marked fibrosis.

AV Bundle, Branching

This showed marked fibrosis. The branching bundle was situated on the left ventricular side (Fig. 8-170).

AV Bundle, Bifurcating

This bifurcated in the central fibrous body on the left side. This again showed marked fibrosis.

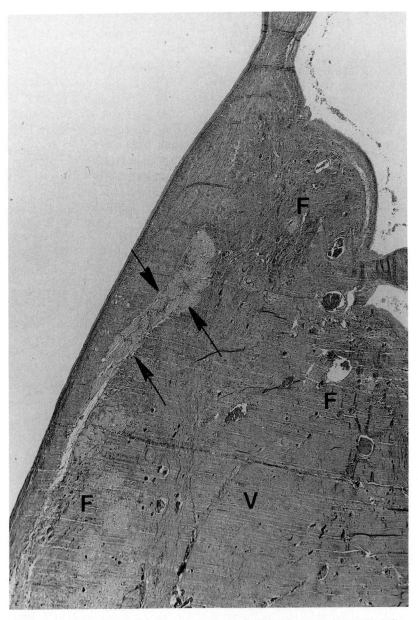

Figure 8-170: Fibrosis of the ventricular septum and left-sided bundle. Weigert-van Gieson stain ×22.5. F = fibrosis; V = ventricular septum. The arrows point to the left-sided bundle with fibrosis.

Left Bundle Branch

The left bundle branch was pushed down into the ventricular septum by ventricular muscle. This showed marked fibrosis and fragmentation (Figs 8-171, 8-172).

Right Bundle Branch

This showed marked fibrosis of the first and second parts. It then proceeded through the fibrotic area on the right side, showing marked fibrosis.

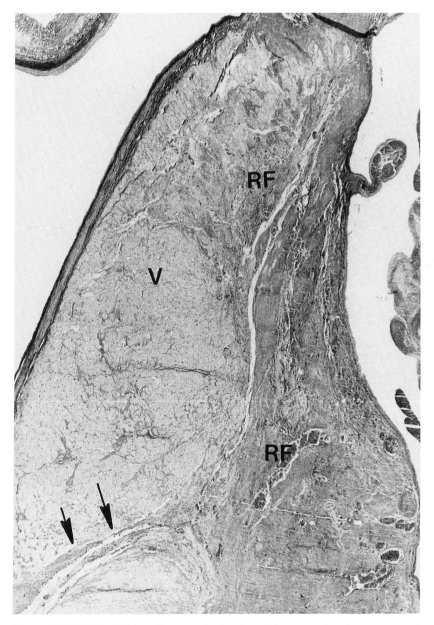

Figure 8-171: The left bundle branch displaced downward and compressed by ventricular septal muscle. Weigert-van Gieson stain ×22.5. V = ventricular septal muscle; RF = marked fibrosis of the right side of the septum. The arrows point to the fibrosed left bundle branch being compressed by the ventricular septal muscle.

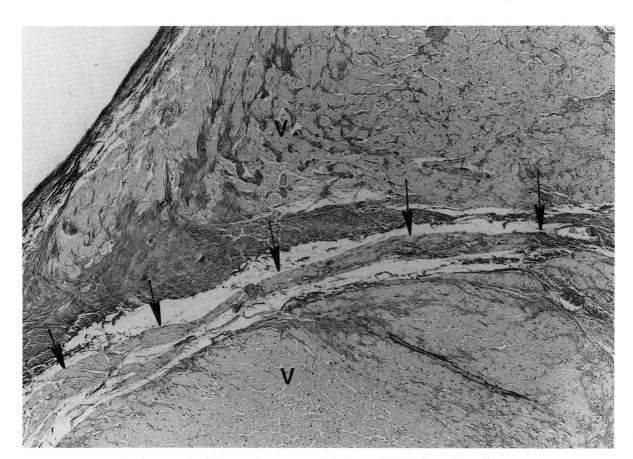

Figure 8-172: The left bundle branch being compressed by the ventricular septal muscle. Higher power view of Figure 8-171. Weigert-van Gieson stain ×60. V = ventricular septal muscle. The arrows point to the fibrosed left bundle branch.

Discussion

The node-like cells from the mitral valve which joined the atrial septum probably were responsible for junctional tachycardia. In addition, the bundle was left-sided and fibrosed. The marked inflammatory changes surrounding the suture in the atria could conceivably have formed a milieu for arrhythmogenicity following the surgical ablation and the previous several attempts at ablation.

Thus, in three cases of junctional tachycardia, there were anatomic abnormalities of the AV junction. This strongly suggests that there is an anatomic base for this type of arrhythmia.

CASE #60

A healthy 31-year-old woman, gravida II, para 0, delivered a full-term stillborn infant 3 days prior to the estimated due date. The day before the delivery, the mother had colicky abdominal pain and catheterized urinalysis showed hematuria, pyuria, and bacteremia. Liver enzymes showed increased alkaline phosphatase of 243 and increased SGOT of 120. The pain resolved. The clinical diagnosis included possible hepatitis, pre-eclampsia, or pyelonephritis. Fetal heart tones were 140 the day before delivery. Seven hours before delivery, fetal heart tones were not found.

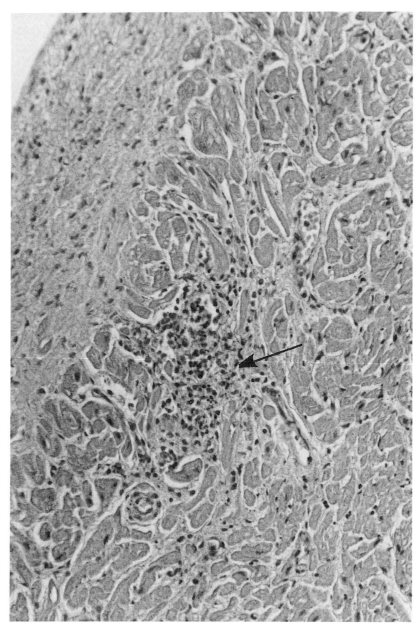

Figure 8-173: Myocarditis. Hematoxylin-eosin stain ×300. The arrow points to myocarditis.

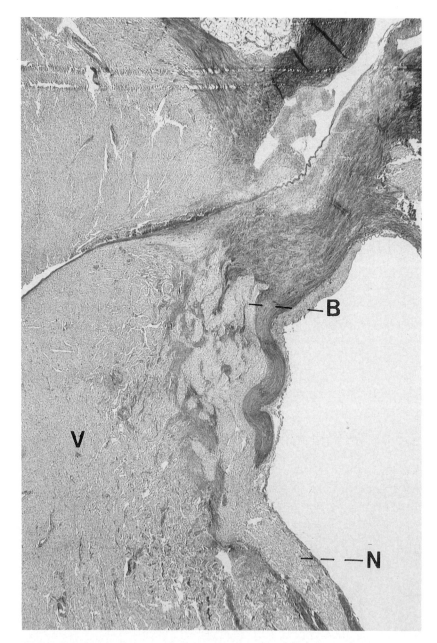

Figure 8-174: Marked lobulation and fragmentation of the bundle. Weigert-van Gieson stain ×30. V = ventricular septal muscle; B = bundle showing fragmentation; N = AV node.

Pathology: Gross

No evidence of anomalies or gross anatomic cause of death were found in this normal-term stillborn. The heart was greatly enlarged, weighing 248 grams (normal full-term, 17 grams).

Microscopic Examination: Positive Findings

Acute myocarditis (Fig. 8-173) with atypical abscesses with massive hemorrhages along the coronary arteries was found. There was marked lobulation and fragmentation of the bundle (Fig. 8-174).

Discussion

The cause of death in this fetus was probably myocarditis. However, the marked lobulation and fragmentation of the bundle of His cannot be overlooked.

CASE #61

A 6-year-old black female was brought to the emergency room by a rescue team after having been found unresponsive for 4 to 5 minutes at school. In the emergency room, she was sleepy but awake.

ECG

Ventricular tachycardia was revealed and the tachycardia degenerated into fibrillation, and she died.

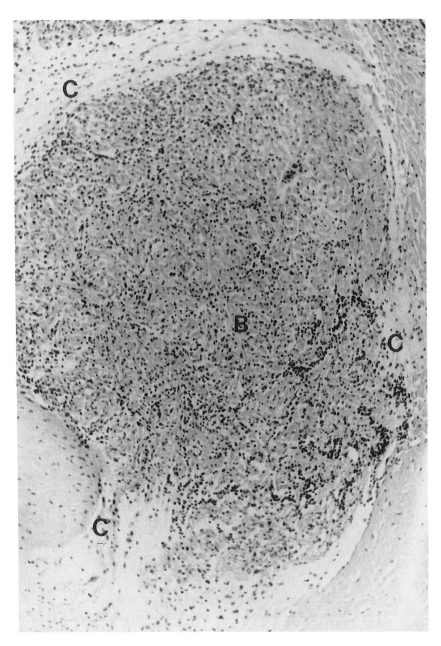

Figure 8-175: Penetrating bundle showing frank myocarditis. Hematoxylin-eosin stain ×120. B = penetrating bundle; C = central fibrous body.

Pathology: Gross

Bilateral pleural effusion, ascites, and marked congestion of lungs, liver, spleen, and kidneys were present. The heart was enlarged, weighing 145 grams.

Microscopic Examination: Positive Findings

Approaches to the AV Node

A real myocarditis was present.

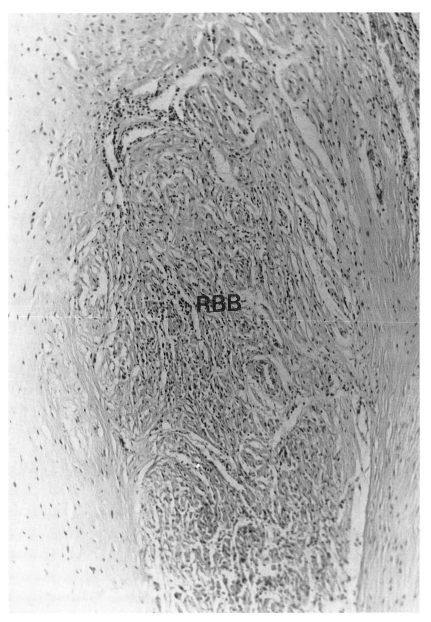

Figure 8-176: Right bundle branch showing frank myocarditis. Hematoxylin-eosin stain ×120. RBB = right bundle branch.

AV Node, Bundle, and Bundle Branches

A frank myocarditis was present (Figs. 8-175, 8-176).

Summit of the Ventricular Septum

Intense myocarditis was present.

Both Ventricles

An intense myocarditis was present.

Discussion

This child died suddenly with a severe myocarditis involving the ventricles, ventricular septum, and the conduction system. Ventricular arrhythmias are known to occur in myocarditis.

CASE #62

This case was a 17-year-old healthy Marine who died suddenly while talking to his girlfriend on the telephone. It was reported that there was a storm with lightening at the time when he was talking on the telephone, and therefore the question of electrocution was raised. The heart was sent to us in blocks, with some pieces of the tissue.

Microscopic Examination: Positive Findings

Approaches to the AV Node

Fibrosis was present.

Atrioventricular Node

This was partly embedded in the tricuspid annulus.

Bundle of His, Bifurcation

Fatty metamorphosis on the right side up to the right bundle branch was noted. Fibrosis of the penetrating bundle was present. Hemorrhage in the left side of the bifurcation was in evidence (Figs. 8-177, 8-178).

Left Bundle Branch

Hemorrhage in the left bundle branch was in evidence. The Purkinje fibers were distinctly smaller than normal (Fig. 8-178).

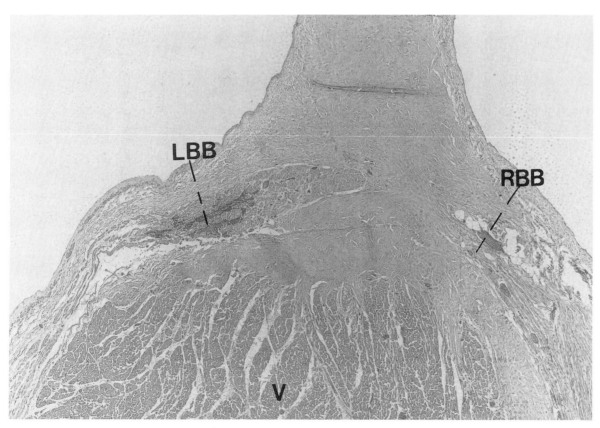

Figure 8-177: Bifurcation showing hemorrhage in the left bundle branch and fatty metamorphosis of the right bundle branch. Hematoxylin-eosin stain ×45. LBB = left bundle branch; RBB = right bundle branch; V = ventricular septal muscle.

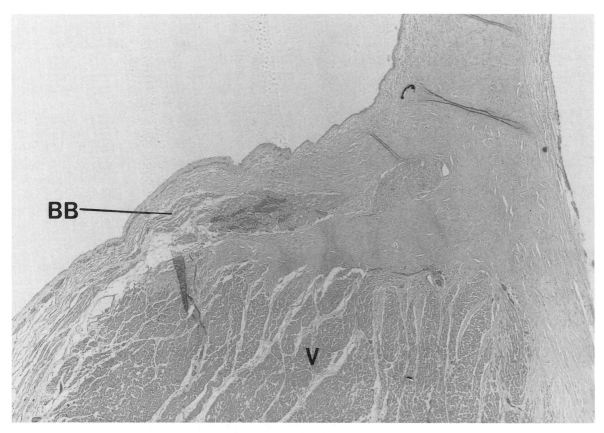

Figure 8-178: Left bundle branch showing hemorrhage and smallness of cells. Hematoxylin-eosin stain ×45. BB = branching bundle; V = ventricular septal muscle.

Summit of the Ventricular Septum

There was focal degeneration of cells.

Myocardium

Hemorrhage was present in the epicardium. There was fibrosis of the trabecular area of the right ventricle and ventricular septum.

Discussion

The hemorrhage in the left bundle branch may be incriminated in the sudden death of this Marine. However, one cannot overlook (1) the partial embedding of the AV node in the tricuspid valve annulus, (2) the fibrosis of the AV node, and (3) the fatty metamorphosis of the first part of the right bundle branch. It is possible that the hemorrhage occurred as a result of electrocution. It is also possible that the above pathological findings made the conduction system vulnerable for electrocution and/or arrhythmia.

CASE #63

A 24-year-old male was found dead lying on the couch. He had been watching television while lying on the couch, and he appeared normal. He had a history of pharyngitis and tonsillitis 2 years earlier, and had herpes a year before, as well as genital herpes and venereal warts. A complete toxicology screen was negative for any drugs or alcohol.

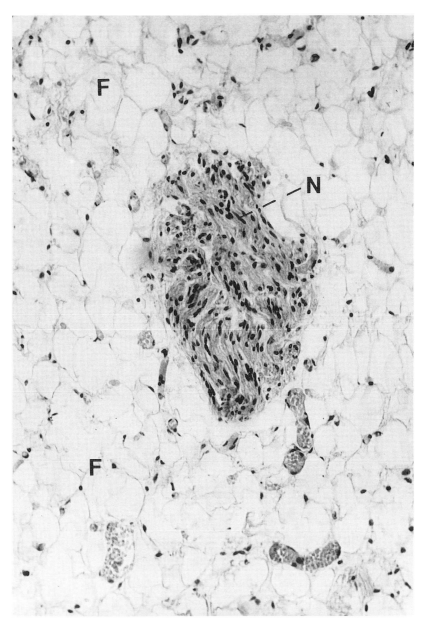

Figure 8-179: The nerve near the SA node showing inflammation. Hematoxylin-eosin stain ×120. N = nerve; F = fat tissue.

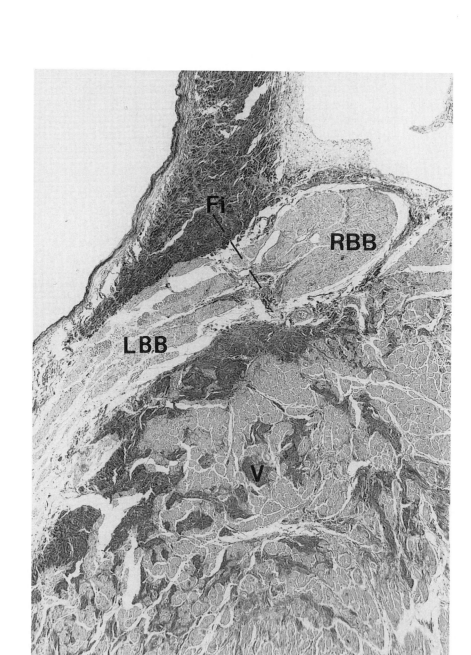

Figure 8-180: Marked fibrosis of the junction of the right bundle branch side of bifurcation with the left. Note also the marked fibrosis of the summit of the ventricular septum. Weigert-van Gieson stain × 48. LBB = left bundle branch; RBB = right bundle branch; V = ventricular septal muscle; Fi = fibrosis.

Pathology: Gross

The gross pathology was unremarkable. The heart weighed 360 grams.

Microscopic Examination: Positive Findings

Approaches to the SA Node

Neuritis was seen (Fig. 8-179).

Branching Bundle

Marked fibrosis of the junction of the right bundle branch side of bifurcation with the left was present (Fig. 8-180).

Left Bundle Branch

This showed fibrosis at the beginning.

Summit of the Ventricular Septum

Marked patchy fibrosis was seen.

Discussion

The main features of this case are the neuritis and the marked fibrosis of the summit of the ventricular septum. The marked fibrosis of the summit can effect the bifurcating part of the bundle.

CASE #64

This healthy 15-year-old youngster had an appendectomy and did well throughout the surgery. Following the surgical procedure, he opened his eyes, was responsive, and was extubated. In the recovery room, there was a brief period of hypotension and the patient was found to be not breathing and could not be resuscitated.

Pathology: Gross

The gross pathology was unremarkable. The heart was enlarged, weighing 434 grams. There was an accessory tricuspid orifice with possible tricuspid insufficiency. The left coronary ostium emerged higher than usual. The ventricular septum presented a bulge at the region of the septal leaflet.

Microscopic Examination: Positive Findings

SA Node and Its Approaches

These showed inflammatory cells around the SA node.

Approaches to the AV Node and the AV Node

Fatty infiltration was present in the approaches. The AV node showed many mononuclear cells (Fig. 8-181).

AV Bundle, Penetrating Portion

This was segmented (Fig. 8-182).

AV Bundle, Branching Portion

This part was abbreviated and markedly segmented with marked hemorrhage (Fig. 8-183) and was divided into two large components. The larger one on the right joined the right side of the ventricular septum. Further down, both the right and left components joined together. What was situated to the right became the right bundle branch.

Left Bundle Branch

In the beginning, the bundle had three components which came together. This showed marked hemorrhage (Fig. 8-184).

Right Bundle Branch

The right bundle branch was quite large and intramyocardial and was divided into two large segments.

Summit of the Ventricular Septum

This showed marked fibrosis on the left side with arteriolosclerosis (Fig. 8-182) and myocardial disarray.

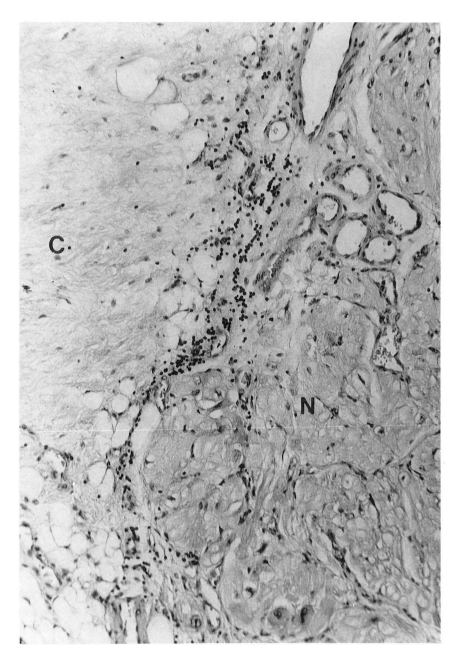

Figure 8-181: Inflammatory cells surrounding the AV node. Hematoxylin-eosin stain ×120. N = AV node; C = central fibrous body.

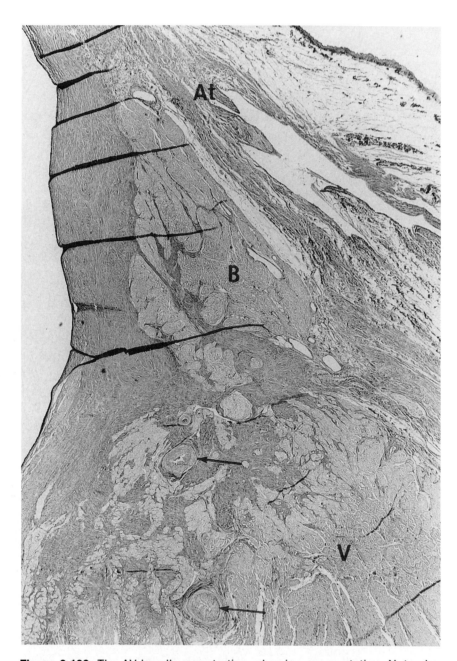

Figure 8-182: The AV bundle, penetrating, showing segmentation. Note also the fibrosis and arteriolosclerosis of the left side of the summit of the ventricular septum. Weigert-van Gieson stain ×30. B = AV bundle; At = atrial musculature; V = ventricular septal muscle. The arrows point to the arteriolosclerosis.

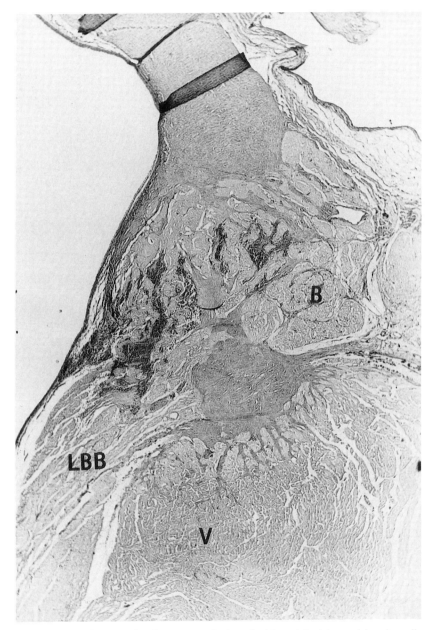

Figure 8-183: The markedly segmented and abbreviated branching bundle showing marked hemorrhage. Weigert-van Gieson stain ×36. B = branching bundle with marked hemorrhage; LBB = large posterior radiation of left bundle branch showing hemorrhage; V = ventricular septal muscle.

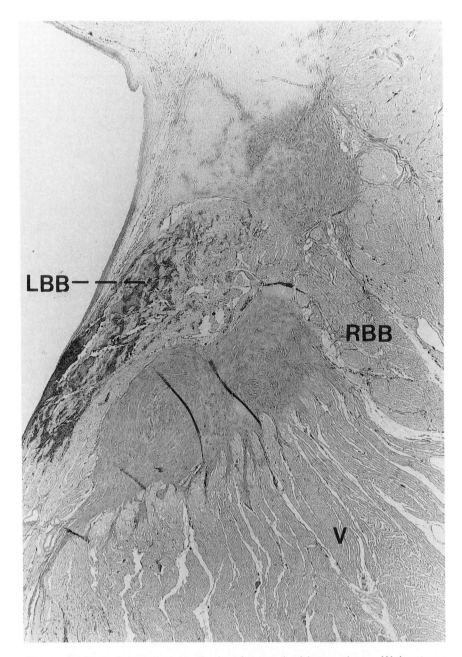

Figure 8-184: Left bundle branch showing marked hemorrhage. Weigert-van Gieson stain ×36. LBB = posterior radiation of left bundle branch showing marked hemorrhage; RBB = right bundle branch; V = ventricular septal muscle.

Discussion

There was an abnormally formed branching bundle and large posterior radiation. Both of these showed marked hemorrhage. In addition, the AV nodal area and perinodal area showed mononuclear cells. These could have been related to sudden death.

CASE #65

This case was a 25-year-old police officer who, while running along the boardwalk in New Jersey, collapsed and died suddenly. A few months previously, he had taken the departmental test and passed with a perfect score. He was considering a move to Florida and needed a certification for running 12 minutes. After several minutes of warm-up, he ran for 1¼ miles in 9.37 minutes. Then he slowed down, fell backwards, and collapsed. Despite immediate cardiopulmonary resuscitation, he died.

He had been a diabetic since the age of 2 years and was on insulin. It was indicated in his history that his diabetes was not well controlled. In addition, he had some marital problems.

Pathology: Gross

Pulmonary edema and congestion and cerebral edema and congestion were found. The heart weighed 440 grams. The tricuspid and the mitral valves were redundant, thickened, and large, with probable tricuspid and/or mitral insufficiency, with mild to moderate segmental coarctation of the aorta.

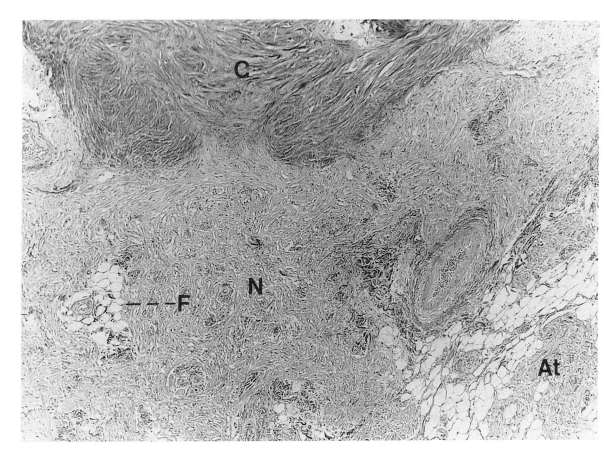

Figure 8-185: The AV node showing fatty infiltration of the approaches and in the node. Weigert-van Gieson stain ×45. N = AV node showing fatty metamorphosis; At = atrial musculature; C = central fibrous body; F = fatty metamorphosis.

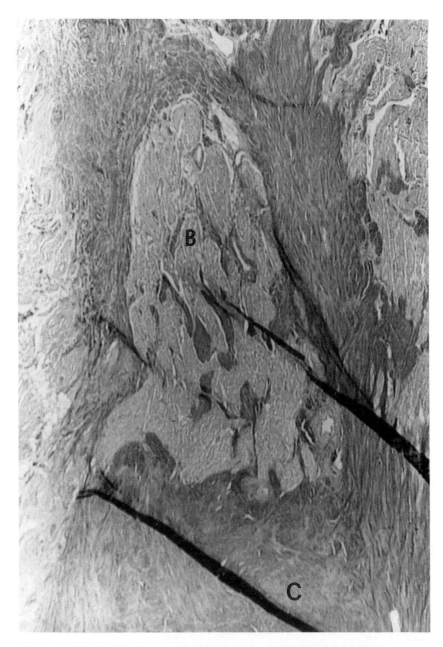

Figure 8-186: Markedly septated bundle of His. Weigert-van Gieson stain ×45. B = AV bundle; At = atrial musculature; V = ventricular septal muscle.

Microscopic Examination: Positive Findings

AV Node and Its Approaches

Fatty infiltration was present in and around the AV node with a tenuous connection to the surrounding atrial muscle (Fig. 8-185).

AV Bundle, Penetrating Portion

This was markedly septated (Fig. 8-186).

AV Bundle, Branching Portion

This was on the left side and showed fibrosis.

Summit of the Ventricular Septum

Arteriolosclerosis was apparent.

Discussion

The significant finding is the marked fatty infiltration of the atrioventricular node, creating loop-like formation within the node. The septated bundle may also be implicated in the sudden death.

CASE #66

This 31-year-old black female was a schizophrenic inmate at the Graystone Park Psychiatric Hospital, New Jersey, and was found unconscious and unresponsive on the bathroom floor by a patient. During the immediate resuscitative attempts, she was found to be in ventricular fibrillation with idioventricular rhythm, and despite defibrillation, she could not be resuscitated.

She had a history of drug abuse and her schizophrenia had been attributed to "angel dust." She had been on Thorazine, 200 mg tid for some time and also Symmetrel (amantadine hydrochloride) for only one day. She had spoken to her family shortly before going to the bathroom and was her normal self at that time. She had showed no evidence of an overdose of either Thorazine or of a "hard drug."

Pathology: Gross

The patient was obese. The heart weighed 300 grams. There was right atrial enlargement with diffuse thickening of the tricuspid valve.

Microscopic Examination: Positive Findings

Atrial Septum

Fatty infiltration was evident.

AV Node

Chronic myocarditis was evident (Figs. 8-187, 8-188).

AV Bundle, Penetrating

In the beginning, there was a moderate infiltration of mononuclear cells with moderate fibrosis and fatty infiltration (Fig. 8-189).

AV Bundle Branching

This showed moderate to marked fibrosis (Fig. 8-190).

Left Bundle Branch

Fibrosis was in evidence. The cells in the beginning were small with degeneration and fibrosis.

Ventricular Walls

There was a moderate infiltration of mononuclear cells.

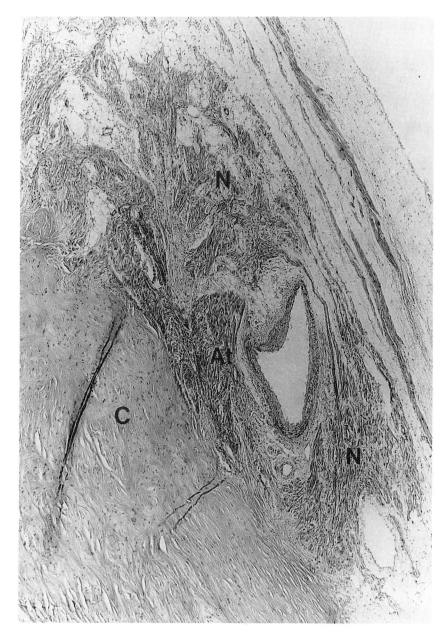

Figure 8-187: Myocarditis of the AV node. Hematoxylin-eosin stain ×45. N = AV node; At = atrial musculature; C = central fibrous body.

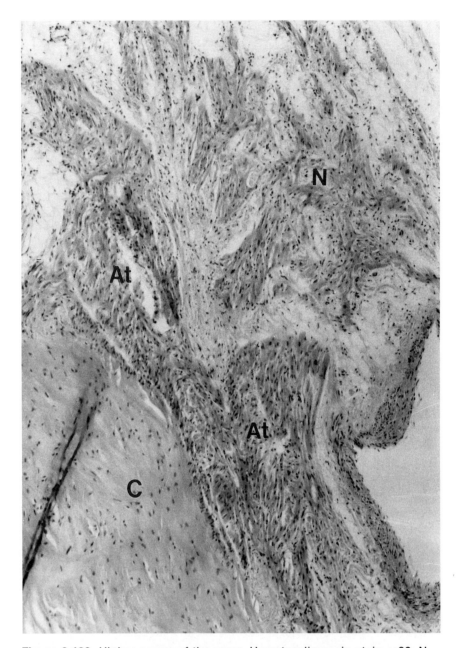

Figure 8-188: Higher power of the same. Hematoxylin-eosin stain ×90. N = AV node; At = atrial musculature; C = central fibrous body.

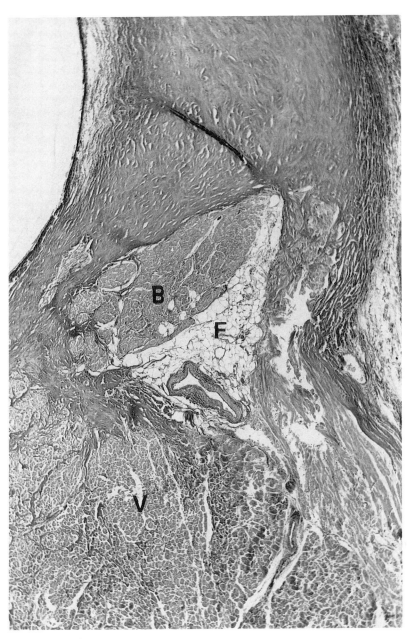

Figure 8-189: Penetrating bundle showing fatty infiltration. Hematoxylin-eosin stain ×45. B = bundle; F = fat tissue; V = ventricular septal muscle.

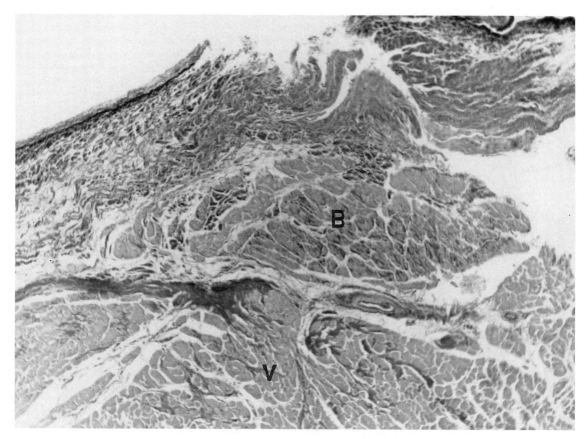

Figure 8-190: Branching bundle showing moderate fibrosis. Weigert-van Gieson stain ×75. B = bundle; V = ventricular septal muscle.

Discussion

This is an abnormal conduction system with a myocarditis of the AV node and ventricular walls with fibrosis of the AV bundle. The effect of "drug abuse" and the medications upon the conduction system is not known today.

CASE #67[208]

A 44-year-old active businessman who played racquetball and walked 1 to 2 miles per day died suddenly. Earlier, during a routine physical examination, he was noted to have left bundle branch block and occasional 2:1 atrioventricular block. He had been treated with hydrochlorothiazide and propranolol (20 mg qid) for hypertension. His father died at the age of 48 of what was thought to be a heart attack.

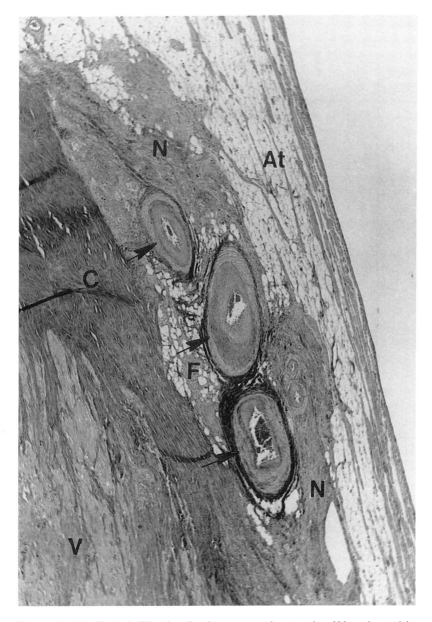

Figure 8-191: Fatty infiltration in the approaches to the AV node and in the AV node, with marked arteriolosclerosis of the branches of the ramus septi fibrosi. Weigert-van Gieson stain ×30. N = AV node; V = ventricular septal muscle; C = central fibrous body; At = atrial myocardium converted into fat; F = fatty tissue. The arrows point to arteriolosclerotic vessels.

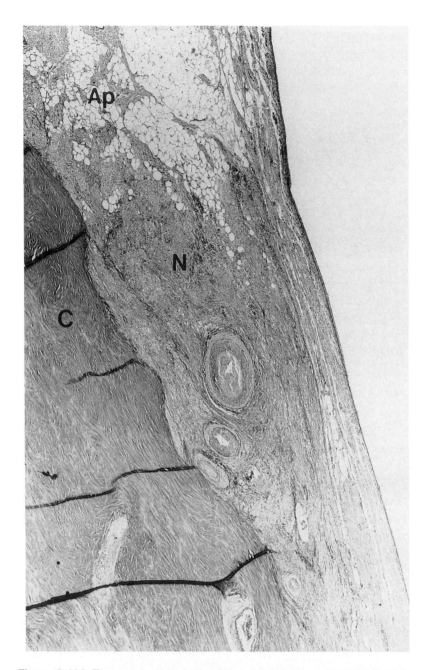

Figure 8-192: The approaches to the AV node and the node. Note the fatty metamorphosis of the approaches and of the node and the atherosclerosis of the branches of the ramus septi fibrosi. Weigert-van Gieson stain ×30. N = node showing fibrosis, atherosclerosis, and fatty metamorphosis; C = central fibrous body; Ap = approaches showing fatty metamorphosis.

ECG

This revealed a PR of 0.28 sec, a QRS of 0.17 sec, a QT of 0.42 sec, and a pattern of left bundle branch block. A review of rhythm strips revealed sinus pauses compatible with sinoatrial exit block.

Coronary angiography revealed coronary artery irregularity with no stenosis. An inferior wall hypokinesis and ejection fraction of 0.50 and a normal left ventricular end-diastolic volume index were found in the ventricular angiography.

An endomyocardial biopsy was performed

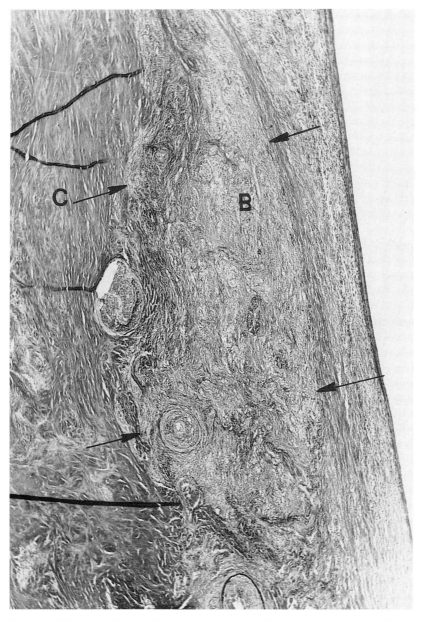

Figure 8-193: The AV bundle showing marked fibrosis with chronic inflammation. Weigert-van Gieson stain ×45. B = penetrating AV bundle showing fibrosis and arteriolosclerosis; C = central fibrous body. The arrows demarcate the penetrating bundle.

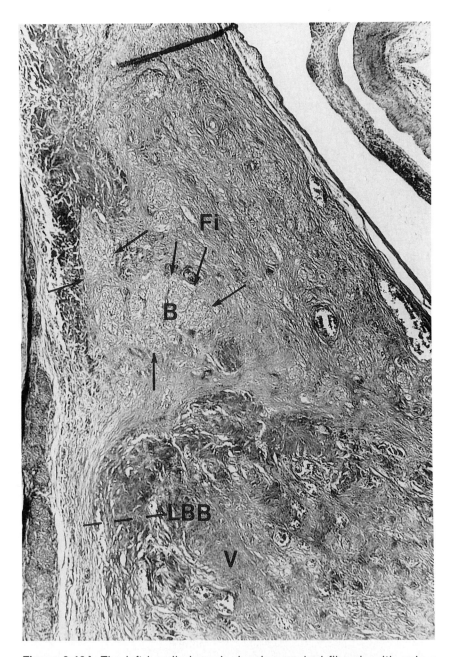

Figure 8-194: The left bundle branch showing marked fibrosis with only a remnant of bundle remaining. Weigert-van Gieson stain ×30. LBB = left bundle branch; B = branching bundle; Fi = fibrotic replacement of bundle; V = ventricular septal muscle showing marked fibrosis. The arrows point to the remainder of the bundle.

which showed solitary granuloma with central necrosis and giant cells and lymphocytes. Subsequent staining and culture for acid bacilli and fungi were not remarkable.

EPS

This revealed prolonged AH time with a normal HV interval (40 ms). There was spontaneous sinoatrial pauses compatible with sinoatrial exit block. Right ventricular extrastimulus testing induced two repetitive ventricular responses.

Because of the granuloma and a reduced left ventricular performance, the patient was started on prednisone, 16 mg per day, and this was tapered to 20 mg per day. One month later, while asymptomatic, the patient had a

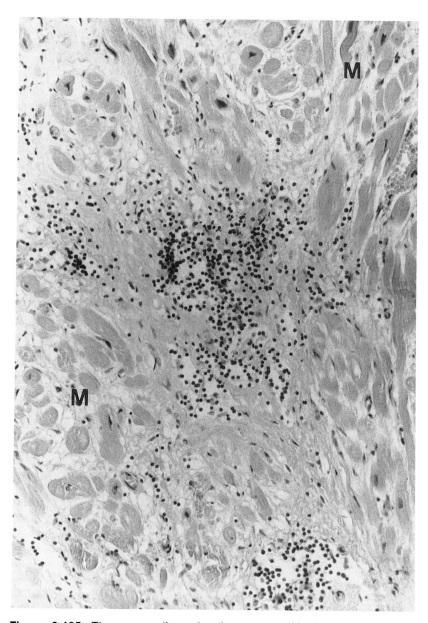

Figure 8-195: The myocardium showing myocarditis. Hematoxylin-eosin stain ×225. M = myocardium.

repeat Holter monitor which revealed three to four beat runs of ventricular ectopic beats. The PR interval was 0.21 seconds and there were no sinoatrial pauses or AV block demonstrated. Two months later, the patient was due back for a repeat biopsy and electrophysiological studies when he died suddenly.

Pathology: Gross

The heart was enlarged, weighing 450 grams. There were whitish scar areas in the anterior wall of the right ventricle and along the interventricular septum and posterior wall of the left ventricle.

Microscopic Examination: Positive Findings

SA Node and Its Approaches

The SA node was replaced by fibrous tissue and fat.

Atrial Septum

The right side showed fibrosis.

AV Node and Its Approaches

Fatty infiltration was evident in the approaches. There was marked arteriosclerosis of the branches of the ramus septi fibrosi. The node showed marked fibrosis and fatty metamorphosis (Figs. 8-191, 8-192).

AV Bundle

This showed marked fibrosis with chronic inflammation (Fig. 8-193).

Right Bundle Branch

Marked fibrosis was also seen here, with practically no right bundle remaining.

Left Bundle Branch

The left bundle branch was partially fibrotic (Fig. 8-194).

Myocardium

Chronic inflammation of the entire myocardium (Fig. 8-195) was in evidence both in the right and the left ventricles with fibrosis.

Discussion

This patient had multiple abnormalities such as fat, myocarditis, fibrosis, and arteriolosclerosis in the conduction system. This ultimately led to his death.

CASE #68²⁰⁸

This 22-year-old active, healthy, full-time college student died suddenly in his classroom. His medical history was unremarkable except that he had a history of palpitations. The cause of the symptoms had never been documented and he had never been treated. There was no history of drug use or abuse. His father and brother also had palpitations. His brother is 21-year-old and at age 15 was seen by his pediatrician for some chest discomfort; the electrocardiogram was normal. A follow-up of this patient is given below.

ECG

A year later, the electrocardiogram revealed frequent ventricular and supraventricular premature beats with couplets and triplets. The PR and QRS and QT intervals of his sinus beats were normal. He was given a trial of beta blockade (atenolol, 50 mg per day). A 24-hour rhythm monitoring, while on this drug, revealed three to five beat episodes of wide QRS tachyarrhythmias with some variation in RR intervals, the shortest being 380 ms. While on the beta blockade medication, there were episodes of atrial premature beats without ventricular response, of sinus pauses that were as long as 2½ seconds, sinus beats with no ventricular capture (Mobitz type II AV block could not be excluded on occasion), and paroxysmal episodes of atrial fibrillation with repeated 3–6 second pauses.

Cardiac Catherization

Because his brother had died suddenly, a cardiac catherization was done which revealed normal angiography and pressures.

An endomyocardial biopsy was performed which revealed no evidence of inflammation, hypertrophy, or fiber necrosis. There was some mild variation in size and shape of the nuclei. The electrophysiological testing showed no evidence of distal conduction system abnormalities nor was there any evidence of abnormal conduction distal to the His bundle.

Pathology: Gross

The heart was enlarged, weighing 417 grams. The tricuspid orifice was enlarged and the medial and inferior leaflets were divided off into several segments, and there was considerable thickening of the valve.

Microscopic Examination: Positive Findings

AV Bundle

This showed arteriolosclerosis.

Bundle Branches

Moderate fibrosis was present here.

Summit of the Ventricular Septum

There was marked fibrosis with arteriosclerosis and arteriolosclerosis, especially on the right side (Fig. 8-196).

Atria

These showed fibrosis with neuritis (Fig. 8-197).

Myocardium

Fatty infiltration, chronic inflammation, and fibrosis of the conus musculature of the right ventricle were in evidence (Fig. 8-198).

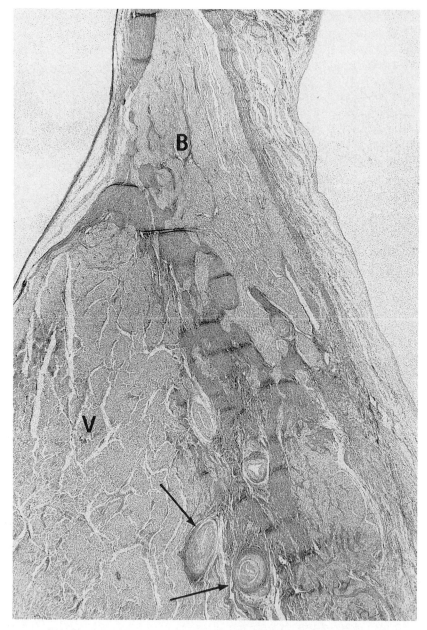

Figure 8-196: Summit of the ventricular septum showing marked fibrosis and arteriolosclerosis on the right side. Weigert-van Gieson stain ×19.5. B = bundle of His; V = ventricular septal muscle. The arrows point to arteriolosclerosis and fibrosis.

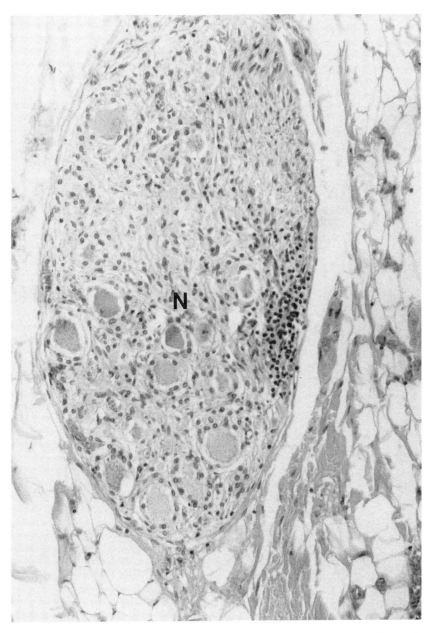

Figure 8-197: A nerve in the atrium showing inflammation. Hematoxylin-eosin stain ×150. N = nerve.

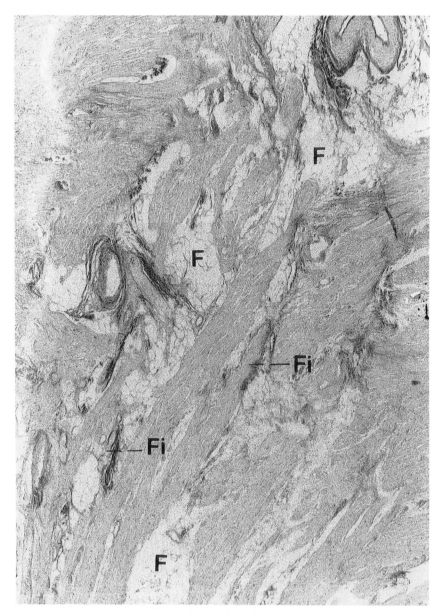

Figure 8-198: Fatty metamorphosis of the conus musculature of the right ventricle. Weigert-van Gieson stain ×30. F = fatty infiltration; Fi = fibrosis.

Discussion

This is a case of an individual coming from a family with palpitations. Outstanding is the fibrosis of the right side of the summit of the ventricular septum, the neuritis, and the fatty metamorphosis of the conal musculature. The familial history of palpitations, and the pathological findings of fibrosis of the summit of the ventricular septum on the *right side* suggest a genetically abnormally formed myocardium and/or the nerves.

CASE #69[208]

A 6-year-old female child with a history of ventricular dysrhythmia died suddenly.

She was born to a methadone mother who had evidence of intrauterine postnatal chaotic ventricular dysrhythmia which included paroxysmal ventricular tachycardia, ventricular fibrillation, varying degrees of AV block, and a prolonged QT interval. The infant was managed by transvenous ventricular pacing which controlled the rhythm disturbance by overdrive suppression. A permanent epicardial unipolar VVI pacemaker was implanted at 1 week of age. The patient had a stable course subsequently, with evidence of sinus rhythm.

EPS

This revealed normal AH, HV, sinus node recovery time at rest an on atrial pacing. Hemodynamic study was normal. Development of complete right bundle branch block with the left axis deviation was suggestive of a bifascicular disease. Seizures occurred with fever at age 5. Holter studies demonstrated normal pacemaker function and capture and no ventricular ectopy. Two weeks prior to her sudden death, a short self-terminated run of ventricular tachycardia was noted.

Pathology: Gross

Generalized visceral congestion, severe lymphadenopathy (and abdominal) marked lymphoid hypoplasia of the terminal ilium and appendix were also noted.

The heart was enlarged. The membranous part of the ventricular septum was quite abbreviated. The demand pacemaker unit was intact with no evidence of battery dysfunction. The hypertrophy involved both atria and the left ventricle. The left ventricle showed fibroelastosis.

Microscopic Examination: Positive Findings

Approaches to the SA Node

Mononuclear cells were adjacent to the SA node. Nerves were infiltrated with mononuclear cells.

Approaches to the AV Node

Nerves were infiltrated with mononuclear cells.

AV Node

This was situated in the central fibrous body (Fig. 8-199).

AV Bundle, Penetrating

The bundle was lobulated and showed moderate fibrosis and considerable space formation (Fig. 8-200).

AV Bundle, Branching

This showed moderate to marked fibrosis.

Bundle Branches

Moderate fibrosis was noted with space formation in the left bundle branch (Figs. 8-201, 8-202).

Summit of the Ventricular Septum

Fibrosis was present here.

Atrial Septum

Neuritis was noted here.

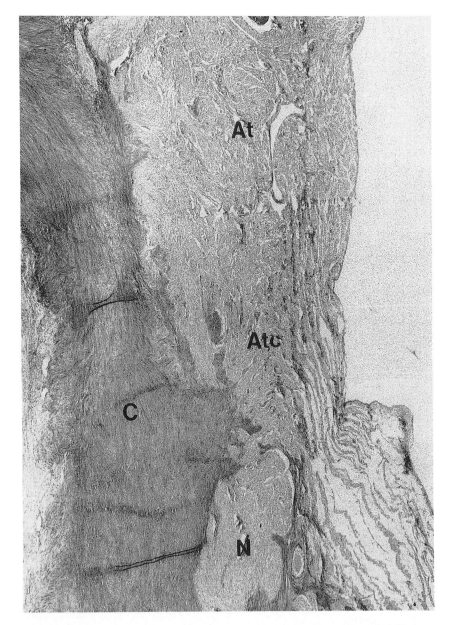

Figure 8-199: The AV node lying in the central fibrous body. Weigert-van Gieson stain ×30. At = atrial septal musculature; Atc = atrial muscle in the central fibrous body; N = AV node in the central fibrous body; C = central fibrous body.

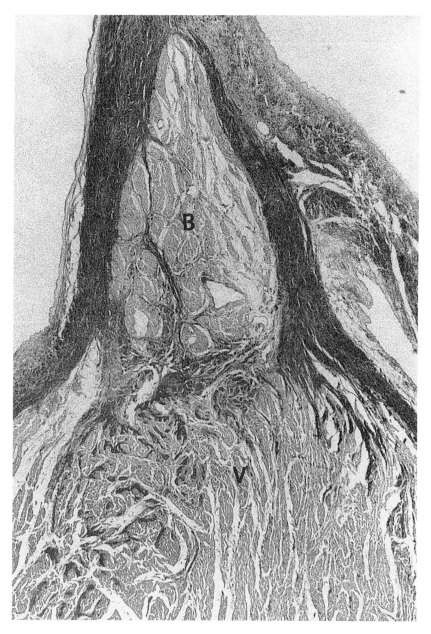

Figure 8-200: Penetrating bundle showing lobulation, moderate fibrosis and space formation. Weigert-van Gieson stain ×45. B = bundle; V = ventricular septal musculature.

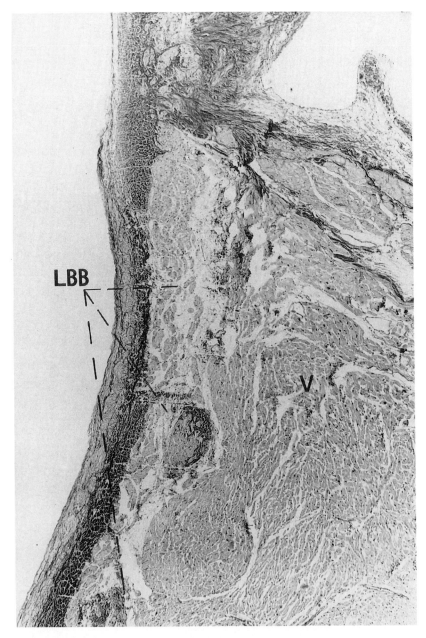

Figure 8-201: Left bundle branch showing fibrosis and space formation. Weigert-van Gieson stain ×45. LBB = left bundle branch; V = ventricular septal musculature.

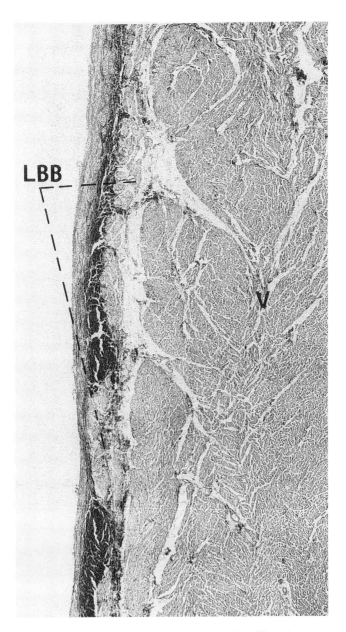

Figure 8-202: More distal area of LBB showing fibrosis and space formation. Weigert-van Gieson stain ×45. LBB = left bundle branch; V = ventricular septal muscle.

Discussion

This patient was the daughter of a mother on methadone. The abnormalities in the conduction system that may be related to her sudden death are: (1) the presence of the AV node in the central fibrous body; (2) the lobulation and space formation in the penetrating bundle; and (3) the fibrosis and space formation in the left bundle branch. The relationship of these abnormalities to the methadone addiction of the mother is unknown.

CASE #70[208]

This case was a 14-year-old female who was asymptomatic and died suddenly on the street while running with friends. She had a 6-year history of paroxysmal ventricular tachycardia, normal electrophysiological studies, and was free of ventricular dysrhythmia with propranolol therapy.

A brother with an identical condition had documented clinical and electrophysiological studies that showed evidence of catechol-induced ventricular premature beats and tachycardia.

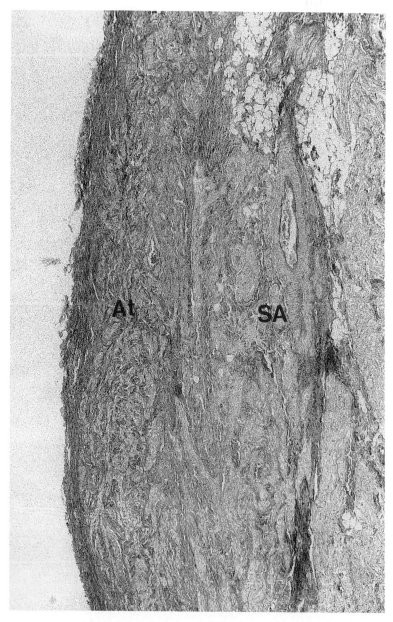

Figure 8-203: SA node showing marked fibrosis. Weigert-van Gieson stain ×45. SA = SA node; At = atrial musculature.

Pathology: Gross

The heart weighed 184 grams. There was a small aneurysm of the fossa ovalis. The membranous part of the ventricular septum extended more posteriorly than usual. The tricuspid valve was divided off into several segments. The anterolateral papillary muscle likewise was divided into several segments.

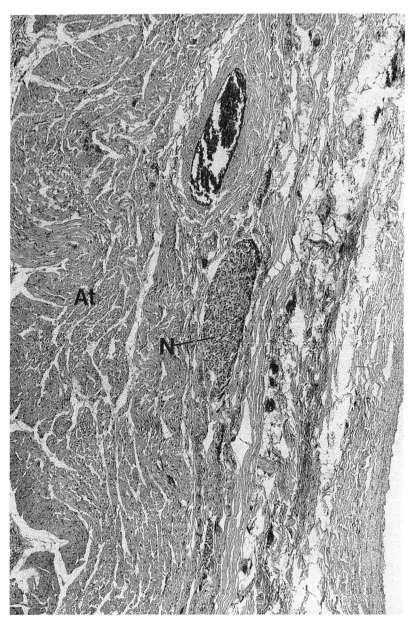

Figure 8-204: Chronic neuritis in atria. Hematoxylin-eosin stain ×61.5. N = nerve showing neuritis; At = atrial musculature.

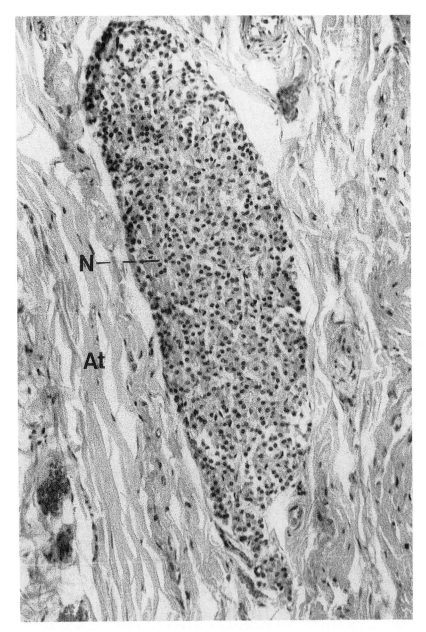

Figure 8-205: Higher power of nerve showing neuritis. Hematoxylin-eosin stain ×225. N = nerve; At = atrial musculature.

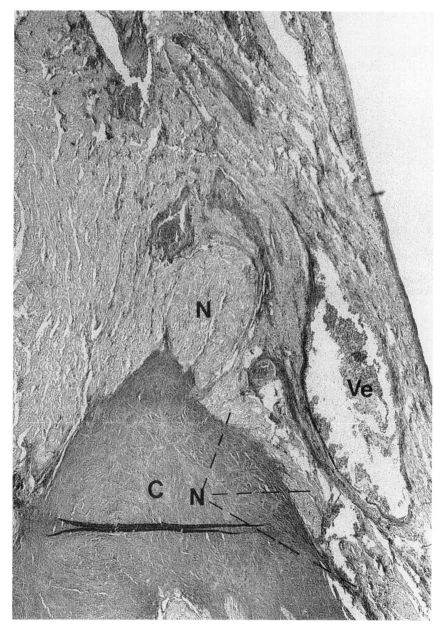

Figure 8-206: Probable pressure of the dilated vein upon the AV node. N = atrioventricular node; C = central fibrous body; Ve = dilated vein.

Microscopic Examination: Positive Findings

SA Node and Its Approaches

These showed fibrosis (Fig. 8-203).

Preferential Pathways and Atria

Fibrosis was present with chronic neuritis (Figs. 8-204, 8-205).

Approaches to the AV Node

The veins were dilated. There was possible pressure on the AV node (Fig. 8-206). Chronic epicarditis of the atria was also present.

AV Bundle, Branching

Moderate fatty metamorphosis with slight fibrosis was noted.

Left Bundle Branch

There was focal necrosis and narrowing of the diameter of some of the Purkinje cells.

Summit of the Ventricular Septum

Increased fibrosis of the left side of the summit was evident.

Myocardium

Basophilic degeneration of the aorta and mitral valve was seen.

Discussion

The thing that stands out in this case is the neuritis of the atria and the epicarditis of the atria. We do not know the cause of the ventricular tachycardia that she and her brother had. It is possible that they both showed the same neuritis. It is becoming apparent that the familial occurrence of abnormalities of the conduction system must be emphasized as a concept in itself. Since the brother showed evidence of catechol-induced ventricular premature beats, there might be a genetic tendency for susceptibility of the sympathetic nervous system which might have played a role in the sudden death of this child.

CASE #71

A 27-year-old medical student collapsed while jogging. Immediate resuscitative methods showed that he was in ventricular fibrillation. After defibrillation, he went into asystole and could not be resuscitated.

In the last year, he had complained of vague chest pains and was seen by a cardiologist. This consisted of dull sternal chest discomfort which usually occurred at rest. There was no association with eating, and the pain would last for 2 hours. He was given some antacids which seemed to help the chest discomfort. In the last 1½ years, he had had several episodes. One such episode occurred while he was in class. This was accompanied by a feeling of light-headedness and some numbness of the left hand. A similar episode occurred a week earlier when he was driving.

An echocardiogram revealed mitral valve prolapse with normal left ventricular size and function. No other abnormalities were noted. Treadmill examination was negative for the diagnosis of ischemic heart disease and the patient demonstrated an excellent exercise tolerance 1½ years earlier. It is of interest that he had separated from his wife and was going through a stressful divorce.

Pathology: Gross

Aside from the congestion of the organs, there were no abnormal findings.

The heart weighed 410 grams. There was an accessory tricuspid orifice and the space of His was aneurysmally dilated. The mitral valve was markedly thickened, irregular, nodose, and floppy. In addition, the summit of the ventricular septum showed distinct thickening.

Microscopic Examination: Positive Findings

SA Node and Its Approaches

The nerves showed fibrosis adjacent to the SA node.

Atrial Septum

Fatty infiltration was evident.

AV Node and Its Approaches

The AV node was located in the aortic-mitral annulus. It was slightly to moderately fibrosed (Fig. 8-207).

AV Bundle, Penetrating

This showed moderate fibrosis (Fig. 8-208).

AV Bundle, Branching

This showed distinct fibrosis (Figs. 8-209, 8-210).

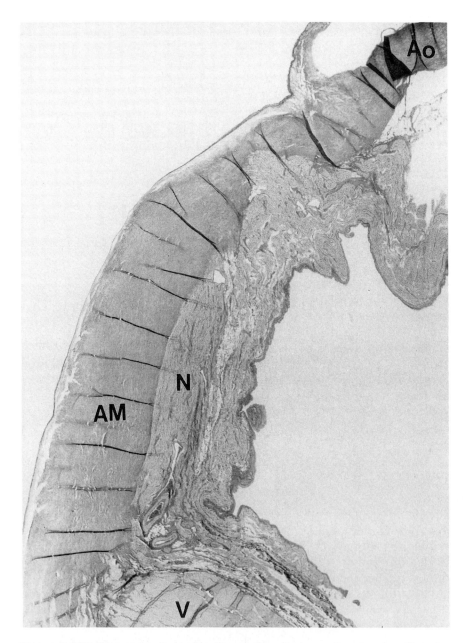

Figure 8-207: The node situated in the aortic-mitral annulus showing fibrosis. Weigert-van Gieson stain × 13.5. N = AV node; AM = aortic-mitral annulus; Ao = aorta; V = ventricular septal muscle.

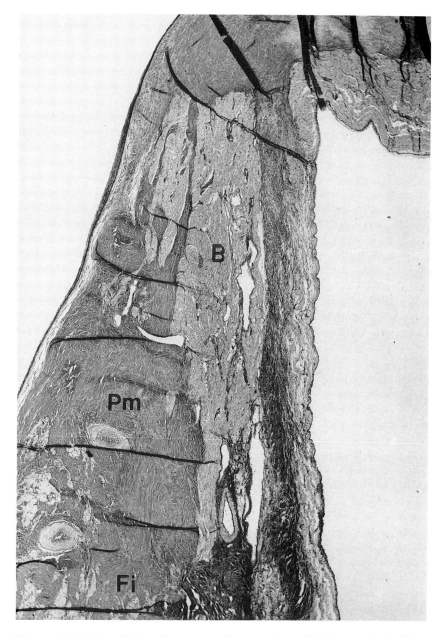

Figure 8-208: The AV bundle, penetrating, showing slight to moderate fibrosis. Weigert-van Gieson stain ×30. B = AV bundle; Fi = fibrosis at top of ventricular septum; Pm = pars membranacea.

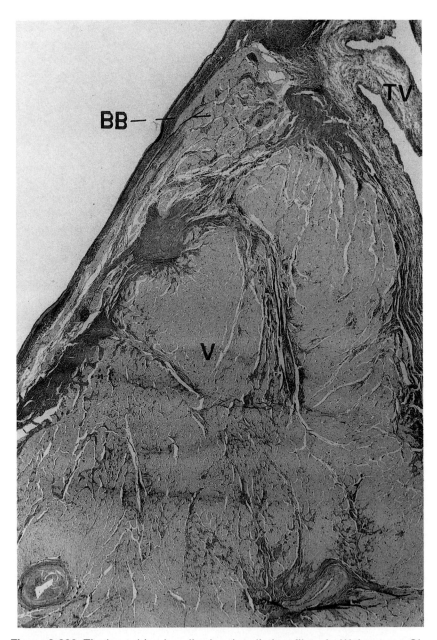

Figure 8-209: The branching bundle showing distinct fibrosis. Weigert-van Gieson stain ×30. BB = branching bundle; V = ventricular septal muscle; TV = tricuspid valve.

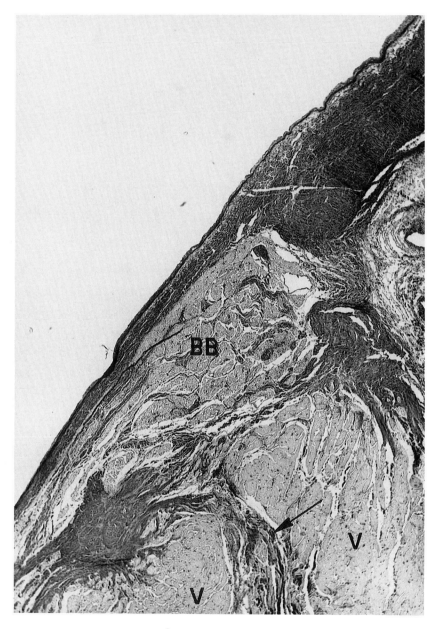

Figure 8-210: Higher power view of Figure 8-209. Weigert-van Gieson stain ×40. BB = branching bundle; V = ventricular musculature. The arrow points to the fibrosis.

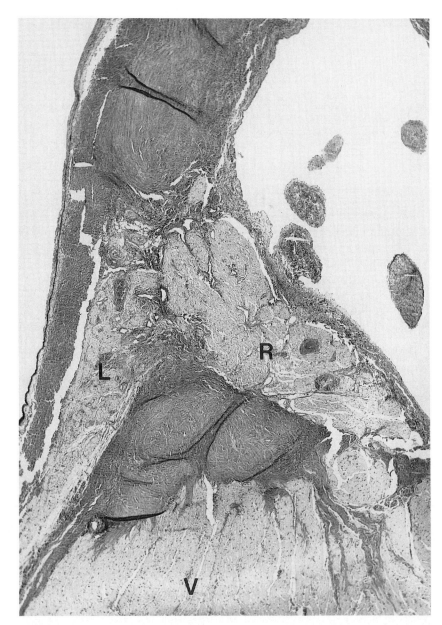

Figure 8-211: Bifurcation showing fibrosis and arteriolosclerosis. Weigert-van Gieson stain ×30. L = left side; R = right side; V = ventricular septal muscle.

AV Bundle, Bifurcation

Distinct fibrosis was noted in this part (Fig. 8-211).

Bundle Branches

Arteriolosclerosis was in evidence with fibrosis. Hemorrhage in the left bundle branch was also noted (Fig. 8-212).

Myocardium

Fibrosis of the nerves was evident, especially adjacent to the SA node (Fig. 8-213).

Summit of the Ventricular Septum

Moderate fibrosis was evident with arteriolosclerosis (Fig. 8-209).

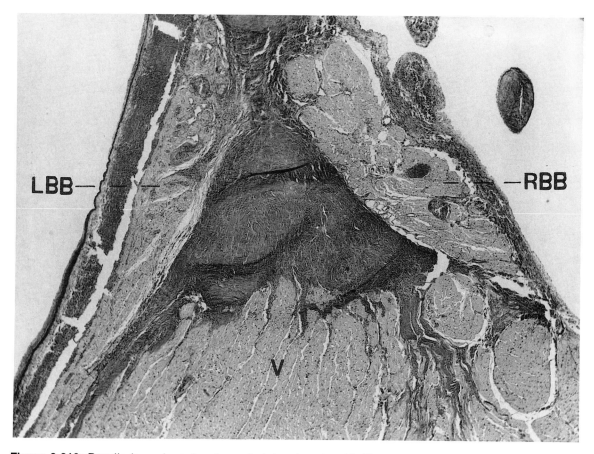

Figure 8-212: Bundle branches showing arteriolosclerosis with fibrosis. Hemorrhage was also noted in the left bundle branch. Weigert-van Gieson stain ×45. LBB = left bundle branch; RBB = right bundle branch; V = ventricular septal muscle.

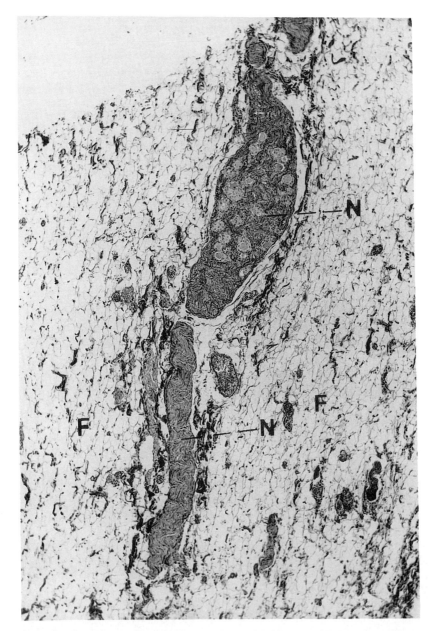

Figure 8-213: Fibrosis of nerves adjacent to the SA node. Weigert-van Gieson stain ×63. F = fat; N = nerve.

Discussion

The conduction system of this patient showed: (1) abnormal placement of the AV node with fibrosis, (2) fibrosis of the AV bundle, both penetrating and branching, associated with arteriolosclerosis, and (3) fibrosis of the nerves around the SA node. We do not know whether any of these are related to the cause of sudden death. It is clear, however, that we are dealing with an abnormal conduction system.

CASE #72

A 22-year-old black football player collapsed suddenly and was in seizure while relaxing in a bar. During the immediate resuscitative attempts, he was found to have a carotid pulse of 56/minute and the initial monitor showed sinus bradycardia with wide QRS complexes. He could not be resuscitated despite all attempts.

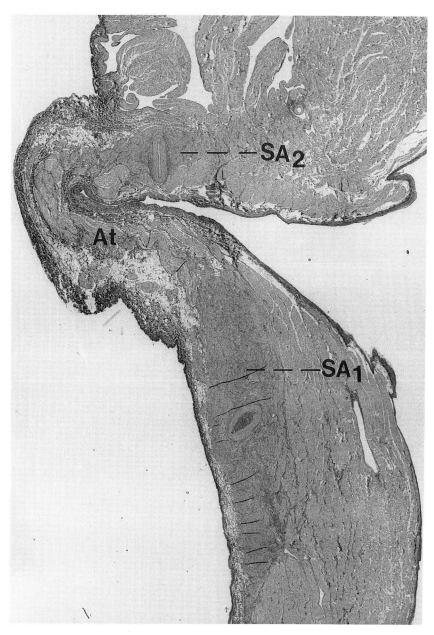

Figure 8-214: Division of the SA node into two components. Weigert-van Gieson stain ×12. SA$_1$ = body of the SA node; SA$_2$ = head of the SA node; At = atrial muscle.

There was vague history of a cardiac murmur in high school, but he was cleared to play football. In addition, he had junctional tachycardia (a long time ago) which disappeared after exercise.

Pathology: Gross

The patient was found to have diplomyelia (double spinal cord).

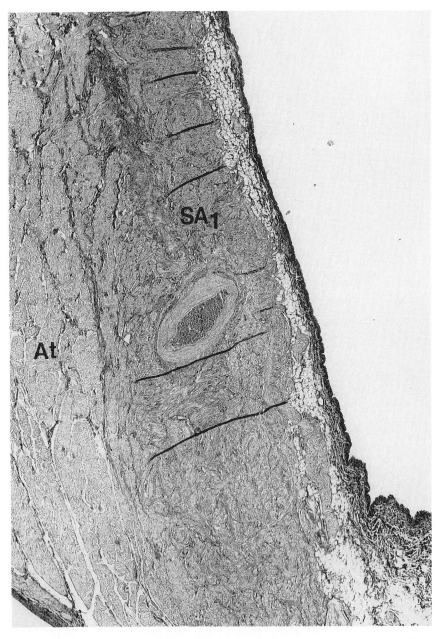

Figure 8-215: Division of the SA node into two components. Weigert-van Gieson stain ×30. SA₁ = body of the SA node; At = atrial muscle.

The heart weighed 380 grams. The right atrium and the right ventricle were hypertrophied and enlarged. The atrial and tricuspid portions of the heart were abnormally formed. The posterior crest was abnormal. The attachment of the medial leaflet of the tricuspid valve was upward in the right atrium and it formed a bulge in the distal part of the atrial septum. This bulge corresponded to the noncoronary cusp of the aortic valve on the left side.

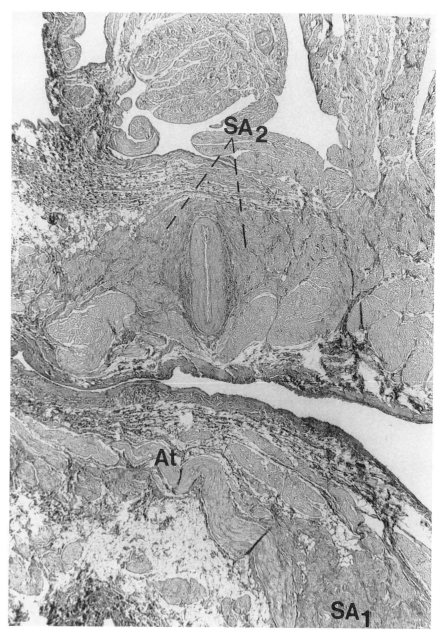

Figure 8-216: Division of the SA node into two components. Weigert-van Gieson stain ×30. SA₁ = body of the SA node; SA₂ = head of the SA node; At = atrial muscle.

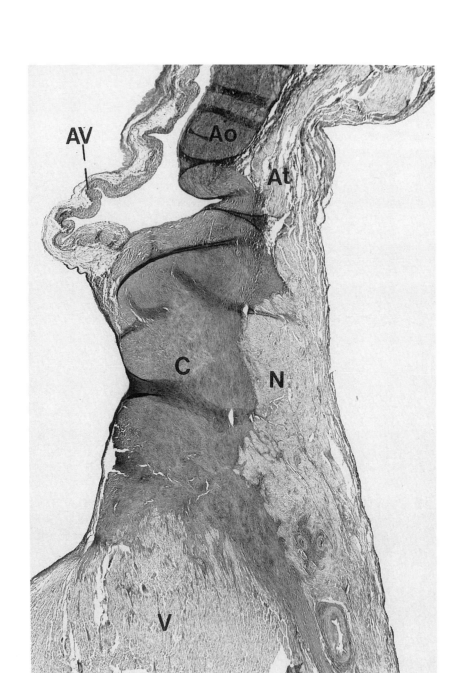

Figure 8-217: The AV node situated adjacent to the aorta with mild to moderate focal fibroelastosis. Weigert-van Gieson stain ×13.5. N = AV node; Ao = aorta; C = central fibrous body; V = ventricular septal myocardium; At = atrial muscle; AV = aortic valve.

Microscopic Examination: Positive Findings

SA Node

In the beginning, this was situated in the atrial appendage with its vessel. It then made a curve into the atrial appendage. As it did so, atrial muscle intervened, producing a tenuous connection between the head of the node and the body of the node. This resulted in the division of the node into two distinct components (Figs. 8-214, 8-215, 8-216).

Approaches to the SA Node

Fibrosis of nerves and degeneration of nerves were present. In addition, epicarditis and fibrosis were noted.

AV Node

Fatty infiltration in and around the node with partial separation of the node from the surrounding atrial approaches was present. The AV nodal artery was narrowed. The node was situated adjacent to the aorta with mild to moderate focal fibroelastosis (Fig. 8-217).

Central Fibrous Body

This was markedly deformed from the aortic sinus of Valsalva, with a long tricuspid component.

Pars Membranacea

This was short and thick.

AV Bundle, Penetrating

This was located close to the aortic valve, with fibrosis and some hemorrhage.

Left Bundle Branch

This showed moderate fibrosis.

Right Bundle Branch

This was intramyocardial from the beginning with moderate to marked fibrosis.

Discussion

This case depicts the division of the SA node into two portions. The effect of this on conduction is unknown. In addition, the AV node is close to the aorta.

The theme which is developing is that the central fibrous body, the eustachian and thebesian valves, the mitral annulus and the tricuspid and aortic annulus, and the summit of the ventricular septum are all connected with the position and pull on the conduction system. We do not know how this produces arrhythmias and dysrhythmias.

One may hypothesize that impulse generation and propagation might have occurred simultaneously from both SA nodes which might have collided and created a milieu for arrhythmogenicity.

CASE #73

A 13-year-old boy died suddenly and unexpectedly. There was a strong history of familial sudden death. In addition, there was a suggestion that some of the family members may have prolonged QT syndrome.

Pathology: Gross

The heart was enlarged and weighed 270 grams. The coronary vein entered very close to the AV nodal region. There was thickening of the septal leaflet of the tricuspid valve with focal fibrosis of the right ventricle. Marked thickening and fibrosis of the summit of the ventricular septum in the region of the His bundle and beginning of the left bundle branch was in evidence. The posterior leaflet of the mitral valve was redundant and floppy.

Microscopic Examination: Positive Findings

SA Node

This showed a moderate amount of inflammatory cells in and around the node. There was fatty infiltration of the approaches to the SA node.

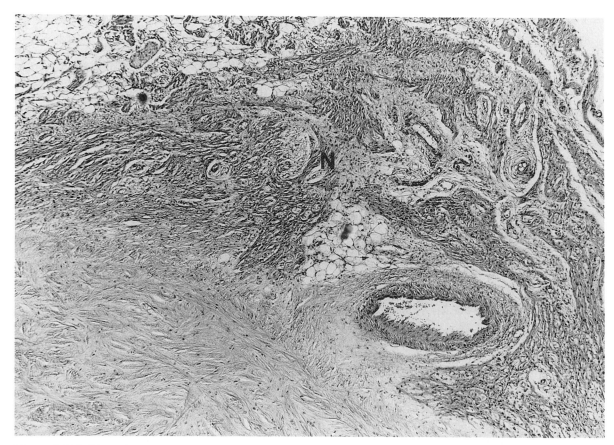

Figure 8-218: The AV node showing inflammatory cells in and around the node. Hematoxylin-eosin stain ×63. N = AV node.

Atrial Septum

Marked fatty infiltration with moderate infiltration of cells was noted.

Approaches to the AV Node

There was a moderate infiltration of mononuclear cells with moderate fatty infiltration.

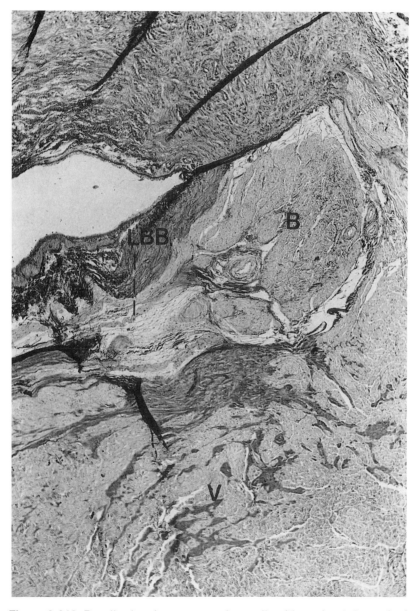

Figure 8-219: Bundle showing mononuclear cells with moderate to marked fibrosis. Weigert-van Gieson stain ×45. B = AV bundle; V = ventricular septal myocardium; LBB = left bundle branch with loss of fibers.

AV Node

Marked infiltration of mononuclear cells and slight fatty infiltration were present (Fig. 8-218).

Penetrating Bundle

A moderate amount of mononuclear cells was seen, with moderate to marked fibrosis.

AV Bundle, Branching

Slight to moderate fibrosis with arteriolosclerosis was noted (Fig. 8-219).

Bifurcating Bundle

This was distinctly pressed on by the bulbar muscle which produced fibrosis of the bifurcating bundle. In addition, there was arteriolosclerosis.

Left Bundle Branch

In the beginning, loss of cells was quite marked (Fig. 8-219).

Summit of the Ventricular Septum

The architecture of the junction of the bulbar muscle with the ventricular myocardium was bizarre with arteriolosclerosis. Marked fatty metamorphosis was present on the right side.

Right Ventricle and Left Ventricle

A scattered amount of mononuclear cells was present.

Discussion

Distinct myocarditis of the AV node, distinct pressure upon and fibrosis of the bifurcating bundle, and loss of the beginning of the left bundle branch fibers were present. In addition, marked fatty metamorphosis of the approaches of the AV node was noted. How this produced sudden death is speculation.

CASE 74

A 13-year-old girl died suddenly at home. She was known to have diffuse conduction disease since birth, and manifested sick sinus syndrome and intraventricular conduction delay with wide QRS tachycardia as well as supraventricular tachycardia. She had a pacemaker insertion several years ago and was reasonably active and living normally.

Pathology: Gross

The heart weighed 365 grams and was greatly enlarged. There was marked fatty infiltration of the AV and interventricular sulci. The space of His was aneurysmally dilated. The right aortic cusp was markedly fenestrated and had two coronary ostia. There was diffuse fibroelastosis of all the chambers.

Microscopic Examination: Positive Findings

Sinoatrial Node

This was small and located endocardially with an increase in fibrous tissue (Fig. 8-220).

Approaches to the SA Node

There was marked fatty infiltration.

AV Node (First)

There was a node-like structure that developed immediately proximal to the markedly disarrayed pattern of the right ventricular side of the ventricular septum. This structure was within the ventricular mass and slowly climbed close to the central fibrous body, with marked fibrosis and fat within the node (Figs. 8-221, 8-222).

Central Fibrous Body

This was quite abnormal. The tendon of Todaro did not join the central fibrous body.

Second Atrioventricular Node

This developed abruptly from the center part of the atrial septum (or the mid-portion between the two components of the central fibrous body). This node hardly made any connection with the atrial tissue (Figs. 8-223, 8-224). There was marked fatty infiltration close to this nodal tissue on the atrial side and fibrosis. The node showed lobulations, fragmentations, and formed a markedly fragmented His bundle.

His Bundle

The His bundle, penetrating portion, was markedly segmented, being divided into almost 10 small pieces. The segments occasionally joined together, tenuously at times, but mostly remained as small fractions (Fig. 8-225).

AV Node 1

The first AV node fused with the right ventricular side of the ventricular myocardium.

Branching Bundle

This was dispersed and circled a piece of a septal musculature. In addition, the branching bundle showed marked space formation (Fig. 8-226).

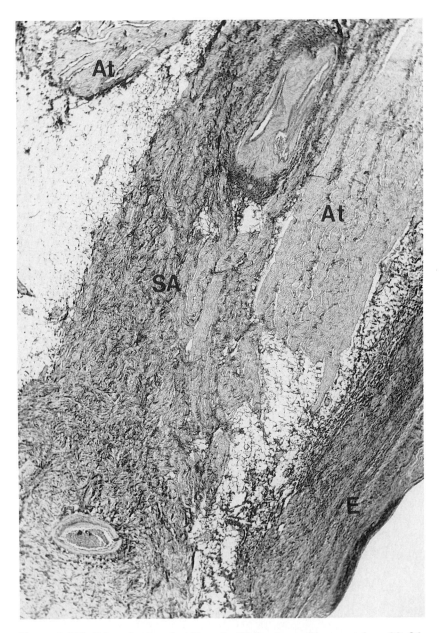

Figure 8-220: SA node showing fibrosis. Weigert-van Gieson stain ×30. SA = SA node; At = atrial musculature; EE = endocardium.

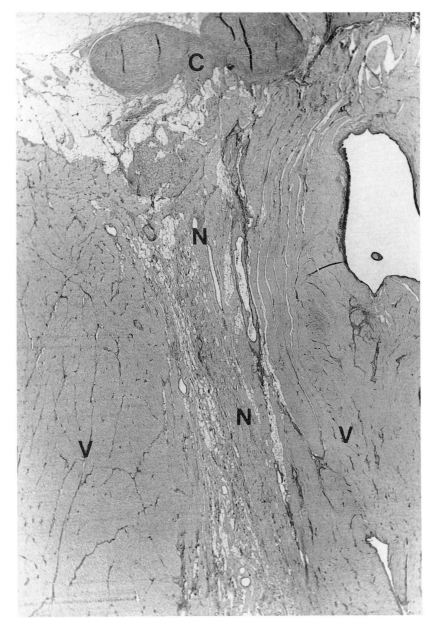

Figure 8-221: AV node 1, situated within the ventricular mass showing marked fibrosis and fatty metamorphosis. Weigert-van Gieson stain ×30. N = node-like structure; V = ventricular septal myocardium; C = central fibrous body.

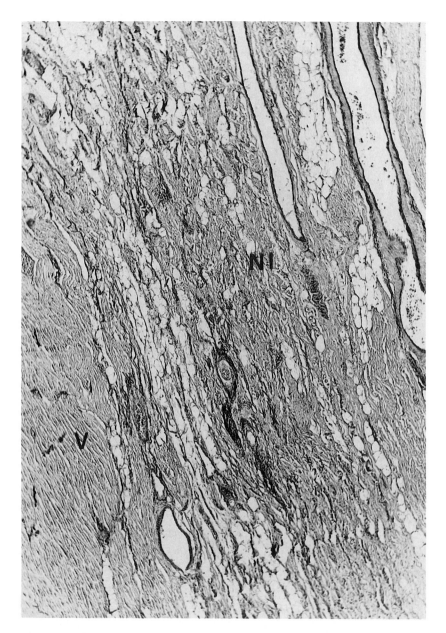

Figure 8-222: Another view of AV node 1 described in Figure 8-221. Weigert-van Gieson stain ×63. N1 = possible AV node 1; V = ventricular septal muscle.

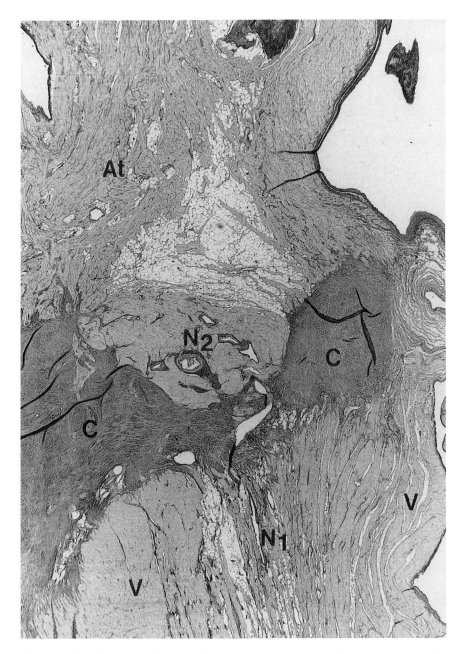

Figure 8-223: Second AV node with tenuous connection with atrial muscle, with marked fatty metamorphosis, lobulation, and fragmentation, situated within the central fibrous body. Weigert-van Gieson stain ×16.5. N_2 = regular AV node; C = central fibrous body; N_1 = possible AV node in ventricular muscle; V = ventricular septal myocardium; At = atrial muscle.

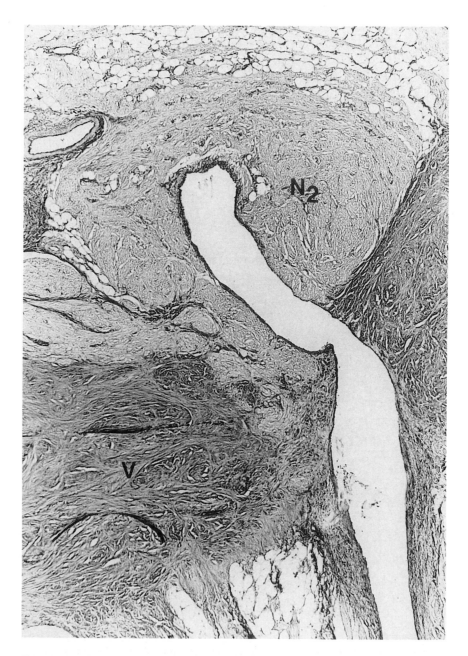

Figure 8-224: Another view of AV node 2 within the central fibrous body. Weigert-van Gieson stain ×63. N₂ = regular AV node; V = ventricular septal muscle.

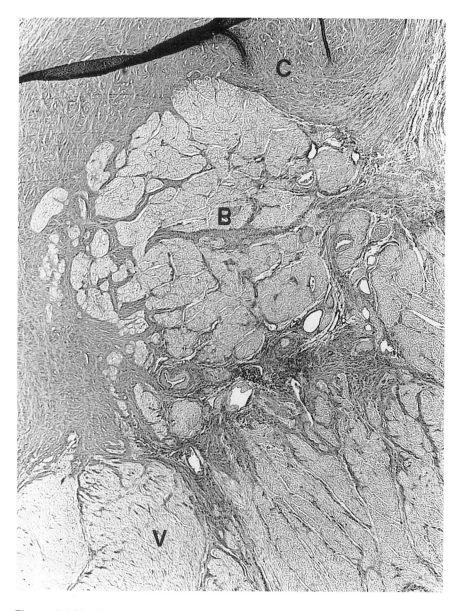

Figure 8-225: AV bundle showing marked fragmentation. Weigert-van Gieson stain ×45. B = bundle of His; V = ventricular septal myocardium; C = central fibrous body.

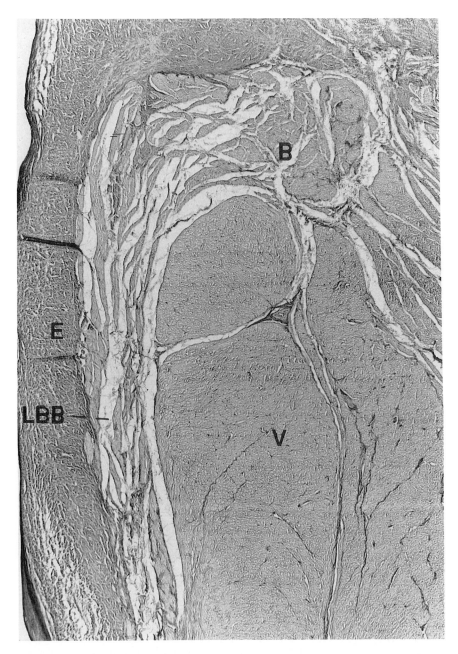

Figure 8-226: Branching bundle showing space formation and fibrosis. Weigert-van Gieson stain ×45. B = bundle; V = ventricular septal muscle; E = endocardium of left ventricle; LBB = left bundle branch.

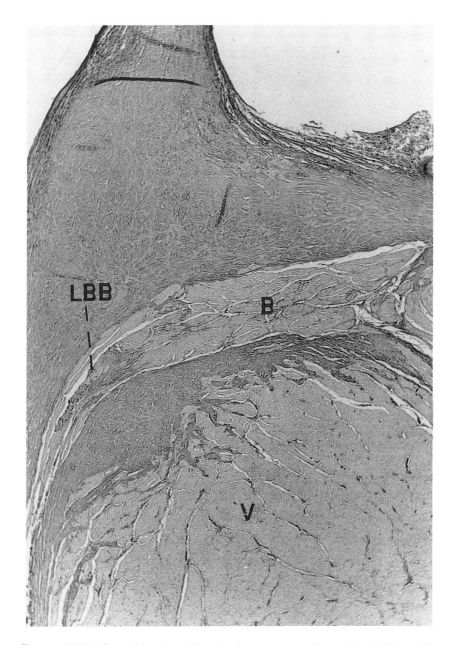

Figure 8-227: Branching bundle showing compression of the left bundle branch with fibrosis of endocardium and subendocardium. Weigert-van Gieson stain ×63. B = branching bundle; V = ventricular musculature; LBB = left bundle branch.

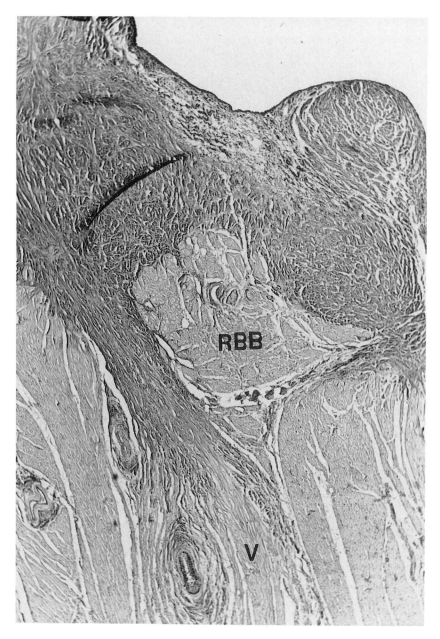

Figure 8-228: Right bundle branch showing fibrosis. Weigert-van Gieson stain ×45. RBB = right bundle branch; V = ventricular septal muscle.

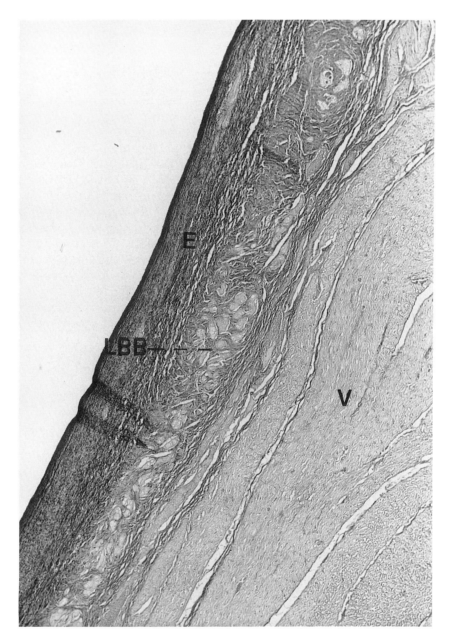

Figure 8-229: Left bundle branch more distally showing marked fibrosis of the peripheral Purkinje fibers, compressed by endocardial and subendocardial fibrosis. Weigert-van Gieson stain ×63. LBB = left bundle branch; V = ventricular septal muscle; E = left ventricular endocardium.

Bifurcating Bundle

There was considerable fibrosis.

Left Bundle Branch

This immediately formed large Purkinje cells. There was considerable fibrosis of the endocardium and subendocardium compressing the Purkinje cells (Fig. 8-227) and the left bundle branch showed marked fibrosis more peripherally.

Right Bundle Branch

This first divided into two and then joined together and immediately became intramuscular. Practically the entire course of the right bundle branch was intramuscular and showed marked fibrosis. It then divided into two parts many times and joined again. The third part of the right bundle branch showed fibrosis (Fig. 8-228). The left bundle branch more distally showed marked fibrosis (Fig. 8-229).

Discussion

This is a case of a sick sinus disease with segmented bundle of His, double AV node, and abnormal bundle branches. The SA node was mostly intramyocardial. Likewise, the first AV node was within the ventricular myocardium on the right side. The second AV node was within the abnormally developed central fibrous body and had very little contact with the surrounding atrial musculature. Most of the course of the right bundle branch was intramuscular. Thus, we are fundamentally dealing with an abnormally developed conduction system. One can speculate about several mechanisms for arrhythmogenicity and sudden death in this case. Obviously, the diffuse conduction disease is related to the cause of death.

CASE #75

A 42-year-old man had a cardiac arrest at home sleeping in bed. Despite the emergency treatment, the patient remained comatose and died 6 days later.

Eleven years earlier, his electrocardiogram demonstrated conduction delay. Ten months prior to his death, he had cardiac arrest while in California and was resuscitated from ventricular fibrillation by paramedics. Three to four days following the cardiac arrest, he had regained his normal mental status.

Cardiac Catheterization and Coronary Arteriography

These studies revealed normal coronaries and normal ventricular performance.

EPS

EPS demonstrated a slight increase in the HV interval with pacing and the patient developed polymorphic ventricular tachycardia. An implantable defibrillator was recommended. Before this could be carried out, the patient developed pulmonary embolism and was treated until his second cardiac arrest.

Pathology: Gross

The heart weighed 410 grams. The space of His was aneurysmally dilated. The summit of the ventricular septum revealed aging changes.

Microscopic Examination: Positive Findings

Approaches to the AV Node and the AV Node

This showed marked fatty infiltration. In addition, there were large areas of fibrosis in the atrial septum. There was marked arteriolosclerosis with narrowing. The AV node was quite small and was in part within the atrial septum, and separated in many areas from the atria by fat.

AV Bundle, Penetrating

This was quite small and showed some fatty infiltration.

AV Bundle, Branching

This was situated on the left side of the ventricular septum.

Left Bundle Branch

This showed moderate fibrosis and falling out of cells.

Bifurcating Bundle

This occurred intramuscularly.

Right Bundle Branch

The second part of the right bundle branch was intramuscular. There was considerable fibrosis of the right bundle branch, with almost complete obliteration.

Summit of the Ventricular Septum

There was marked fibrosis and disarray on the left side. Further anteriorly, the fibrosis was more centrally located.

Mitral and Tricuspid Valves

These revealed marked thickening.

Right Ventricle

There was marked fatty infiltration.

Left Ventricle

There were large areas of degeneration which were acute in nature, with infiltration of mononuclear cells.

Posterior Septum Apex

This showed mononuclear cells.

Pathological Diagnosis

1. Fibrosis and acute degeneration of the atrial musculature with fatty metamorphosis.
2. Marked arteriolosclerosis with narrowing of the branches of the AV nodal artery.
3. Fatty metamorphosis of the approaches to the AV node and within the AV node.
4. Moderate elastosis and fatty metamorphosis of the AV bundle.
5. Branching bundle on the left side of the ventricular septum.
6. Moderate fibrosis, space formation, and falling out of cells of the left bundle branch.
7. Intramuscular part of the first part of the right bundle branch.
8. Marked fibroelastosis and complete obliteration of the right bundle branch.
9. Fatty metamorphosis of the right ventricle.
10. Increased fibrosis of the summit of the ventricular septum.
11. Focal acute degeneration of the myocardium of the left ventricle.
12. AV node, bundle, and bundle branches, relatively small structures.

Discussion

The cause of sudden death in this patient is related to: (1) the marked fatty infiltration of the approaches to the AV node and the AV node; (2) the fibrosis and falling out of cells in the left bundle branch; (3) the fibrosis of the right bundle branch; (4) the fibrosis of the summit of the ventricular septum; (5) the fatty infiltration of the right ventricle; and (6) the large areas of degeneration of the left ventricle. As one views the cases of sudden death, one is impressed by the fatty metamorphosis of the atrial septum.

Chapter 9

Analysis of Our Work

Analysis of Our Material

We have divided our cases of sudden death into the following categories:

1. Sudden unexpected death with no known disease entity responsible for the death.
2. Sudden unexpected death with a known disease probably responsible for the death.
3. Sudden death occurring in families.
4. Sudden death occurring in athletes.
5. Sudden Infant Death Syndrome.
6. Sudden death in which autopsy revealed a mitral valve prolapse.
7. Sudden death many months or years following surgical treatment of congenital heart disease.
8. Sudden death many months or years after the knowledge of the presence of congenital heart disease without surgical intervention.
9. Sudden death associated with a known presence of heart block or other conduction abnormalities (cardiac rhythm abnormalities).
10. Sudden death related to the presence of myocarditis.
11. Sudden death after catheter or surgical ablation of part of the conduction system in cases of intractable arrhythmias.
12. Sudden death in which autopsy revealed mild downward displacement of the tricuspid valve.
13. The relationship of neuritis or fibrosis of the nerves to sudden death.

Category I: Sudden Death with No Known Disease Entity Responsible for the Death

Thirty cases fell into this category. There were 17 males and 13 females. The age ranged from 6 months to 59 years, with the maximum number of cases falling into the first three decades of life. Most hearts were moderately or slightly hypertrophied and enlarged.

The Conduction System

The sinoatrial node was not often involved. Where it was involved, it was infiltrated by fat. At times it was separated in part from the atrium by fat. The atrial preferential pathways were at times likewise infiltrated by fat. Such involvement was also present in the approaches to the AV node, producing a tenuous connection between the atrial musculature and the AV node.

The most prominent finding in the AV node was that it was often embedded within the central fibrous body, all of it or in part. In some cases, fatty metamorphosis was present in the node. Occasionally, the node was displaced into the tricuspid annulus.

The bundle of His was often segmented or fragmented with the formation of loops. In some cases, the bundle showed hemorrhage within its branching or penetrating portion or in both. At the region of bifurcation, the bundle often showed degenerative changes on both sides of the bifurcation. Often the branching bundle was on the left side of the ventricular septum.

The Summit of the Ventricular Septum

This, in almost all cases, demonstrated an increase in fibrosis, either on the left or on the right side. The bundle branches often showed

fibrosis on either side, at times with hemorrhage present mostly on the left side.

Category II: Sudden Death with a Known Disease Entity Probably Responsible for Sudden Death

In this group, there were various diseases that were associated with sudden death.

A. In a 16-year-old male, there was a small ventricular septal defect. The heart was hypertrophied and enlarged. The atrial septum was abnormally formed with fibrosis of the atria. The approaches to the SA node revealed an increase in connective tissue. The approaches to the AV node showed marked swelling of the cells. The AV bundle was septated and the left bundle branch was focally cut off from the bundle.

B. In a group of cases, the coronary arteries were narrowed.

1. In a 35-year-old female, the left circumflex coronary artery was narrowed, and the SA and AV nodal arteries were thickened and narrowed. Hemorrhage was occasionally present in the SA node. The heart was hypertrophied and enlarged.

2. In a 40-year-old female, the anterior descending coronary artery was narrowed to the extent of 60%. The heart was hypertrophied and enlarged. The approaches to the AV node were a seat of fatty metamorphosis. The AV bundle lay within the tricuspid annulus. The summit of the ventricular septum showed patchy fibrosis.

3. In a 24-year-old male, there was thickening of the AV nodal artery associated with chronic myocarditis. Fatty metamorphosis was present in the approaches to the SA and AV nodes. The penetrating bundle was lobulated with loop formation. The branching bundle lay on the left side. The right bundle branch revealed marked fibrosis, while the left bundle branch showed moderate fibrosis. The summit to the ventricular septum presented an in-

crease in connective tissue with arteriosclerosis.

4. In a 16-year-old female, there was thickening of the AV nodal artery (ramus septi fibrosi) associated with a hypertrophied and enlarged heart. In the approaches to the SA node, the large arterioles were thickened and narrowed. The penetrating portion of the bundle of His showed fatty metamorphosis and the branching portion was infiltrated with mononuclear cells. The left bundle branch revealed degenerative changes. The summit of the ventricular septum showed fibrosis and arteriolosclerosis and an infiltration of mononuclear cells.

5. In a 25-year-old female, there was moderate narrowing of the ramus septi fibrosi. The heart was hypertrophied and enlarged. At the approaches to the SA node, the large arterioles were narrowed. The penetrating and branching portions of the bundle revealed moderate fibrosis. The summit of the ventricular septum was the seat of marked fibrosis.

6. In a 32-year-old male, there was severe coronary disease with distinct calcification and fenestration of the aortic valve, and localized narrowing of the left circumflex and anterior descending coronary arteries. The SA node showed fibroelastosis and the approaches to the node were the seat of fatty metamorphosis. The penetrating portion of the bundle revealed fatty metamorphosis while the branching part showed fibromuscular changes with spaces. The right bundle branch showed fibrosis of the first part and the left bundle branch was the seat of space formation. The summit of the ventricular septum revealed a moderate increase in fibrosis.

7. In a 4½-year-old male with Kawasaki disease, associated myocarditis was evident.

8. In a 1½-month-old male with DiGeorge syndrome and hypertensive pulmonary venous disease, the whole heart was hypertrophied. This was associated with truncus communis, a bicuspid and dysplastic truncal valve and incomplete cortriatriatum dexter. Here the AV node showed chronic inflammation.

9. In a 74-year-old male, the left circumflex coronary artery was narrowed and completely occluded by a thrombus. This was as-

sociated with an adenocarcinoma of the ascending colon with metastasis to the liver. There was a recent infarct in the proximal two-thirds of the posterior septum. The SA node showed early necrosis and arteriolosclerosis. The approaches to the SA node revealed fibrosis, elastosis, and arteriolosclerosis. The approaches to the AV node showed fatty metamorphosis and arteriolosclerosis. The AV node revealed chronic inflammation with proliferation of sheath cells. The penetrating bundle showed focal degeneration of cells. The bifurcating bundle revealed fatty metamorphosis on the left side. The summit of the ventricular septum was increased in fibrosis of the left and right side.

Category III: Sudden Death Occurring in Families

There were eight cases in which there were familial trends; four were male and four female. Their ages ranged from 4½ years to 41 years. All hearts were hypertrophied and enlarged. One case was a familial lipidemia. Three cases had mitral valve prolapse. One had severe coronary disease.

The SA node of four cases showed fibrosis. One case showed an organizing thrombus in the SA node. The approaches to the SA node revealed fatty metamorphosis, fibrosis, and neuritis. In one case, node-like cells of the mitral valve entered the central fibrous body and joined the AV node.

Category IV: Sudden Death Occurring in Athletes

There were 13 cases, all males, in this group. They were engaged in basketball, cycling, football, socker, skiing, or all-around sports. Their age ranged from 14 to 47 years. All the hearts were hypertrophied and enlarged. Occasionally, an accessory tricuspid valve was present.

The SA node was, in one case, divided, and in another it was replaced by fibrous tissue. The approaches to the SA node showed fatty metamorphosis. The AV node was almost always in part or mostly situated in the central fibrous body, and occasionally partly embedded in the tricuspid annulus or in the aortic-mitral annulus. The ramus septi fibrosi was frequently thickened and narrowed. The posterior mitral leaflet was frequently enlarged, redundant, and, at times, floppy. The eustachian valve was often a thick or enlarged membrane. The atrium and the approaches to the SA and AV nodes were frequently infiltrated with fat. In one case, the aortic valve was fenestrated and calcified. The penetrating portion of the bundle was frequently lobulated with loop formation. The branching bundle was often fibrosed. The summit of the ventricular septum always showed an increase in fibrosis, either on the left or on the right side.

Category V: Sudden Infant Death Syndrome (SIDS)

The conduction system in 23 hearts were examined without knowing which individual heart belonged to the sudden infant death group and which belonged to the control group. There were 15 hearts belonging to the SIDS group and eight to the control group. The AV node was situated, in part, in the central fibrous body in both the control group and in the SIDS cases. The branching portion of the bundle was located on the left side in 8 of the 15 cases of SIDS and in only two in the control group.

We hypothesize that a left-sided His bundle may be prone to injury during the transition from the relative predominance of the right ventricle at term to the relative predominance of the left ventricle at 2 to 4 months of age. The increase in left ventricular pressure after birth may influence the His bundle, which is in a subendocardial position in some, and may be responsible for arrhythmia and sudden

death. The effect of the presence of the AV node in part in the central fibrous body, the fragmentation of the His bundle, and the presence of neuritis in the atria cannot be evaluated.

Category VI: Sudden Death in Mitral Valve Prolapse

In this category, there were nine cases: seven males and two females. The hearts of all except one were hypertrophied and enlarged. The posterior leaflet of the mitral valve was redundant in all cases. In one case, it was nodose and calcified. In one case, the eustachian and thebesian valves were also enlarged, and in another case, the membranous septum was likewise enlarged. In still another case, the pars membranacea and the aortic valve were thickened. In one case, node-like cells of the mitral valve entered the central fibrous body and joined the AV node.

In one case, the SA node showed an increase in connective tissue. In another, the node was separated from the right atrium by fat. In still another, there was a thrombus in the SA node. In three cases, the AV node was partly embedded in the central fibrous body. In one case, the node was in the aortic-mitral annulus. In still another case, the AV node was compressed by an enlarged left atrium and the calcification in the mitral valve and central fibrous body.

Concerning the AV bundle, one case had a connection between the bundle with the atrium (atrio-Hisian). Here the bundle was lobulated with loop formation. The branching bundle in this case was left-sided. In another case, the penetrating bundle showed fatty metamorphosis, while the branching bundle demonstrated linear degeneration on the left side with fatty metamorphosis. In all cases, the summit of the ventricular septum revealed marked fibrosis. Both bundle branches likewise showed degenerative changes.

Category VII: Sudden Death in Congenital Heart Disease Following Surgery

There were 10 cases who died suddenly a varying time after surgery.

Two children, both males, one a 5-year-old and one a 5-month-old, suddenly died 3 years and 2½ years, respectively, following the Mustard procedure for complete transposition. The first child demonstrated sinus rhythm alternating with junctional rhythm the last year of life. The second child, 2 months before death, had first-degree AV block which progressed to second-degree block with 2:1 conduction alternating with the junctional rhythm with AV dissociation.

The conduction system in both cases showed the approaches to the SA node and AV node to be markedly fibrosed. In addition, there were sutures interrupting the SA node in one case and marked fibrosis of the SA node in the other. The arrhythmias that were present clinically and the possible cause of sudden death in both cases may be related to the surgical injury to the approaches to the SA node and the AV node, and the involvement of the SA node itself.

In two cases, the anomaly operated on was an atrial septal defect, secundum type. The first case was that of a 6½-year-old female. In addition to the chronic foreign body granulomas present in the atria, there was an increased amount of fibrosis in the summit of the ventricular septum. The second case was that of a 47-year-old female who died 2½ years after closure of an atrial septal defect. In addition to the sutures in the atrial septum, there was fatty metamorphosis in the approaches to the SA node, in the AV node, and in the penetrating and branching portion of the bundle of His. The bundle branches likewise showed fibrosis. The ventricular septum showed an increase in fibrosis on the left side.

There was one case of an ostium primum defect in a 30-year-old female. The defect was closed at the age of 13. The heart was hypertrophied and enlarged, with fibrosis being present in the atria. Fatty metamorphosis was present in the approaches to the SA and AV nodes and in the atria. A sclerotic, narrowed artery compressed the AV node, which was, in part, present in the central fibrous body. The AV bundle showed marked fatty metamorphosis and both bundle branches showed fibrosis. The summit of the ventricular septum showed an increase in fibrosis.

A 23-year-old male with a history of tetralogy of Fallot and pulmonary atresia had a heterotopic valve placed between the right ventricle and the pulmonary trunk. The heart was hypertrophied and enlarged. Fibrosis and fatty metamorphosis were present in the approaches to the SA and AV nodes, and the AV node showed edema. The penetrating bundle was lobulated and the branching bundle showed fibrosis and fatty metamorphosis, as did the right bundle branch. The summit of the ventricular septum revealed marked fibrosis and arteriolosclerosis.

A 9-year-old boy who was diagnosed as having double outlet left ventricle had a patch closure of the defect and a Hancock prosthesis placed from the right ventricle to the pulmonary artery. He died 4 years after the operation. He was totally asymptomatic. The SA node showed diffuse inflammation and the atrial preferential pathways revealed marked fibrosis. The penetrating bundle showed moderate fibrosis with lobulation. The summit of the ventricular septum showed an increase in fibrosis with a myocarditis.

A 21-month-old male child who had a Senning procedure for complete transposition done at 6 months of age died suddenly 15 months later. The heart was hypertrophied and enlarged and there was fibroelastosis of both atria. There was chronic myocarditis with maximum involvement of the infundibulum of the right ventricle and the AV node, with a left-sided His bundle. In addition, there was an accessory anterior AV node.

A 38-year-old male with first-degree AV block with a familial history of atrial septal defect and first-degree AV block died suddenly 8 years following closure of the atrial septal defect. Here the SA node could not be identified. Where we would expect the SA node to be, there was a marked foreign body reaction with fibrosis and sutures. There was marked fatty metamorphosis in the atrial preferential pathways, in the approaches to the AV node, and within the node itself. This extended to the region of the penetrating and branching bundle and the left bundle branch. The right bundle branch could not be identified and in its stead there were large Purkinje-like cells throughout the subendocardium of the right ventricle.

Category VIII: Congenital Heart Disease without Surgery

There were three congenitally abnormal hearts that did not have surgical correction. The first case was that of a 15-year-old male. The basic anomaly was a quadricuspid pulmonic valve. The heart was hypertrophied and enlarged and all leaflets in the tricuspid valve were markedly thickened. The atrial preferential pathways and the approaches to the AV node showed moderate fatty metamorphosis with distinct fibrosis of nerves. The summit of the ventricular septum showed moderate to marked fatty metamorphosis.

The second case was that of a 64-year-old male who had a large sinus venosus atrial septal defect with pacemaker insertion for syncopal attacks. Here the conduction system showed considerable fatty infiltration and degenerative changes, as well as extensive arteriolosclerosis of the summit of the ventricular septum involving the right side.

The third case was that of a 1½-year-old male child with DiGeorge syndrome and hypertensive pulmonary vascular disease. He had a truncus communis associated with an incomplete cortriatriatum dexter and a tricuspid dysplastic truncal valve. There was myocarditis of the AV node in this case. This was also included in category II.

Category IX: Cases with Varying Degrees of Atrioventricular Block

There was a group of hearts that demonstrated various degrees of AV block.

A. In a 16-year-old female with complete AV block, there was a mesothelioma which replaced the AV node.

B. In a 67-year-old male, complete AV block was present. The heart was hypertrophied and enlarged. The mitral valve was calcified at its base. The pars membranacea, the central fibrous body, and the base of the mitral valve were thickened. The approaches to the SA node and the atrial preferential pathways showed fatty metamorphosis. The approaches to the AV node revealed fibrosis. The AV node demonstrated marked calcification in both the line of closure and the edges. The ramus septi fibrosi was thickened. The right bundle branch revealed fibrosis and the left bundle branch was separated from the bundle. The summit of the ventricular septum showed calcification.

C. A 25-year-old male was stabbed in the chest, producing a ventricular septal defect and complete AV block. The heart was hypertrophied and enlarged. He died suddenly 3 years later. The AV bundle was markedly fibrosed. The bifurcation was destroyed as was the beginning of the bundle branches. The summit to the ventricular septum showed a marked increase in fibrosis.

Category X: Myocarditis

Several cases showed myocarditis, which is a well-known cause of sudden death. A 31-year-old female gave birth to a stillborn baby with myocarditis. A 6-year-old female with a hypertrophied and enlarged heart likewise died suddenly with myocarditis, as did a 46-year-old female with a hypertrophied and enlarged heart. A 4½-year-old male had Kawasaki disease associated with a generalized myocarditis. This was also included in category II.

Category XI: Sudden Death after Catheter or Surgical Ablation of Part of the Conduction System in Cases of Intractable Arrhythmias

A 59-year-old female with recurrent atrial fibrillation refractory to treatment with beta blockers, digoxin, verapamil, and other medications had AV junctional ablation with two shocks of 500 joules which resulted in complete AV block. A permanent pacemaker was implanted. She died suddenly 6 weeks later. Histologically, a partially fibrosed atrio-Hisian connection was present. There was marked fatty infiltration of the approaches to the AV node and the AV node with tremendous chronic inflammatory changes in the atrial septum and summit of the ventricular septum.

A 22-year-old female had intractable junctional tachycardia with intervening normal sinus rhythm since 1 week of age. She subsequently had attacks of sick sinus syndrome. Accordingly, catheter ablation was performed at the AV junction. The heart was hypertrophied and enlarged. The atrial preferential pathways showed fibrosis and fatty metamorphosis. The approaches to the AV node were surgically ablated. There were small node-like cells from the mitral annulus which joined the atrial musculature. The penetrating bundle was left-sided and showed fibrosis. The branching bundle was intramuscular. The first and second part of the right bundle branch revealed fibrosis, as did the left bundle branch.

These two cases illustrate that congenital abnormalities of the conduction system may be elusive in nature and may not be amenable for ablative procedures in some. Furthermore, the inflammatory changes following the ablation may itself form a nidus for future arrhythmic events resulting in sudden death in some.

Category XII: Sudden Death in Other Diseases

A. A 13-year-old female had pre-excitation. The heart was hypertrophied and en-

larged with fibroelastosis of the left ventricle. The SA node and its approaches showed fatty infiltration, as did the approaches to the AV node. Fibrosis was present at the junction of the bundle with the left bundle branch and in both bundle branches. The left side of the summit of the ventricular septum showed fibrosis. There were two small bypass tracts in the anterolateral wall of the right atrioventricular rim.

B. A 34-year-old male presented with third-degree AV block and had generalized sarcoidosis, which was present throughout the entire heart.

C. A 72-year-old male had Monckeberg's sclerosis. The heart was hypertrophied and enlarged. The approaches to the SA node revealed marked fibrosis, elastosis, and arteriolosclerosis. The penetrating bundle showed fatty metamorphosis. The right bundle branch was a seat of fibroelastosis. The left bundle branch had a disruption of its connection with the bundle. The summit of the ventricular septum showed marked fibrosis and arteriolosclerosis.

D. This was a case of myotonia dystrophica. A 36-year-old female had a hypertrophied and enlarged heart. The atrial preferential pathways and the approaches to the AV node presented fatty metamorphosis. The penetrating bundle was lobulated. The bundle branches showed marked fibrosis and disruption. The summit of the ventricular septum revealed marked fibrosis on both sides.

E. There was also a 36-year-old male with Kearns-Sayre disease. The heart was markedly hypertrophied and enlarged. The atrial preferential pathways and the approaches to the AV node revealed fatty metamorphosis. The bundle of His and the right bundle branch showed marked fatty metamorphosis. The posterior radiation of the left bundle branch was replaced by a linear formation. The summit of the ventricular septum showed marked fibrosis and fatty metamorphosis.

F. A hypertensive, diabetic 64-year-old male developed complete heart block. He possessed a large sinus venosus atrial septal defect. The SA node showed fibroelastosis, and the approaches to the node were partially separated from the atrium by fat. The branching bundle showed fibrosis, as did the bundle branches. The summit of the ventricular septum revealed increased fibrous tissue.

G. A 25-year-old male had diabetes since 2 years of age, which was not well controlled by insulin. The tricuspid and mitral valves were redundant, thickened, and were probably insufficient. He also had segmental coarctation of the aorta.

The approaches to the AV node and the AV node itself presented fatty metamorphosis with loop formation. The penetrating bundle was on the left side and showed fibrosis. The summit of the ventricular septum showed arteriolosclerosis.

H. A 31-year-old female schizophrenic and drug abuser had a hypertrophied and enlarged heart. The tricuspid valve was diffusely thickened. Fatty infiltration was present in the atrial musculature. The AV node showed chronic myocarditis. The penetrating bundle revealed a moderate infiltration of mononuclear cells. The branching bundle showed marked fibrosis.

I. A 44-year-old male had left bundle branch block and occasional 2:1 AV block. The heart was hypertrophied and enlarged. The SA node was replaced by fibrous tissue and fat. The atrial preferential pathways showed fibrosis, while the approaches to the AV node revealed marked fatty metamorphosis with marked arteriolosclerosis of the ramus septi fibrosi. The AV node revealed marked fibrosis and fatty metamorphosis. The AV bundle showed marked fibrosis and chronic inflammation. The right bundle branch was the seat of marked fibrosis, while the left bundle branch showed partial fibrosis.

J. A 22-year-old male had diplopia. The heart was hypertrophied and enlarged. The atria and tricuspid valve were abnormally formed. The SA node was divided into two parts. The approaches to the SA node showed fibrosis and degeneration of nerves. The AV node was the seat of fatty metamorphosis with partial separation from the approaches. The AV nodal artery was narrowed. The central fi-

brous body was markedly deformed with a long tricuspid component. The penetrating bundle was close to the aortic valve, with fibrosis and hemorrhage. The right bundle branch showed marked fibrosis. The left bundle branch revealed moderate fibrosis.

K. A 42-year-old male at 11 years of age showed a conduction delay with the space of His aneurysmally dilated. The atrial preferential pathways showed large areas of fibrosis. The approaches to the AV node revealed marked fatty metamorphosis with arteriolosclerosis, with the normal AV node and separated by fat from the atrial musculature. The AV bundle was small with fatty metamorphosis. The branching bundle was on the left side. The bifurcating bundle was intramuscular. The right bundle branch showed fibrosis and almost obliteration. The left bundle branch revealed fibrosis with fatty metamorphosis. The summit of the ventricular septum showed marked fibrosis with disarray on the left side.

L. There was a slight downward displacement of the medial leaflet of the tricuspid in a 21-year-old male. The heart was hypertrophied and enlarged. There was a small aneurysm of the fossa ovalis. The eustachian valve was prominent with marked fenestrations. The approaches to the AV node showed fibroelastosis. The AV node was in part within the central fibrous body. The penetrating bundle showed lobulation with loop formation. The branching bundle was on the left side. The summit of the ventricular septum revealed fibrosis more on the left side.

Category XIII: The Relationship of Neuritis or Fibrosis of the Nerves to Sudden Death

In many cases, the nerves, especially around the sinoatrial node, showed either neuritis or fibrosis. The functional aspects of these pathological changes are not known today.

Chapter 10

Conclusions and Future Work

The purpose of this study was to ascertain whether changes in the conduction system of the heart might be related to sudden unexpected death. The following positive findings stand out as important:

1. The heart was hypertrophied and enlarged in practically all cases.

2. The epicardial coronary arteries were usually normal, except in category IIB.

3. The conduction system was abnormal in *all* cases studied.

4. The maximum changes were found in the bundle of His, but were not limited to the bundle. These changes consisted of fibrosis, septation, fragmentation, lobulation, and at times loop formation in the bundle. The changes were sometimes in the penetrating portion, less frequently in the branching portion, and sometimes at the bifurcation.

5. Changes in the bundle branches were also present, but were not as frequent as in the bundle. These consisted of fibrosis of various parts.

6. The changes in the summit of the ventricular septum were almost universal. These consisted of fibrosis, sometimes on the right side, sometimes on the left side. This was almost always associated with atherosclerosis or arteriosclerosis.

7. There are congenital abnormally formed conduction systems that might result in sudden death, especially in the young, during an altered physiological or metabolic state. Among these abnormalities are:

A. Double SA node.
B. SA node intramyocardially situated in part.

C. AV node situated in the tricuspid valve annulus.

D. AV node situated in the mitral valve annulus.

E. AV node situated close to the aorta (left side).

F. AV node may be divided into two components.

G. Two AV nodes may be present (one on the left and one on the right).

H. Anterior AV node may be well developed in some.

I. Node-like cells from the mitral valve may join the AV node.

J. Atrial muscle may be trapped within the central fibrous body and join the AV node.

K. Branching bundle and bifurcating bundle and the beginning of the left and right bundle branch may be present in the pars membranacea and not on the summit of the septum.

8. The penetrating or branching bundle may be in the tricuspid valve annulus. The branching bundle may be on the left or the right side of the ventricular septum. It may be surrounded or compressed by a left-sided or right-sided hypertrophied ventricular septal muscle.

9. Atrio-Hisian connections may be present (from the left or right atrium).

10. The bundle may wind around a piece of the ventricular septum at its summit.

11. In many cases, the atrial septum is the seat of fatty metamorphosis.

12. Frank myocarditis was noted in only a few cases.

13. Fibrosis of nerves was found in many cases in the approaches to the SA and AV nodes.

14. The AV node was housed in the central fibrous body in many cases.

15. All postoperative congenital heart disease cases who died suddenly, regardless of the type of surgery and the interval between the time of surgery and the time of death, demonstrated foreign body reaction, fat, fibrosis, and mononuclear cells to a varying degree.

16. In addition to these findings, in several cases the SA node was surrounded by an ep-icarditis. The effect of this on the SA node is unknown.

17. There are distinct disease entities such as Uhl's anomaly and mitral valve prolapse seen in this series. Other disease entities such as sarcoidosis, amyloidosis, Kearns-Sayre syndrome, myotonia dystrophica, Kawasaki disease, tumor of the AV node, etc., made their appearance. The effect of these on the myocardium of the heart and/or the conduction system are in general quite marked pathologically. Thus, there are several disease entities that may affect the myocardium and/or the conduction system to a varying degree and thereby form a milieu for arrhythmogenicity. These disease entities are usually progressive in nature and have a fatal outcome sooner or later. However, some of them, although pathologically severe in nature, may be completely asymptomatic for a long period of time or may disable the young individual to a mild or moderate degree, nevertheless permitting survival with a more or less normal life pattern.

18. Another theoretical consideration emerges that may affect part or all of the conduction system. These structures lie in an anatomical background, which acts on the function of the conduction system. The anatomical background consists of the eustachian valve, the tendon of Todaro, the fibrous extension of the aorta to the central fibrous body, the central fibrous body itself, the fibrous base of the tricuspid and mitral valves, the ventriculo-ventricular component of the membranous septum, the left ventriculo-right atrial part of the membranous septum, and the summit of the ventricular septum. The push or pull of any of these structures due to diseases may affect the functioning of the contained structures and lead to fatal arrhythmias.

Limitations of Our Study:

1. Because of the double-embedding techniques, immunohistochemical studies were not done.

2. New soft-tissue imaging techniques should be developed to identify these

abnormalities in the living, by means of high technology, which may form a basis for detecting biochemical alterations at the molecular level in the abnormal structure itself.

3. Where there is a definite history of tendency for sudden death in families or in the young, these families should be examined thoroughly prospectively, and very carefully at the molecular, genetic, and immunological levels by means of highly sophisticated techniques.

4. The above may give a clue as to the possible cause of one type of etiogenesis of sudden death in the young which triggers an arrhythmic event and may end fatally.

5. The 21st century is emerging as a health-conscious era with emphasis on lowering of cholesterol, getting rid of excess fat, and increasing exercise levels. We make no attempt to enter into the polemics of these highly debatable controversial issues. However, since we have studied the conduction system in a fair number of young athletes who died suddenly while playing their favorite sport, we wish to state the following.

All of the young athletes showed *marked* pathological changes in and around the conduction system with hypertrophied and enlarged hearts. The abnormalities varied from congenital to acquired in nature. Therefore, the questions we ask ourselves are:

1. What is *normal* physiological hypertrophy of cardiac muscle as a result of exercise in the age group of 7 to 70 years?

2. The biochemical and histochemical changes of the structurally altered cell and its function are not known today. For example, the calcium, the potassium, the magnesium, and other constituents of the pathological cell have not yet been defined.

3. The immune response of the conduction system to aging and injury is totally unknown today.

4. The genetic constitution of the conduction system cells has yet to be explored.

5. The reaction of the conduction tissue to emotion has to be studied.

6. Nervous impulses and other unknown factors that act on the physiological state may be responsible for triggering an arrhythmia, and may create abnormal re-entry mechanisms, or fractionization of an impulse, or abnormal automaticity which could be responsible for bradytachyarrhythmias and sudden death.

7. Electron microscopy studies of the conduction system should be instituted in all cases.

Added Conclusive Thoughts

1. Although all cases demonstrated histological abnormalities in the conduction system and/or the surrounding myocardium which were in the form of subtle to remarkable changes, these changes apparently had no effect on the individual before the sudden death in many cases, and had permitted the individual to live a "more or less normal life" for a considerable period of time. Some had arrhythmias.

2. What is normal physiological hypertrophy of cardiac muscle following exercise beyond the age group of 17 to 25 years?

3. What is normal physiological hypertrophy of cardiac muscle following exercise with each decade of life from 30 to 70 years?

4. How do disease states such as mild diabetes and mild hypertension react to the above three conditions mentioned?

In order to understand the physiological event of sudden cardiac death in young and healthy individuals, a prospective study of sports medicine and sudden death in the young and healthy should be undertaken at the national level. This should include not only the various parameters at the clinical level, such as invasive and noninvasive techniques, imaging, biochemical, genetic, immune complexes, etc. A thorough pathological study of the hearts must be undertaken as well. At least two or three centers are necessary for the study of the conduction system as detailed as we have described in our work. If all centers find the pathological changes *in all cases* as we have, we may then get into the statistical analysis of the predictability of sudden death in the young and healthy in a given population. We strongly believe that the *pathological* findings might have made the individual susceptible to an arrhythmic event and sudden death.

Chapter 11

References

1. Lev M, McMillan JB: A semiquantitative histopathologic method for the study of the entire heart for clinical and electrocardiographic correlations. *Am Heart J* 1959; 58:140–158.

2. McMillan JB, Lev M: The aging heart: I. Endocardium. *J Gerontol* 1959; 14:268–283.

3. Lev M, McMillan JB: Ageing changes in the heart. In: *Structural Aspects of Ageing.* Edited by GH Bourne. London, Pitman Medical Publishing Co., Ltd., 1961, pp. 325–349.

4. McMillan JB, Lev M: The aging heart: myocardium and epicardium. In: *Biological Aspects of Aging.* Edited by NW Shock. New York/London, Columbia University Press, 1962, pp. 163–173.

5. Lev M, Widran J, Erickson EE: A method for the histopathologic study of the AV node, bundle and branches. *AMA Arch Pathol* 1951; 52:73–83.

6. Widran J, Lev M: The dissection of the human AV node, bundle and branches. *Circulation* 1951; 4:863–867.

7. Lev M, Watne AL: Method for routine histopathologic study of the sinoatrial node. *Arch Pathol* 1954; 57:168–177.

8. Lev M, Lerner R: The theory of Kent: a histologic study of the normal atrioventricular communications of the human heart. *Circulation* 1955; 12:176–184.

9. Lev M, Bharati S: Lesions of the conduction system and their functional significance. In: *Pathology Annual 1974.* Edited by SC Sommers. NY, Appleton-Century Crofts, 1974; 9:157–208.

10. Lev M, Bharati S: A method of study of the pathology of the conduction system for electrocardiographic and His bundle electrogram correlations. *Anatomical Record* 1981; 201:43–49.

11. Bharati S, Lev M: The anatomy and histology of the conduction system. In: *Ar-*

tificial Cardiac Pacing: Practical Approach, Second Edition. By EK Chung. Baltimore, Williams & Wilkins Co, 1984, Chap. 2, pp. 12–27.

12. Lev M, Bharati S: Anatomic basis for impulse generation and atrioventricular transmission. In: His Bundle Electrocardiography and Clinical Electrophysiology (from "An International Symposium on Recent Advances in Clinical Electrophysiology: His Bundle Electrocardiography," Miami, Florida, 1/9–11/74). Edited by OS Narula. Philadelphia, FA Davis Co, 1975, pp. 1–17.

13. Bharati S, Lev M: The anatomy and pathology of the conduction system. In: Cardiac Pacing, 2nd Edition. Edited by P Samet, N El-Sherif. NY, Grune & Stratton, Inc., 1980, Chap. 1, pp. 1–35.

14. Lev M, Bharati S: Anatomical basis for preexcitation. In: Cardiac Arrhythmias: Electrophysiology, Diagnosis and Management. Edited by O Narula. Baltimore, Williams & Wilkins, 1979, Chap. 29, pp. 556–564.

15. Lev M, Bharati S: The anatomy of the conduction system in normal and congenitally abnormal hearts. In: Cardiac Arrhythmias in the Neonate Infant and Child. Edited by N Roberts, H Gelband. NY, Appleton-Century Crofts, 1977, Chap. 2, pp. 29–54.

16. Lev M: Aging changes in the human sinoatrial node. J Gerontol 1954; 9:1–9.

17. Erickson EE, Lev M: Aging changes in the human atrioventricular node, bundle, and bundle branches. J Gerontol 1952; 7:1–12.

18. Lev M, Bharati S: The fibrous skeleton of the heart. In: Update IV: The Heart. Edited by J Willis Hurst. NY, McGraw Hill, 1981, Chap. 2, pp. 7–17.

19. Lev M: The conduction system. In: Pathology of the Heart and Blood Vessels, 3rd Edition. Edited SC Gould. Springfield, Illinois, Charles C. Thomas, 1968, pp. 180–220.

20. Lev M, Bharati S: Embryology of the heart and pathogenesis of congenital malformations of the heart. In: Pediatric Surgery, Vol. 1, Third Edition. Edited by MM Ravitch, KJ Welch, CD Benson, E Aberdeen, JG Randolph. Chicago/London, Year Book Medical Publishers, Inc., 1979, Chap. 49, pp. 582–590.

21. Bedford THB: The pathology of sudden death: a review of 198 cases "brought in dead." J Pathol Bacteriol 1933; 36:333–347.

22. Koppisch E: On the causes of sudden death in Puerto Rico: an analysis of 61 cases studied postmortem. Puerto Rico J Public Health Trop Med 1934; 9:328–345.

23. Allen AC: Eosinophilia of the spleen associated with sudden death. Arch Pathol 1944; 37:20–23.

24. Helpern M, Rabson SM: Sudden and unexpected natural death: general considerations and statistics. New York J Med 1945; 45:1197–1201.

25. Moritz, AR, Zamcheck N: Sudden and unexpected deaths of young soldiers. Arch Pathol 1946; 42:459–494.

26. Richards R: A note on the causation of sudden death. Br Med J 1947; 2:51–53.

27. Majoska AV: Sudden death in Filipino men: an unexplained syndrome. Hawaii Med J 1948; 7:469–473.

28. Evans W: Familial cardiomegaly. Br Heart J 1949; 11:68–82.

29. Sta Cruz JZ: The pathology of "Bangungut." J Philippine Med Assoc 1951; 27:476–481.

30. Teare D: Asymmetrical hypertrophy of the heart in young adults. Br Heart J 1958; 20:1–8.

31. Sugai M: A pathological study on sudden and unexpected death, especially on the cardiac death autopsied by medical examiners in Tokyo. Acta Pathologica Japonica 1959; 9:(Suppl)723–752.

32. Aponte GE: The enigma of "Bangungut." Ann Intern Med 1960; 52:1258–1263.

33. Burch GE, DePasquale NP: Sudden, unexpected, natural death. *Am J Med Sci* 1963; 249:112–123.

34. Fraser GR, Froggatt P, James TN: Congenital deafness associated with electrocardiographic abnormalities, fainting attacks and sudden death. *Q J Med* 1964; 33:361–384.

35. James TN, Rupe CE, Monto RW: Pathology of the cardiac conduction system in systemic lupus erythematosus. *Ann Intern Med* 1965; 63:402–410.

36. Kuller L, Lilienfeld A, Fisher R: Sudden and unexpected deaths in young adults. *JAMA* 1966; 198:248–252.

37. James TN, Monto RW: Pathology of the cardiac conduction system in thrombotic thrombocytopenic purpura. *Ann Intern Med* 1966; 65:37–43.

38. James TN, Birk RE: Pathology of the cardiac conduction system in polyarteritis nodosa. *Arch Intern Med* 1966; 117:561–567.

39. Kuller L, Lilienfeld A, Fisher R: An epidemiological study of sudden and unexpected deaths in adults. *Medicine* 1966; 46:341–361.

40. James TN, Froggatt P, Marshall TK: Sudden death in young athletes. *Ann Intern Med* 1967; 67:1013–1021.

41. Luke JL, Helpern M: Sudden unexpected death from natural causes in young adults: a review of 275 consecutive autopsied cases. *Arch Pathol* 1968; 85:10–17.

42. James TN: Sudden death in babies: new observations in the heart. *Am J Cardiol* 1968; 22:479–506.

43. Green JR Jr, Korovetz MJ, Shanklin DR, DeVito JJ, Taylor WJ: Sudden unexpected death in three generations. *Arch Intern Med* 1969; 124:359–363.

44. James TN: Pathogenesis of arrhythmias in acute myocardial infarction. *Am J Cardiol* 1969; 24:791–799.

45. Anderson WR, Edland JF, Schenk EA: Conduction system changes in the sudden infant death syndrome. *Scientific Proceedings* 1970; 35a (72).

46. Goodwin JF: Congestive and hypertrophic cardiomyopathies. *Lancet* 1970; 1:731–739.

47. James TN: Cardiac conduction system: fetal and postnatal development. *Am J Cardiol* 1970; 25:213–226.

48. Schwartz CJ, Walsh WJ: The pathologic basis of sudden death. *Prog Cardiovasc Dis* 1971; 13:465–481.

49. Haerem JW: Platelet aggregates in intramyocardial vessels of patients dying suddenly and unexpectedly of coronary artery disease. *Atherosclerosis* 1972; 15:199–213.

50. Ferris JAJ: Hypoxic changes in conducting tissue of the heart in sudden death in infancy syndrome. *Br Med J* 1973; 2:23–25.

51. Valdes-Dapena MA, Greene M, Basavarand N, Catherman R, Truex RC: The myocardial conduction system in sudden death in infancy. *N Engl J Med* 1973; 289:1179–1180.

52. Friedman M, Manwaring JH, Rosenman RH, Donlon G, Ortega P, Grube SM: Instantaneous and sudden deaths: clinical and pathological differentiation in coronary artery disease. *JAMA* 1973; 225:1319–1328.

53. Anderson RH, Bouton J, Burrow CT, Smith A: Sudden death in infancy: a study of cardiac specialized tissue. *Br Med J* 1974; 2:135–139.

54. Ferris JAJ, Kendeel SR: Sudden death in infancy. *Br Med J* 1974; 2(5918):559–560.

55. James TN, Armstrong RS, Silverman J, Marshall TK: De subitaneis mortibus VI: two young soldiers. *Circulation* 1974; 44:1239–1246.

56. Marshall CE, Shappell SD: Sudden death and the ballooning posterior leaflet syndrome: detailed anatomic and histochemical investigation. *Arch Pathol* 1974; 98:134–138.

57. Ferris JAJ: Conducting tissue changes in

sudden death. *Med Sci Law* 1974; 14:36–39.

58. James TN, Marshall ML, Craig MW: De subitaneis mortibus VII: disseminated intravascular coagulation and paroxysmal atrial tachycardia. *Circulation* 1974; 50:395–401.

59. Shah PM, Adelman AG, Wigle ED, Gobel FL, Burchell HB, Hardarson T, Curiel R, de la Calzada C, Oakley CM, Goodwin JF: The natural (and unnatural) history of hypertrophic obstructive cardiomyopathy. *Circulation Res* 1974; 34 & 35(Suppl):11, 179–195.

60. Pruitt RD: Death as an expression of functional disease. *Mayo Clin Proc* 1974; 9:627–634.

61. Abildskov JA: The nervous system and cardiac arrhythmias. *Circulation* 1975; 51 & 52(Suppl):III-116–119.

62. Lie JT: Histopathology of the conduction system in sudden death from coronary heart disease. *Circulation* 1975; 51:446–452.

63. Lie JT, Titus JL: Pathology of the myocardium and the conduction system in sudden coronary death. *Circulation* 1975; 51 & 52(Suppl):III-41–52.

64. James TN, Marshall TK: Asymmetrical hypertrophy of the heart. *Circulation* 1975; 51:1149–1166.

65. James TN, Marilley RJ Jr, Marriott HJL: De subitaneis mortibus XI: young girl with palpitations. *Circulation* 1975; 51:743–748.

66. Gotoh K: A histopathological study on the conduction system of the so-called "Pokkuri disease" (sudden unexpected cardiac death of unknown origin in Japan). *Japn Circ J* 1976; 40:753–768.

67. Lie JT, Rosenberg HS, Erickson EE: Histopathology of the conduction system in the sudden infant death syndrome. *Circulation* 1976; 53:3–8.

68. James TN, Marshall TK: Persistent fetal dispersion of the atrioventricular node and His bundle within the central fibrous body. *Circulation* 1976; 53:1026–1034.

69. Doyle JT: Mechanisms and prevention of sudden death. *Mod Concepts Cardiovas Dis* 1976; 45:111–116.

70. James TN, Marshall TK: Multifocal stenoses due to fibromuscular dysplasia of the sinus node artery. *Circulation* 1976; 53:736–742.

71. Brechenmacher C, Coumel P, James TN: Intractable tachycardia in infancy. *Circulation* 1976; 53:377–381.

72. Voigt J: Reflections on the value of histological examination of the cardiac conduction system in cases of natural unexpected death. *Forensic Sci* 1976; 8:29–31.

73. Gillette PC, Yeoman MA, Mullins CE, McNamara DG: Sudden death after repair of tetralogy of Fallot: electrocardiographic and electrophysiologic abnormalities. *Circulation* 1977; 56:566–571.

74. James TN, Galakhov I: Fatal electrical instability of the heart associated with benign congenital polycystic tumor of the atrioventricular node. *Circulation* 1977; 56:667–678.

75. James TN, Jackson DA: Histological abnormalities in the sinus node, atrioventricular node and His bundle associated with coarctation of the aorta. *Circulation* 1977; 56:1094–1102.

76. James TN: Sarcoid heart disease. *Circulation* 1977; 56:320–326.

77. Lown B, Verrier RL, Rabinowitz SH: Neural and psychologic mechanisms and the problem of sudden cardiac death. *Am J Cardiol* 1977; 39:890–902.

78. Branch CE, Robertson BT, Beckett SD, Waldo AL, James TN: An animal model of spontaneous syncope and sudden death. *J Lab Clin Med* 1977; 90:592–603.

79. James TN, Froggatt P, Atkinson WJ Jr, Lurie PR, McNamara DG, Miller WW, Schloss GT, Carroll JF, North RL: Observations on the pathophysiology of the long QT syndromes with special reference to the neuropathology of the heart. *Circulation* 1978; 57:1221–1231.

80. James TN: Apoplexy of the heart. *Circulation* 1978; 57:385–391.

81. Thiene G, Valente M, Rossi L: Involvement of the cardiac conducting system in panarteritis nodosa. *Am Heart J* 1978; 95:716–724.

82. Fontaine G, Guiraudon G, Frank R, Vedel J, Grosgogeat Y, Cabrol C: Modern concepts of ventricular tachycardia: the value of electrocardiological investigations and delayed potentials in ventricular tachycardia of ischemic and nonischemic etiology (31 operated cases). *Eur J Cardiol* 1978; 8:565–580.

83. Meierhenry EF, Liu S: Atrioventricular bundle degeneration associated with sudden death in the dog. *JAMA* 1978; 172:1418–1422.

84. Haerem JW: Sudden unexpected coronary death: the occurence of platelet aggregates in the epicardial and myocardial vessels of man. *Acta Pathol Microbiol Scand* 1978; (Suppl No. 265):1–47.

85. Davies MJ, Popple A: Sudden unexpected cardiac death: a practical approach to the forensic problem. *Histopathology* 1979; 3:255–277.

86. Okada R: Pathology of sudden cardiac death in the young. Cardiology, International Congress Series No. 470. *Proceedings of the VI World Congress of Cardiology 1978.* Edited by Hayase S, Murano S. Amsterdam, Exerpta Medica, 1979, pp. 487–493.

87. Lahiri A, Balasubramanian V, Raftery EB: Sudden death during ambulatory monitoring. *Br Med J* 1979; 1:1676–1678.

88. Lown B: Cardiac death: the major challenge confronting contemporary cardiology. *Am J Cardiol* 1979; 3:313–328.

89. Southall DP, Arrowsmith WA, Oakley JR, McEnery G, Anderson RH, Shinebourne EA: Prolonged QT interval and cardiac arrhythmias in two neonates: sudden infant death syndrome in one case. *Arch Dis Child* 1979; 54:776–779.

90. Kulbertus HE, Wellens HJJ: *Sudden Death: Developments in Cardiovascular Medicine 4.* The Hague/Boston/London, Martinus Nijhoff, 1980.

91. Maron BJ, Roberts WC, McAllister HA, Rosing DR, Epstein SE: Sudden death in young athletes. *Circulation* 1980; 62:218–229.

92. Morales AR, Romanelli R, Boucek RJ: The mural left anterior descending coronary artery, strenous exercise and sudden death. *Circulation* 1980; 62:230–237.

93. Waller FB, Roberts WC: Sudden death while running in conditioned runners: coronary disease is the culprit. *Am J Cardiol* 1980; 45:423.

94. James TN, Pearce WN, Givhan EG: Sudden death while driving. *Am J Cardiol* 1980; 45:1095–1102.

95. James TN, MacLean WAH: Paroxysmal ventricular arrhythmias and familial sudden death associated with neural lesions in the heart. *Chest* 1980; 78:24–30.

96. Krikler DM, Davies MJ, Rowland E, Goodwin JF, Evans RC, Shaw DB: Sudden death in hypertrophic cardiomyopathy: associated accessory atrioventricular pathways. *Br Heart J* 1980; 43:245–251.

97. Kuller LH: Sudden death: definition and epidemiologic considerations. *Prog Cardiovasc Dis* 1980; 23(1):1–12.

98. Rossi L: Occurrence and significance of coagulative myocytolysis in the specialized conduction system: clinicopathologic observations. *Am J Cardiol* 1980; 45:757–761.

99. Cheitlin MD: The intramural coronary artery: another cause for sudden death with exercise? (editorial). *Circulation* 1980; 62:238–239.

100. Pedersen PK: Poor results in attempting to demonstrate the cause of death by examination of the conduction system of the heart in cases of sudden death. *Forensic Sci Int* 1980; 16:281–282.

101. Davies MJ: Pathologic view of sudden cardiac death. *Br Heart J* 1981; 45:88–96.

102. Anderson KR, Bowie J, Dempster AG, Gwynne JF: Sudden death from occlu-

sive disease of the atrioventricular node artery. *Pathology* 1981; 13:417–421.

103. Fitchett DH, MacArthur CG, Oakley CM, Krikler DM, Goodwin JF: Right ventricular cardiomyopathy. *Br Heart J* 1981; 45:354.

104. Smeeton DH, Anderson KR, Ho SY, Davies MJ, Anderson RH: Conduction tissue changes associated with enlarged membranous septum: a cause of sudden death? *Br Heart J* 1981; 46:636–642.

105. Rossi L, Thiene G: Recent advances in clinicohistopathologic correlates of sudden cardiac death. *Am Heart J* 1981; 102:478–484.

106. Gallagher JJ, Smith WM, Kasell JH, Benson DW Jr, Sterba R, Grant AO: Role of Mahaim fibers in cardiac arrhythmias in man. *Circulation* 1981; 64:176–189.

107. Marinato GP, Thiene G, Menghetti L, Buja GF, Nava A, Cecchetto A, Rossi L: Clinicopathologic assessment of arrhythmias: a case of scleroderma heart disease with sudden death. *Eur J Cardiol* 1981; 12:321–331.

108. Virmani R, Robinowitz M, Clark MA, McAllister HA Jr: Sudden death and partial absence of the right ventricular myocardium: a report of three cases and a review of the literature. *Arch Pathol Lab Med* 1982; 106:163–167.

109. Marcus FI, Fontaine GH, Guiraudon G, Frank R, Laurenceau JL, Malergue C, Grosgogeat Y: Right ventricular dysplasia: a report of 24 adult cases. *Circulation* 1982; 65:384–398.

110. Hinkle LE Jr: Short-term factors for sudden death. *Ann NY Acad Sci* 1982; 382:22–38.

111. Schroeder P, Lyons C: A possible role of the specialized conduction system in the conversion of ventricular tachycardia to ventricular fibrillation. *PACE* 1982; 5:683–687.

112. Lown B: Mental stress, arrhythmias and sudden death. *Am J Med* 1982; 72:117–180.

113. Schwartz PJ, Montemerlo M, Facchini U, Salice P, Rosti D, Poggio G, Giorgetti R: The QT interval throughout the first six months of life: a prospective study. *Circulation* 1982; 66:496–501.

114. Rossi L: Pathologic changes in the cardiac conduction and nervous system in sudden coronary death. *Ann NY Acad Sci* 1982; 382:50–68.

115. Vesterby A, Markil Gregersen M: Sudden unexpected death due to coronary heart disease: postmortem coronary angiography and histological investigation of the heart conduction system. *Acta Med Leg Soc* 1982; 32:65–69.

116. Wellens HJJ, Brugada P, Frits Bar WHM: The role of intraventricular conduction disorders in precipitating sudden death. *Ann NY Acad Sci* 1982; 382:136–142.

117. Davies MJ, Anderson RH, Becker AE: *Sudden Death and the Conduction System in the Conduction System of the Heart.* London, Butterworths, 1983, Chap. 13, pp. 301–323.

118. Rossi L: The pathologic basis of cardiac arrhythmias. *Cardiol Clin* 1983; 1:13–37.

119. Sakurai T, Kawai C: Sudden death in idiopathic cardiomopathy. *Japan Circ J* 1983; 47:581–585.

120. Baron RC, Thacker SB, Gorelkin L, Vernon AA, Taylor WR, Choi K: Sudden death among Southeast Asian refugees: an unexplained nocturnal phenomenon. *JAMA* 1983; 250:2947–2951.

121. James TN: Chance and sudden death. *J Am Coll Cardiol* 1983; 1:164–183.

122. Garson A Jr, Porter CJ, Gillette PC, McNamara DG: Induction of ventricular tachycardia during electrophysiologic study after repair of tetralogy of Fallot. *J Am Coll Cardiol* 1983; 1:1493–1502.

123. Thiene G, Pennelli N, Rossi L: Cardiac conduction system abnormalities as a possible cause of sudden death in young athletes. *Human Pathol* 1983; 14:704–709.

124. Okada R, Kawai S: Histopathology of the conduction system in sudden cardiac death. *Japan Circ J* 1983; 47:573–580.

125. Rossi L, Thiene G: Mild Ebstein's anomaly associated with supraventricular tachycardia and sudden death: clinicomorphologic features in three patients. *Am J Cardiol* 1984; 53:332–334.

126. Furlanello F, Bettini R, Cozzi F, Del Favero A, Disertori M, Vergara G, Durante GB, Guarnerio M, Inama G, Thiene G: Ventricular arrhythmias and sudden death in athletes. *Ann NY Acad Sci* 1984; 427:253–279.

127. Rossi L, Piffer R, Turolla E, Frigerio B, Coumel P, James TN: Multifocal Purkinje-like tumor of the heart occurrence with other anatomic abnormalities in the atrioventricular junction of an infant with junctional tachycardia, Lown-Ganong-Levine syndrome, and sudden death. *Chest* 1985; 87:340–345.

128. Fuster V, Steele PM, Chesebro JH: The role of platelets and thrombosis in the clinical complications of coronary atheroscelerotic disease including sudden death. *J Am Coll Cardiol* 1985; 5(Suppl):175B–184B.

129. James TN: Normal variations and pathologic changes in structure of the cardiac conduction system and their functional significance. *J Am Coll Cardiol* 1985; 5:71B–78B.

130. Driscoll DJ, Edwards WD: Sudden unexpected death in children and adolescents. *J Am Coll Cardiol* 1985; 5:118B–121B.

131. Joshi NC: Cardiac arrhythmias in infants and children. *Indian J Pediatr* 1985; 52:569–577.

132. Meijler FL, Van Der Tweel I, Herbschleb JN, Hauer RN, Robles de Medina EO: Role of atrial fibrillation and atrioventricular conduction (including Wolff-Parkinson-White syndrome) in sudden death. *J Am Coll Cardiol* 1985; (Suppl)17B–22B.

133. Surawicz B: Ventricular fibrillation. *J Am Coll Cardiol* 1985; 5:43B–54B.

134. Kirschner RH, Eckner FAO, Baron RC: The cardiac pathology of sudden unexplained nocturnal death in Southeast Asian refugees. *JAMA* 1986; 256:2700–2705.

135. Gavaghan TP, Kelly RP, Kuchar DL, Hickie JB, Campbell TJ: The prevalence of arrhythmias in hypertrophic cardiomyopathy: role of ambulatory monitoring and signal-averaged electrocardiography. *Aust NZ J Med* 1986; 16:666–670.

136. Shah VK, Pahalajani DB, Gandhi MJ, Pandey BJ, Punjabi AH: Arrhythmias in mitral valve prolapse. *Indian Heart J* 1986; 38:404–408.

137. Northcote RJ, Flannigan C, Ballantyne D: Sudden death and vigorous exercises: a study of 60 deaths associated with squash. *Br Heart J* 1986; 55:198–203.

138. Vikhert AM, Tsiplenkova VG, Cherpachenko NA: Alcoholic cardiomyopathy and sudden cardiac death. *J Am Coll Cardiol* 1986; 8:3A–11A.

139. Shvalev VN, Vikhert AM, Stropus RA, Sosunov AA, Pavlovich ER, Kargina-Terentyeva RA, Zhuchkova NI, Anikin AYU, Maryan, KL: Changes in neural and humoral abnormalities of the heart in sudden death due to myocardial abnormalities. *J Am Coll Cardiol* 1986; 8:55A–64A.

140. James TN: Degenerative lesions of a coronary chemoreceptor and nearby elements in the hearts of victims of sudden death. *J Am Coll Cardiol* 1986; 8:12A–21A.

141. James TN, Vikert AM: The fourth USA/USSR symposium on sudden cardiac death. *J Am Coll Cardiol* 1986; 18:1A–109A.

142. Coumel P, Leclercq JF, Leenhardt A: Arrhythmias as predictors of sudden death. *Am Heart J* 1987; 114:929–937.

143. Dimsdale JE, Ruberman W, Carleton RA, DeQuattro V, Eaker E, Eliot RS, Furberg CD, Irvin CW, Lown B, Shapiro AP, Shumaker SA: Task Force 1: sudden cardiac death. Stress and cardiac arrhythmias. *Circulation* 1987; 76:1198–1201.

144. Zipes DP, Levy MN, Cobb LA, Julius S, Kaufman PG, Miller NE, Verrier RL: Task

Force 2: sudden cardiac death. Neural-cardiac interactions. *Circulation* 1987; 76:1202–1207.

145. Corr PB, Pitt B, Natelson BH, Reis DJ, Shine KI, Skinner JE: Task Force 3: sudden cardiac death. Neural-chemical interactions. *Circulation* 1987; 76:1208–1214.

146. Schwartz PJ, Randall WC, Anderson EA, Engel BT, Friedman M, Hartley LH, Pickering TG, Thoresen CE: Task Force 4: sudden cardiac death. Nonpharmacologic intervention. *Circulation* 1987; 76:1215–1219.

147. Bigger JT Jr: Why patients with congestive heart failure die: arrhythmias and sudden cardiac death. *Circulation* 1987; 75(Suppl):28–35.

148. Verrier RL: Mechanisms of behaviorally induced arrhythmias. *Circulation* 1987; 76(Suppl):I-48–56.

149. Kligfield P, Levy D, Devereux RB, Savage DD: Arrhythmias and sudden death in mitral valve prolapse. *Am Heart J* 1987; 113:1298–1307.

150. Wiedermann CJ, Becker AE, Hopferwieser T, Muhlberger V, Knapp E: Sudden death in a young competitive athlete with Wolff-Parkinson-White syndrome. *Eur Heart J* 1987; 8:651–655.

151. Hattori R, Murhohara Y, Yui Y, Takatsu Y, Kawai C: Diffuse triple-vessel coronary artery spasm complicated by idioventricular rhythm and syncope. *Chest* 1987; 92:183–185.

152. Borhani NO: Left ventricular hypertrophy, arrhythmias and sudden death in systemic hypertension. *Am J Cardiol* 1987; 60:131–181.

153. Prystowsky EN, Fananapazir L, Packer DL, Thompson KA: German LD Wolff-Parkinson-White syndrome and sudden cardiac death. *Cardiology* 1987; 2:67–71.

154. Furberg CD: Overview of completed sudden death trials: US experience. *Cardiology* 1987; 2 (Suppl)74:24–31.

155. Amsterdam EZ: Silent myocardial ischemia, arrhythmias and sudden death: are they related? *Am J Cardiol* 1987; 59:919–920.

156. Andreoli A, di Pasquale G, Pinelli G, Grazi P, Tognetti F, Testa C: Subarachnoid hemorrhage: frequency and severity of cardiac arrhythmias. *Stroke* 1987; 18:558–564.

157. Nakamura M, Takeshita A, Nose Y: Clinical characteristics associated with myocardial infarction, arrhythmias, and sudden death in patients with vasospastic angina. *Circulation* 1987; 75:1110–1116.

158. Kennedy GJ, Fisher JD: Aging, stress, and sudden cardiac death. *Mt. Sinai J Med* 1987; 54:56–62.

159. Surawicz B: prognosis of ventricular arrhythmias in relation to sudden cardiac death: therapeutic implications. *Am Coll Cardiol* 1987; 10:435–447.

160. Lehmann, MH, Steinman RT: Preventing sudden cardiac death with electrophysiologic testing and the implantable defibrillator. *Postgrad Med* 1987; 82:36–39, 43–45.

161. Yee ES, Schienman MM, Griffin JC, Ebert PA: Surgical options for treating ventricular tachyarrhythmia and sudden death. *J Thorac Cardiovasc Surg* 1987; 94:866–873.

162. Eldar M, Sauve MJ, Scheinman MM: Electrophysiologic testing and follow-up of patients with aborted sudden death. *J Am Coll Cardiol* 1987; 10:291–298.

163. Gillette PC, Hammill WW: Sudden death in children: prediction and prevention. In: *Cardiac Arrhythmias: Recent Progress in Investigation and Management 1988.* Edited by T Iwa, G Fontaine. Amsterdam/NY, Elsevier, 1988, Chap. 13, pp. 171–176.

164. Okada R, Gotoh K: Pathology of the conduction system in Pokkuri disease (sudden death of unknown etiology in young men). In: *Cardiac Arrhythmias: Recent Progress in Investigation and Management.* Edited by T Iwa, G Fontaine. Amsterdam/NY, Elsevier, 1988, Chap. 16, pp. 177–188.

165. Fontaine G, Fontaliran F, Limares-Cruz E, Chomette G, Grosgogeat Y: The arrhythmogenic right ventricle. In *Cardiac Arrhythmias: Recent Progress in Investigation and Management. Edited by T Iwa, G Fontaine. 1988, Chap. 17, pp. 189–202.*

166. Inoue H, Zipes DP: Cocaine-induced supersensitivity and arrhythmogenesis. *J Am Coll Cardiol* 1988; 11:867–874.

167. Lemery R, Brugada P, Havenith M, Barbour D, Roberts W, Wellens HJJ: Sudden death in hemochromatosis after closed-chest catheter ablation of the atrioventricular junction. *Am J Cardiol* 1988; 61:941–943.

168. Crozier IG, Low CJS, Dow LJ, Ikram H: Cardiac electrophysiological assessment and the natural history of unexplained syncope. *NZ Med J* 1988; 101:106–108.

169. Bhandari AK, Hong R, Au P, McKay CR, Rahimtoola SH: Out-of-hospital cardiac arrest in patients with no overt heart disease: electrophysiologic observations and clinical outcome. *Canadian J Cardiol* 1988; 4:80–84.

170. Skadberg BT, Bruserud O, Karwinski W, Ohm OJ: Sudden death caused by heart block in a patient with multiple myeloma and cardiac amyloidosis. *Act Med Scand* 1988; 233:379–383.

171. Baye's de Luna A, Coumel P, Leclerc JF: Ambulatory sudden cardiac death: mechanisms of production of fatal arrhythmias on the basis of data from 157 cases. *Am Heart J* 1989; 117:151–159.

172. Harris R, Siew S, Lev M: Smoldering myocarditis with intermittent complete AV block and Stokes-Adams syndrome: a histopathologic and electrocardiographic study of "trisfascicular" bundle branch block. *Am J Cardiol* 1969; 24:880–889.

173. Gault JH, Cantwell J, Lev M, Braunwald E: Fatal familial cardiac arrhythmias: histologic observation in the cardiac conduction system. *Am J Cardiol* 1972; 29:548–553.

174. Bharati S, Chervony A, Gruhn J, Rosen KM, Lev M: Atrial arrhythmias related to trauma to sinoatrial node. *Chest* 1972; 61:331–335.

175. Husson GS, Blackman MS, Rogers MC, Bharati S, Lev M: Familial congenital bundle branch system disease. *Am J Cardiol* 1973; 32:365–369.

176. Bharati S, Bicoff JP, Fridman JL, Lev M, Rosen KM: Sudden death caused by benign tumor of the atrioventricular node. *Arch Intern Med* 1976; 136:224–228.

177. Bharati S, Ciraulo DA, Bilitch M, Rosen KM, Lev M: Inexcitable right ventricle and bilateral bundle branch block in Uhl's disease. *Circulation* 1978; 57:636–644.

178. Bharati S, Molthan ME, Veasy LG, Lev M: Conduction system in two cases of sudden death two years after the Mustard procedure. *J Thorac Cardiovasc Surg* 1979; 77:101–108.

179. Bharati S, Lev M, Denes P, Modlinger J, Wyndham C, Bauernfiend R, Greenblatt M, Rosen KM: Infiltrative cardiomyopathy with conduction disease and ventricular dysrhythmia: electrophysiological and pathological correlations. *Am J Cardiol* 1980; 45:163–173.

180. Bharati S, Nordenberg A, Bauernfiend R, Varghese JP, Carvalho AG, Rosen K, Lev M: The anatomic substrate for the sick sinus syndrome in adolescence. *Am J Cardiol* 1980; 46:163–172.

181. Bharati S, McAnulty JH, Lev M, Rahimtoola SH: Idiopathic hypertrophic subaortic stenosis with split His bundle potentials: electrophysiologic and pathologic correlation. *Circulation* 1980; 62:1373–1380.

182. Bharati S, Bauernfiend R, Miller LB, Strasberg B, Lev M: Sudden death in three teenagers: conduction system studies. *J Am Coll Cardiol* 1983; 1:879–886.

183. Bharati S, Feld A, Bauernfiend R, Kattus A Jr, Lev M: A case of hypoplasia of the right ventricular myocardium with ven-

tricular tachycardia. *Arch Pathol Lab Med* 1983; 107:249–253.

184. Bharati S, Lev M: Arrhythmogenic ventricles. *PACE* 1983; 6:1035–1049.

185. Bharati S, Lev M: Cardiac disease in sudden death. Special communication. *Arch Int Med* 1984; 114:1811–1812.

186. Bharati S, Lev M: The pathology of sudden death in sudden cardiac death. In: *Cardiovascular Clinics.* Edited by ME Josephson. Philadelphia, F.A. Davis Company, 1985; Chap. 15, pp. 1–27.

187. Bharati S, Lev M: Sudden death in teenagers. *Primary Cardiol* 1985; 11:73–88.

188. Bharati S, Krongrad E, Lev M: Study of the conduction system in a population of patients with SIDS. *Pediatr Cardiol* 1985; 6:29–40.

189. Bharati S, Dreifus L, Bucheleres G, Molthan M, Covitz W, Isenberg HS, Lev M: The conduction system in cases with prolonged Q-T interval. *J Am Coll Cardiol* 1985; 6:1110–1119.

190. Bharati S, Lev M: Congenital abnormalities of the conduction system in sudden death in young adults. *J Am Coll Cardiol* 1986; 8:1096–1104.

191. Bharati S, Lev M: Conduction system in cases of sudden death in congenital heart disease many years after surgical correction. *Chest* 1986; 90:861–868.

192. Bharati S, Lev M: Positive findings in the conduction system in five more young sudden death victims (abstract). *Circulation* 1986; 74(2):189.

193. Bharati S, Dreifus LS, Chopskie E, Lev M: Conduction system in a trained jogger with sudden death. *Chest* 1988; 93:348–351.

194. Bharati S, Lev M: Conduction system in sudden unexpected death a considerable time after repair of atrial septal defect. *Chest* 1988; 94:142–148.

195. Bharati S, Lev M, Wu D, Denes P, Dhingra R, Rosen KM: Pathophysiologic correlations in two cases of split His bundle potentials. *Circulation* 1974; 49:615–623.

196. Bharati S, Rosen KM, Miller RA, Lev M: Conduction system examination in a case of spontanous heart block in a dog. *Am Heart J* 1974; 88:596–600.

197. Lev M, Bharati S, Hoffman FG, Leight L: The conduction system in rheumatoid arthritis with complete atrioventricular block. *Am Heart J* 1975; 90:78–83.

198. Bharati S, Towne WD, Patel R, Lev M, Rahimtoola SH, Rosen KM: Pathologic correlations in a case of complete heart block with split His potentials resulting from a stab wound of the heart. *Am J Cardiol* 1976; 38:388–393.

199. Bharati S, Bauernfiend R, Scheinman M, Massie B, Cheitlin M, Denes P, Wu D, Lev M, Rosen KM: Congenital abnormalities of the conduction system in two patients with recurrent tachyarrhythmias. *Circulation* 1979; 59:593–606.

200. Bharati S, Granston AS, Liebson PR, Loeb HS, Rosen KM, Lev M: The conduction system in mitral valve prolapse syndrome with sudden death. *Am Heart J* 1981; 101:667–670.

201. Bharati S, Strasberg B, Bilitch M, Salibi H, Mandel W, Rosen KM, Lev M: Anatomic substrate for preexcitation in idiopathic myocardial hypertrophy with fibroelastosis of the left ventricle. *Am J Cardiol* 1981; 48:47–58.

202. Bharati S, Bump T, Bauernfiend R, Lev M: Dystrophica myotonia: correlative electrocardiographic, electrophysiologic and conduction system study. *Chest* 1984; 86:444–450.

203. Bharati S, Scheinman MM, Morady F, Hess DS, Lev M: Sudden death after catheter-induced atrioventricular junctional ablation in the human. *Chest* 1985; 88:883–889.

204. Gallastegui J, Hariman RJ, Handler B, Lev M, Bharati S: Cardiac involvement in the Kearns-Sayre syndrome. *Am J Cardiol* 1987; 60:385–388.

205. Brookfield L, Bharati S, Denes P, Halstead RD, Lev M: Familial sudden death:

report of a case and review of the literature. *Chest* 1988; 94:989–993.

206. Bharati S, Scheinman M, Estes M, Moskowitz W, Lev M: Junctional tachycardia: anatomic substrate and its significance in ablative procedures (abstract). *J Am Coll Cardiol* 1989; 13:175A.

207. Bharati S, Engle MA, Fatica NS, Bussell JB, Sulayman RF, Lev M, Lynfield J: The heart and conduction system in acute Kawasaki disease. Report of fraternal cases: One lethal, one relapsing. *Am Heart J* 1990; 120:359–365.

208. Bharati S, Lev M: Conduction system in 21 cases of sudden unexpected death in the young (abstract). *Circulation* 1989; 80(Suppl II):II–658.

209. Rosen KM, Rahimtoola SH, Gunnar RM, Lev M: Site of heart block as defined by His bundle recording. *Circulation* 1972; 45:965–987.

210. Kaplan BM, Langendorf R, Lev M, Pick A: Tachycardia-bradycardia syndrome (so-called "sick sinus syndrome"): pathology, mechanisms and treatment. *Am J Cardiol* 1973; 31:497–508.

Index